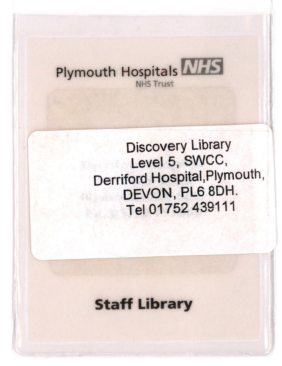

Atlas of Minimally Invasive Surgery

Atlas of Minimally Invasive Surgery

Constantine T. Frantzides, MD, PhD, FACS
Professor of Surgery
Northwestern University Feinberg School of Medicine
Chicago, Illinois
Director, Minimally Invasive Surgery Fellowship Program
Resurrection Healthcare
Evanston, Illinois
Director, Chicago Institute of Minimally Invasive Surgery
Skokie, Illinois

Mark A. Carlson, MD, FACS
Associate Professor of Surgery
University of Nebraska Medical Center
Staff Surgeon
Veterans Administration Medical Center
Omaha, Nebraska

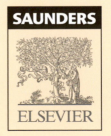

SAUNDERS

ELSEVIER

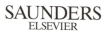

SAUNDERS
ELSEVIER

1600 John F. Kennedy Blvd.
Ste 1800
Philadelphia, PA 19103-2899

ATLAS OF MINIMALLY INVASIVE SURGERY   ISBN: 978-1-4160-4108-5

Notice

Knowledge and best practice in this field are constantly changing. As new research and experience broaden our knowledge, changes in practice, treatment and drug therapy may become necessary or appropriate. Readers are advised to check the most current information provided (i) on procedures featured or (ii) by the manufacturer of each product to be administered, to verify the recommended dose or formula, the method and duration of administration, and contraindications. It is the responsibility of the practitioner, relying on their own experience and knowledge of the patient, to make diagnoses, to determine dosages and the best treatment for each individual patient, and to take all appropriate safety precautions. To the fullest extent of the law, neither the Publisher nor the Editors assumes any liability for any injury and/or damage to persons or property arising out of or related to any use of the material contained in this book.

Library of Congress Cataloging-in-Publication Data
Atlas of minimally invasive surgery / [edited by] Constantine T. Frantzides, Mark A. Carlson.—1st ed.
    p. ; cm.
  Includes bibliographical references.
  ISBN 978-1-4160-4108-5
  1. Endoscopic surgery—Atlases. I. Frantzides, Constantine T. II. Carlson, Mark A.
    [DNLM: 1. Surgical Procedures, Minimally Invasive—methods—Atlases.
  2. Laparoscopy—Atlases. WO 517 A88045 2008]
    RD33.53.A87 2008
    617'.057—dc22
                           2008004008

Acquisitions Editor: Scott Scheidt
Developmental Editor: Jean Nevius
Project Manager: Bryan Hayward
Design Direction: Lou Forgione
Illustrators: Alex and David Baker
Marketing Manager: Brenna Christensen

Printed in Canada
Last digit is the print number: 9 8 7 6 5 4 3 2 1

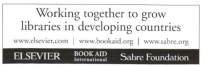

Working together to grow
libraries in developing countries

www.elsevier.com | www.bookaid.org | www.sabre.org

ELSEVIER   BOOK AID
International   Sabre Foundation

Contributors

Basil J. Ammori, MD, FRCS
Consultant General Surgeon and Honorary Senior Lecturer
Manchester Royal Infirmary and University of Manchester
Manchester, United Kingdom

Saleh Baghdadi, MD
Research Fellow
Manchester Royal Infirmary and University of Manchester
Manchester, United Kingdom

Willem A. Bemelman, MD
Professor, Minimally Invasive and Colorectal Surgery
Department of Surgery
Academic Medical Center
Amsterdam, the Netherlands

Malcolm M. Bilimoria, MD, FACS
Assistant Professor of Surgery
Northwestern University Feinberg School of Medicine
Chicago, Illinois
Department of Surgery
Evanston Hospital
Evanston, Illinois

Joseph A. Caprini, MD, MS, FACS, RVT, FACPh
Professor of Surgery
Northwestern University Feinberg School of Medicine
Chicago, Illinois
Louis W. Biegler Chair of Surgery
Senior Attending Surgeon
Evanston Northwestern Healthcare
Professor of Biomedical Engineering
Robert R. McCormick School of Engineering and Applied
    Sciences
Evanston, Illinois

Mark A. Carlson, MD, FACS
Associate Professor of Surgery
University of Nebraska Medical Center
Staff Surgeon
Veterans Administration Medical Center
Omaha, Nebraska

Emery L. Chen, MD
Fellow, Surgical Endocrinology
Rush University Medical Center
Chicago, Illinois

Albert Chi, MD
University of Arizona
Tucson, Arizona

Robert E. Condon, MD, MSc, FACS
Professor of Surgery, Emeritus
Medical College of Wisconsin
Seattle, Washington

Michael J. Demeure, MD, FACS
Professor of Surgery
University of Arizona
Tucson, Arizona
Senior Investigator
Transitional Genomics Research Institute
Translational Drug Development Division
Scottsdale, Arizona

Matthew D. Dunn, MD
Assistant Professor, Aresty Department of Urology
USC/Norris Cancer Hospital
Los Angeles, California

Charles E. Edmiston Jr., PhD, MS, CIC
Professor of Surgery and Hospital Epidemiologist
Director, Surgical Microbiology Research Laboratory
Department of Surgery
Medical College of Wisconsin
Milwaukee, Wisconsin

Eric D. Edwards, MD
Attending, Department of Surgery
St. Mary Medical Center
Langhorne, Pennsylvania

George S. Ferzli, MD, FACS
Chairman, Department of Surgery
Lutheran Medical Center
Brooklyn, New York
Professor, Department of Surgery
Staten Island University Hospital
Staten Island, New York

Morris E. Franklin, Jr., MD, FACS
Director
Texas Endosurgery Institute
San Antonio, Texas

Constantine T. Frantzides, MD, PhD, FACS
Professor of Surgery
Northwestern University Feinberg School of Medicine
Chicago, Illinois
Director, Minimally Invasive Surgery Fellowship Program
Resurrection Healthcare
Evanston, Illinois
Director
Chicago Institute of Minimally Invasive Surgery
Skokie, Illinois

Michel Gagner, MD, FACS
Chairman, Department of Surgery
Mount Sinai Medical Center
Miami, Florida

Frank A. Granderath, MD
Assistant Professor, Laparoscopic and Functional Surgery
Department of General, Visceral and Transplant Surgery
University Hospital
Tuebingen, Germany

Ursula M. Granderath, MD
Laparoscopic and Functional Surgery
Department of General, Visceral and Transplant Surgery
University Hospital
Tuebingen, Germany

Josh Hsu, MD
Aresty Department of Urology
USC/Norris Cancer Hospital
Los Angeles, California

Eric S. Hungness, MD
Assistant Professor of Surgery
Northwestern University Feinberg School of Medicine
Chicago, Illinois

Michael Kent, MD
Cardiothoracic Surgery
Heart, Lung and Esophageal Surgery Institute
University of Pittsburgh Medical Center
Pittsburgh, Pennsylvania

Antonio M. Lacy, MD, PhD
Professor of Surgery
Chief of Gastrointestinal Surgery
Institute of Digestive and Metabolic Diseases
Hospital Clinic
University of Barcelona
Barcelona, Spain

Luis E. Laguna, MD
Member, Chicago Institute of Minimally Invasive Surgery
Surgical Consultants, P.A.
Edina, Minnesota

Daniel A. Lawes, MBBS, MD, FRCS
Surgical Fellow, Division of Colon and Rectal Surgery
Mayo Clinic
Phoenix, Arizona

Cedric S. F. Lorenzo, MD
Fellow, Surgical Endoscopy and Endoluminal Therapy
Department of Surgery
Oregon Health & Science University
Portland, Oregon

Kirk A. Ludwig, MD, FACS
Associate Professor
Department of Surgery
Medical College of Wisconsin
Milwaukee, Wisconsin

James D. Luketich, MD, FACS
Sampson Family Endowed Professor of Surgery
Chief, Division of Thoracic & Foregut Surgery
Heart, Lung and Esophageal Surgery Institute
University of Pittsburgh Medical Center
Pittsburgh, Pennsylvania

Minh Luu, MD
Member, Chicago Institute of Minimally Invasive Surgery
Skokie, Illinois
Fellow, Advanced Laparoscopic and Bariatric Surgery
Evanston, Illinois

Atul K. Madan, MD, FACS
Chief, Division of Laparoendoscopic and Bariatric Surgery
The Dewitt Daughtry Family Department of Medicine
Leonard M. Miller School of Medicine
Miami, Florida

Ronald E. Moore, Jr., MD
Member, Chicago Institute of Minimally Invasive Surgery
Holy Cross Hospital Comprehensive Bariatric Services
Plantation, Florida

Kenric M. Murayama, MD, FACS
Professor of Surgery
John A. Burns School of Medicine
University of Hawaii
Honolulu, Hawaii

Martin Nitsun, MD
Assistant Professor, Anesthesiology
Northwestern University Feinberg School of Medicine
Chicago, Illinois
Evanston Northwestern Healthcare
Evanston, Illinois

Manish Parikh, MD
Instructor of Surgery, Section of Laparoscopic and Bariatric
    Surgery
Frank Glenn Faculty Scholar in Surgery
Joan and Stanford I. Weill Medical College of Cornell University
New York Presbyterian Hospital
New York, New York

Joseph B. Petelin, MD
Shawnee Mission Medical Center
Shawnee Mission, Kansas

George E. Polymeneas, MD, PhD
Associate Professor of Surgery
University of Athens
Athens, Greece

Alfons Pomp, MD, FRCSC, FACS
Associate Professor of Surgery, Section of Laparoscopic and
    Bariatric Surgery
Frank Glenn Faculty Scholar in Surgery
Joan and Stanford I. Weill Medical College of Cornell University
New York Presbyterian Hospital
New York, New York

Guillermo Portillo, MD
Fellow
Texas Endosurgery Institute
San Antonio, Texas

Hubert A. Prins, MD, PhD
Institute of Digestive Diseases
Hospital Clinic
University of Barcelona
Barcelona, Spain

Richard A. Prinz, MD, FACS
Helen Shedd Keith Professor
Chairperson, Department of General Surgery
Rush University Medical Center
Chicago, Illinois

Nathaniel J. Soper, MD, FACS
James R. Hines Professor and Chairman
Department of Surgery
Northwestern University Feinberg School of Medicine
Gastrointestinal and Endocrine Surgery
Chicago, Illinois

Joseph W. Szokol, MD
Vice Chairman, Department of Anesthesia
Evanston Northwestern Healthcare
Evanston, Illinois
Associate Professor
Northwestern University Feinberg School of Medicine
Chicago, Illinois

Tonia M. Young-Fadok, MD, MS, FACS, FACRS
Chair, Division of Colon and Rectal Surgery
Professor of Surgery
Mayo Clinic College of Medicine
Phoenix, Arizona

Tallal M. Zeni, MD
Member, Chicago Institute of Minimally Invasive Surgery
Director, Minimally Invasive and Bariatric Surgery
St. Mary Mercy Hospital
Livonia, Michigan

John G. Zografakis, MD, FACS
Member, Chicago Institute of Minimally Invasive Surgery
Assistant Professor of Surgery
Northeastern Ohio Universities Colleges of Medicine
    (NEOUCOM)
Director, Advanced Laparoscopic Surgical Services
Director, Bariatric Care Center
Summa Health System
Akron, Ohio

Preface

Minimally invasive procedures in general surgery are more amenable to video recording than the previous generation of open procedures, primarily because it is easy to connect a recording device to the laparoscope. As a result, instructional videotapes and DVDs have been available for a variety of minimally invasive procedures since the 1990s. In addition, a number of comprehensive yet conventional operative atlases on laparoscopic general surgical procedures have been published. It seemed only natural to combine these two formats, video and illustrated text, into one instructional format, the DVD-atlas. The *Atlas of Minimally Invasive Surgery* is a product of this union. This multimedia teaching aid consists of a conventional operative atlas combined with a set of DVDs that contain edited video of each procedure described in the book. The *Atlas* differs from earlier instructional video/text presentations in that it contains all of the commonly performed laparoscopic procedures in one presentation, whereas previous attempts at this format were monographic and focused on one procedure or one type of procedure.

The *Atlas of Minimally Invasive Surgery* is not, however, meant to be an encyclopedia of every technique described for every type of procedure. Nor is the *Atlas* intended to be a platform for experimental surgery (e.g., natural orifice procedures). In planning the *Atlas* we generated a list of what we believed to be the most commonly performed laparoscopic procedures; for each we asked a primary author to describe the operation. In truth, there are multiple operative approaches to every procedure in the *Atlas*. Some are more popular than others; some are easier than others; some are more effective than the others; and so forth. Trying to sort out these issues will result in a dialogue that rapidly places the discussants on a "slippery slope" with little controlled data to grab hold to. We admit that our process for selecting operative procedures and their respective authors to include in the *Atlas* was not scientific; it was based on impressions we have acquired while observing the evolution of minimally invasive surgery for the past two decades.

The *Atlas of Minimally Invasive Surgery* is also not intended to be the authority on procedure performance. Since there are few or no controlled data in this area, any claim to such authority, by this product or others, would be nonsensical. The *Atlas is* merely a guide, a collection of "How I Do It," intended as a teaching aid for medical students, surgical residents, and general surgeons. It is also a product that should evolve over time, as newer and/or improved techniques become established. It is our belief, and hope, that the DVD-atlas format of the *Atlas of Minimally Invasive Surgery* will become a favored teaching aid for laparoscopic operations in general surgery.

Constantine T. Frantzides, MD, PhD, FACS
Mark A. Carlson, MD, FACS

Acknowledgments

The authors would like to acknowledge the indispensable contribution of Dr. Robert E. Condon for his narration of the DVD portion of this atlas.

Contents

Esophagus

MICHAEL KENT AND
JAMES D. LUKETICH

Minimally Invasive Esophagectomy

Laparoscopy has become the standard approach for the treatment of a variety of benign esophageal diseases, such as reflux and achalasia. This shift has been driven by the consistent observation that minimally invasive surgery is associated with equal efficacy, less pain, and earlier return to work compared to open surgery. An open approach is still the standard of care, however, for patients with esophageal cancer, because (1) minimally invasive surgery may not be equivalent in terms of nodal clearance and completeness of resection, and (2) a minimally invasive approach may not have a measurable impact on morbidity. We would argue, though, that minimally invasive esophagectomy (MIE) is associated with lower morbidity and mortality rates than the open approach. Two of the more frequent complications following esophagectomy are pneumonia and pulmonary failure; the former complication has a 20% mortality risk. The avoidance of synchronous laparotomy and thoracotomy incisions may reduce the incidence of these complications. Although no randomized studies have been performed, our experience and that of others has suggested that minimally invasive esophagectomy is associated with a lower rate of complications and mortality than that following open esophagectomy.

Another reason to consider minimally invasive surgery is that the morbidity associated with open esophagectomy has led to renewed interest among medical oncologists to treat patients with chemoradiation alone. Two recent studies by Chiu and Stahl (see "Suggested Reading") on squamous cell cancer of the esophagus lend some support to this practice. The impact of these reports has been to recommend nonoperative therapy for marginal surgical candidates, such as the elderly or those with multiple comorbidities. The National Comprehensive Cancer Network, in their recent guidelines, now considers definitive chemoradiation to be an acceptable alternative to esophagectomy. With these challenges, it is incumbent on esophageal surgeons to refine the technique of esophagectomy, in order to offer therapy with lower morbidity, improved survival, or both compared with traditional esophagectomy.

PREOPERATIVE EVALUATION, TESTING, AND PREPARATION

The preoperative evaluation of a candidate for minimally invasive esophagectomy is no different from that for a patient undergoing open esophagectomy. The two primary issues concern whether a patient is resectable and if the patient has sufficient cardiopulmonary reserve to tolerate the operation. Staging of esophageal cancer patients at our center should include an upper endoscopy and computed tomography (CT) scan. Upper endoscopy is performed to identify the proximal and distal extent of the tumor, which may impact on the type of esophagectomy. CT scans primarily are used to rule out distant metastases which, if present, would preclude esophagectomy. CT scanning also is useful to determine the presence of bulky nodal disease within the abdomen. Bulky disease limited to the celiac nodal basin does not preclude esophagectomy, provided there is significant response to induction therapy. We would approach such a patient with a laparotomy in order to ensure a complete dissection of retroperitoneal lymph nodes.

Most patients also undergo endoscopic ultrasound (EUS) and positron emission tomography (PET) scans. The primary benefit of EUS is to determine the degree of invasion of the esophageal wall by tumor. Patients with T3 or N1 disease are usually treated with induction chemotherapy prior to esophagectomy. PET scans also are useful to determine distant disease that is not visualized by CT. We have not found PET particularly helpful in identifying periesophageal nodal disease, as activity within these nodes often is obscured by the primary tumor.

A final staging modality often used at our center is laparoscopy. Typically patients undergo laparoscopy at the time of placement of a port for induction chemotherapy. We have found laparoscopy to be a simple and safe method to identify abdominal metastases (liver or peritoneal) that may not be seen on CT scans. In addition, the presence of bulky nodal disease can be assessed by laparoscopy and confirmed by biopsy. For these patients, additional radiation therapy may be added to the neoadjuvant treatment plan. Laparoscopy usually can be completed within 30 minutes, and patients can be discharged home on the same day.

Patients also should undergo a thorough evaluation to determine medical suitability for operation. This includes a cardiac stress test and, if indicated, coronary angiography. Patients with a significant smoking history also should undergo pulmonary function testing. In addition, the majority of patients with locally advanced cancer will have some degree of dysphagia and weight loss prior to diagnosis. Dysphagia often will improve with induction therapy. If the patient has severe dysphagia, then we will place a jejunostomy tube during laparoscopic staging, although this has not been common for us. We strongly discourage the placement of either an esophageal stent or percutaneous gastrostomy tube for any patient who may be an operative candidate. Esophagectomy may still be performed in these situations, although it is technically more challenging.

OPERATIVE TECHNIQUE

The early efforts with minimally invasive esophageal resection were hybrid approaches, combining thoracoscopic mobilization of the esophagus, an open laparotomy for creation of the gastric tube, and a cervical anastomosis. No conclusive benefit was seen with this approach compared with standard esophagectomy, although the number of patients studied was small. With laparoscopic transhiatal esophagectomy, the entire procedure may be performed in the supine position with a standard single-lumen endotracheal tube. We have found, however, that the disadvantages of this approach far outweigh any benefit. The working space through the hiatus is quite small and allows only limited access to the middle and upper third of the esophagus. As a consequence, any thoracic lymph node dissection is extremely difficult through this approach. We therefore prefer to first mobilize the thoracic esophagus through a right video-assisted thoracscopic surgery (VATS) and then perform laparoscopy to prepare the gastric tube. We now offer minimally invasive esophagectomy to most surgical candidates, including those who have undergone induction chemoradiation therapy. Patients found to have bulky nodal metastases by CT or staging laparoscopy are not candidates for minimally invasive esophagectomy, and consideration is given to either an open operation or definitive chemoradiation. Herein is our technique based on experience with over 600 minimally invasive esophagectomies.

Thoracoscopy

The initial step in minimally invasive esophagectomy is an on-table esophagogastroduodenoscopy (EGD) to confirm the tumor's location and the suitability of the stomach as a conduit for reconstruction. Extension onto the cardia of the stomach often will require a wider gastric margin, and may prevent the construction of a gastric conduit that will reach the neck. For these cases, we prefer a high chest anastomosis, generally performed thoracoscopically (see Minimally Invasive Ivor Lewis Esophagectomy). Laparoscopic staging also may be of use in these patients in order to define the degree of cardia involvement before proceeding with resection.

After endoscopy patients are turned to the left lateral decubitus position for thoracoscopy (Fig. 1-1), the surgeon stands on the right side and the assistant on the left. Four thoracoscopic ports are used (Fig. 1-2). A 10-mm camera port is placed in the seventh or eighth intercostal space, just anterior to the midaxillary line. A 10-mm port is placed at the eighth or ninth intercostal space, posterior to the posterior axillary line, for the ultrasonic coagulating shears. A 10-mm port is placed in the anterior axillary line at the fourth intercostal space, through which a fan-shaped retractor retracts the lung anteriorly to expose the esophagus. The last 5-mm port is placed just anterior to the tip of the scapula, and is used for retraction by the surgeon. For an Ivor Lewis esophagectomy, the inferior port used by the surgeon can be enlarged to allow removal of the specimen and placement of the stapler.

A key step in this procedure is placement of a retraction suture (Endo Stitch, U.S. Surgical, Norwalk, CT) in the central tendon of the right hemidiaphragm (Fig. 1-3). This suture is brought

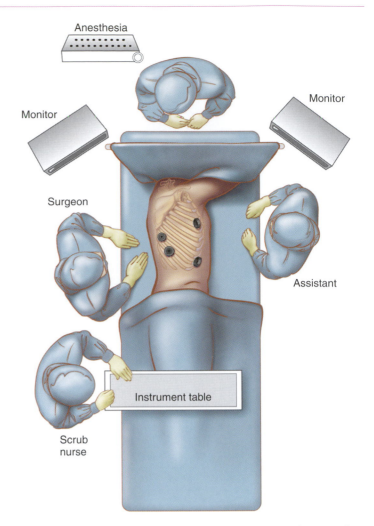

FIGURE 1-1 Operating room setup for the thoracoscopic portion of a minimally invasive esophagectomy.

out percutaneously through a 2-mm nick in the skin near the costophrenic recess anteriorly. Traction on this suture provides an excellent view of the distal thoracic esophagus. The inferior pulmonary ligament is divided to the inferior pulmonary vein, and the mediastinal pleura overlying the esophagus is incised

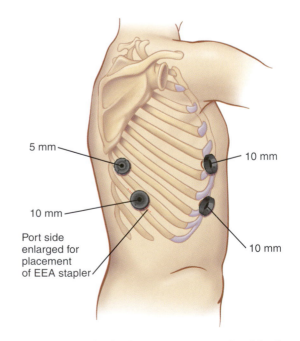

FIGURE 1-2 Port placement for the thoracoscopic portion of a minimally invasive esophagectomy. EEA, end-to-end anastomotic.

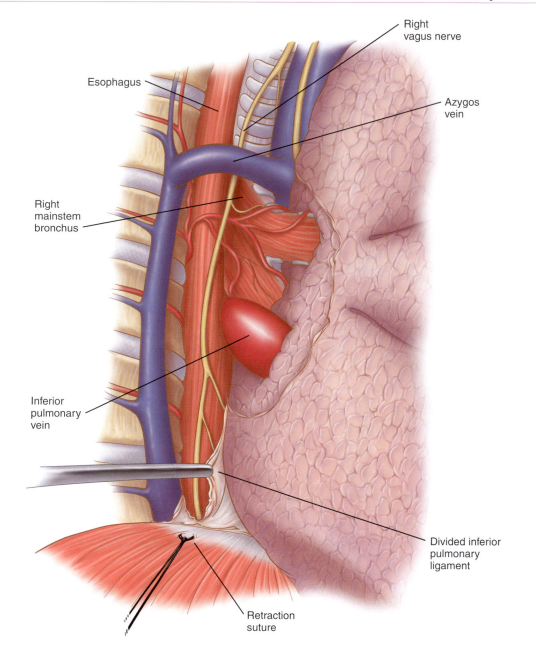

Right
vagus nerve

Esophagus

Azygos
vein

Right
mainstem
bronchus

Inferior
pulmonary
vein

Divided inferior
pulmonary
ligament

Retraction
suture

FIGURE 1-3 Initial thoracic dissection showing the position of the diaphragm retraction suture, division of the pulmonary ligament, and dissection of the posterior mediastinum.

to the level of the azygos vein. The plane between the pericardium and periesophageal area is developed. This plane is developed toward the undersurface of the right mainstem bronchus. All lymph nodes and periesophageal fat are taken en bloc with the esophagus. The dissection plane continues along the pericardium and airway, contralateral pleura, aorta, azygos vein, and thoracic duct. The thoracic duct and azygos vein are not resected. To facilitate the more posterior dissection plane, the mediastinal pleura along the esophagus is opened toward the azygos vein and extended from the azygos vein to the diaphragm.

The azygos vein is ligated using an endoscopic stapler (Fig. 1-4). The mediastinal pleura is preserved above the junction of the azygos vein and the superior vena cava. We believe this pleura maintains the gastric conduit in a mediastinal location and may seal the plane between the stomach and the thoracic inlet, which would minimize downward extension of a cervical anastomotic leak. We then proceed to circumferentially mobilize the esophagus, sweeping all periesophageal nodes and fat into the specimen. Feeder vessels from the aorta to the esophagus are clipped (Fig. 1-5).

We do not include the thoracic duct in the specimen. Any lymphatic branches arising from the duct are carefully clipped and divided in order to prevent chylothorax. A Penrose drain around the esophagus aids in subsequent mobilization. The thoracic esophagus is mobilized from thoracic inlet to the diaphragm. The dissection should not be carried into the peritoneal cavity; this would hinder the creation of pneumoperitoneum during laparoscopy. Also, we keep the dissection close to the esophagus above the azygos vein in order to avoid injury to either the airway or the recurrent laryngeal nerves. It is also important to divide the vagus trunks at or below the level of the azygos vein so that traction injury to the recurrent laryngeal nerves is avoided. After the esophagus has been mobilized, a single 28-F chest tube is placed, and the patient is turned to the supine position for laparoscopy. Prior to turning, we reintubate the patient with a single lumen endotracheal tube. We have found that dissection of the cervical esophagus is more difficult with the larger double-lumen tube in place. In addition, bronchoscopy can be performed through the single-lumen tube prior to extubation.

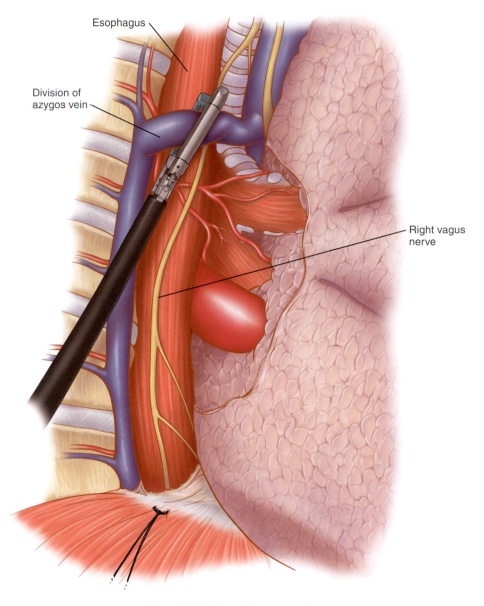

Esophagus

Division of
azygos vein

Right vagus
nerve

FIGURE 1-4 Division of the azygos vein.

Laparoscopy and Cervical Anastomosis

The five abdominal ports used for gastric mobilization are in the same configuration used for benign esophageal cases, although the ports are placed somewhat lower so that the entire stomach may be visualized (Fig. 1-6). The 11-mm port in the right epigastrium is placed first by an open cut-down method. This port will be used for access for stapling devices to create the gastric tube and for suturing. Another 10-mm port is placed on the right lower quadrant (not shown in the figure). This is used for identification of the ligament of Treitz and to facilitate suturing of the feeding jejunostomy tube. The upper abdominal ports should be high enough to be able to reach the upper abdomen with the surgical instruments, but low enough to have a reasonable view of the greater curve of the stomach along with the gastroepiploic arcade and the pylorus.

The left lobe of the liver is retracted upward to expose the esophageal hiatus and held in place with a self-retaining system placed on the left side of the table. The laparoscopic dissection starts by dividing the hepatogastric ligament toward the right crus of the diaphragm (Fig. 1-7). The right crus is exposed and

dissected from the top of the hiatus to the decussation with the left crus. This plane is developed then cephalad along the left crus to develop a retroesophageal window. Unlike other foregut operations, we do not divide the phrenoesophageal ligament until the conclusion of laparoscopy. Care is taken during the early steps of the dissection to avoid entry into the thoracic cavity as this will lead to loss of the abdominal pneumoperitoneum.

The stomach then is mobilized by dividing the short gastric vessels, using either ultrasonic shears or a bipolar coagulating system (Fig. 1-8). The dissection then is taken to the top portion of the esophageal hiatus exposing the left crus. The plane along the greater curve is continued distally, and the gastrocolic omentum is transected (Fig. 1-9). The surgeon should take care to preserve the gastroepiploic arcade (it will supply the gastric tube) without leaving too much fat along the greater curve of the stomach. Dissection in a plane too distal to the stomach will risk injury to the transverse colon. Excess fat along the greater curve may also make it difficult for the gastric tube to ascend through the hiatus into the chest. The dissection along the greater curve continues toward the second portion of the duodenum. Usually

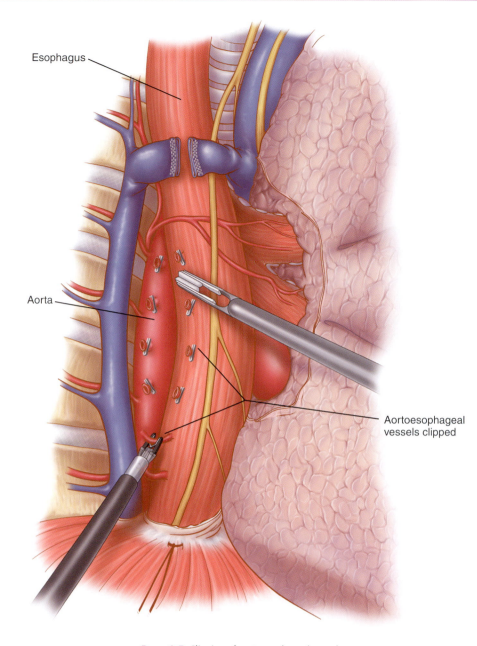

Esophagus

Aorta

Aortoesophageal
vessels clipped

FIGURE 1-5 Clipping of aortoesophageal vessels.

this will allow enough mobility for the pylorus to reach the right crus in a tension-free manner. The lymph nodes and fatty tissue of the celiac axis then are dissected and mobilized upward along the left gastric artery and vein. Once this area is cleared, the stomach is retracted superiorly and the left gastric vessels are divided (Fig. 1-10) using an endoscopic vascular stapler (Endo GIA II, U.S. Surgical).

The pyloroantral area then is mobilized with a Kocher maneuver. During this part of the procedure, we periodically grasp the antrum near the pylorus and carefully lift it toward the diaphragmatic hiatus. When sufficiently mobilized, the pylorus should reach to the right crus without tension. If this cannot be accomplished, then further kocherization is needed. After the Kocher maneuver is complete, a pyloroplasty is performed by opening the pylorus with the ultrasonic shears and closing the pylorus transversely with stitches (Fig. 1-11). In our experience, a laparoscopic pyloromyotomy is difficult to perform and often leads to insufficient gastric emptying. For the pyloroplasty, stay sutures are placed at the top and bottom of the anterior aspect of the muscle. Traction is placed on these sutures and the

pylorus is gently elevated. The muscle is divided along the length of the pyloric channel from the duodenal side until complete division of the muscle is visually evident. The stomach is suctioned clean through the pyloroplasty. The pyloric incision then is closed transversely using nonabsorbable 2-0 sutures applied with an automatic suturing device (Endo Stitch). At this point, the stomach is ready for the creation of the gastric tube.

For the gastric tube, an additional 11-mm port may be placed in the right lower quadrant. This extra port can be used to place downward traction on the antrum of the stomach, while gentle traction is placed on the fundus of the stomach during creation of the gastric tube. An area just above the first two to three arcades of the right gastric artery into the pyloroantral area is chosen for firing the first stapler. The vascular load is used to minimize bleeding. The first few arcades of the right gastric vessels into the pyloroantral area are spared and the stapler is fired in a perpendicular orientation to the lesser curve. As the construction of the gastric tube continues, care is taken to align the stapler parallel to the greater curve arcade (Fig. 1-12). We have found it beneficial to have the first assistant grasp the tip

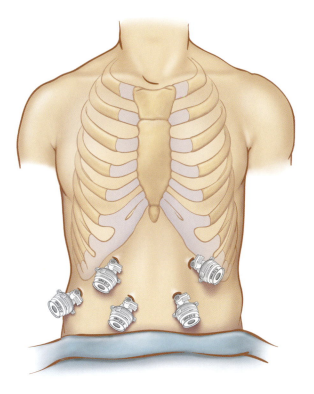

FIGURE 1-6 Port placement for the laparoscopic portion of a minimally invasive esophagectomy.

of the fundus and stretch it toward the spleen, while a second grasper is placed on the antral area for downward retraction. This places the stomach on a slight stretch and facilitates application of a straight staple line which, again, should be parallel to the gastroepiploic arcade. The gastric tube should be 5 to 6 cm in diameter. Early in our experience we created a tube 3 to 4 cm in diameter but had problems with gastric tip necrosis and anastomotic leaks. Again, we continue to apply gentle stretching of the stomach as the tube is constructed. As the gastric tube stapling progresses cephalad, the traction point is changed to the tip of the fundus, along the line of the short gastrics. These manipulations provide for effective tube length and attention to a line parallel to the greater curve avoids spiraling of the tube. The superior portion of the gastric tube then is sutured to the staple line of the resection specimen (Fig. 1-13). These stitches maintain correct orientation of the stomach as it is delivered into the mediastinum and neck.

After the gastric conduit has been completed, a feeding jejunostomy is placed using a needle catheter kit (Compat Biosystems, Minneapolis, MN). A 25-gauge 1.5-inch needle is inserted through the skin into the peritoneal cavity at the chosen entry site. A point approximately 30 cm distal to the ligament is chosen for the jejunostomy tube site, and the relevant limb of jejunum is tacked with a stitch to the anterior abdominal wall at the needle entry site (Fig. 1-14). An additional 10-mm port may be placed in the right lower quadrant to facilitate

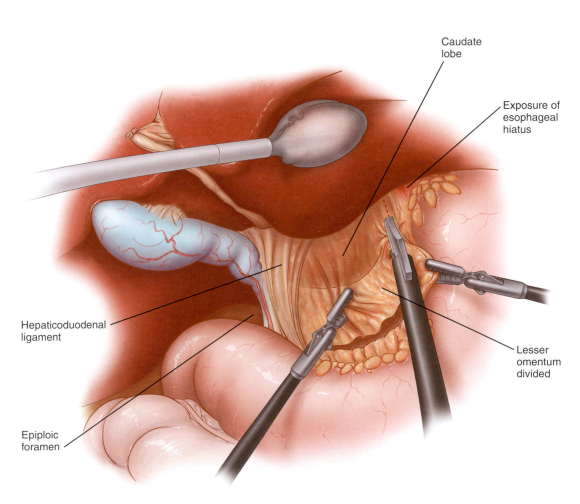

Caudate
lobe

Exposure of
esophageal
hiatus

Hepaticoduodenal
ligament

Lesser
omentum
divided

Epiploic
foramen

FIGURE 1-7 Division of the gastrohepatic ligament.

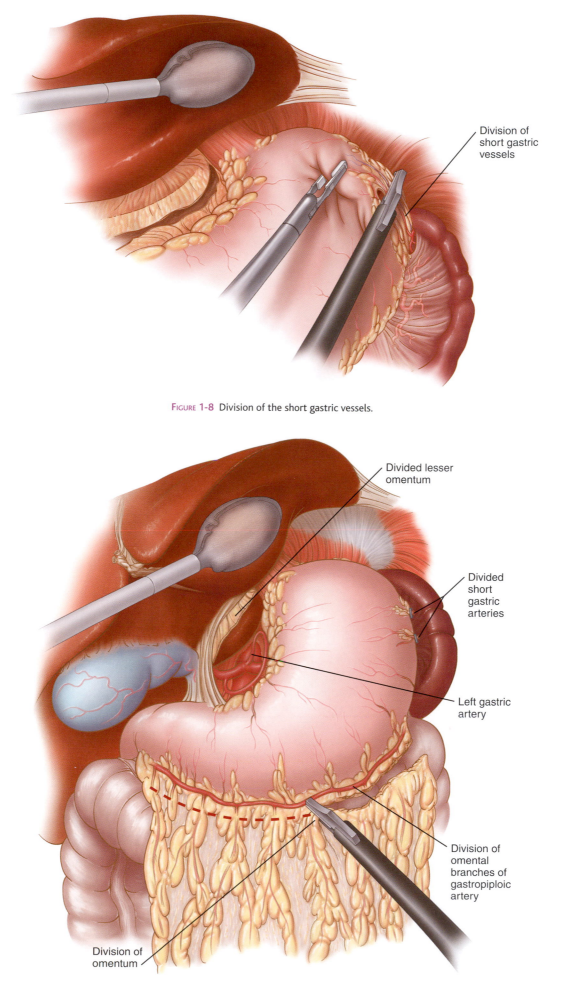

Division of
short gastric
vessels

FIGURE 1-8 Division of the short gastric vessels.

Divided lesser
omentum

Divided
short
gastric
arteries

Left gastric
artery

Division of
omental
branches of
gastropiploic
artery

Division of
omentum

FIGURE 1-9 Division of the gastrocolic omentum.

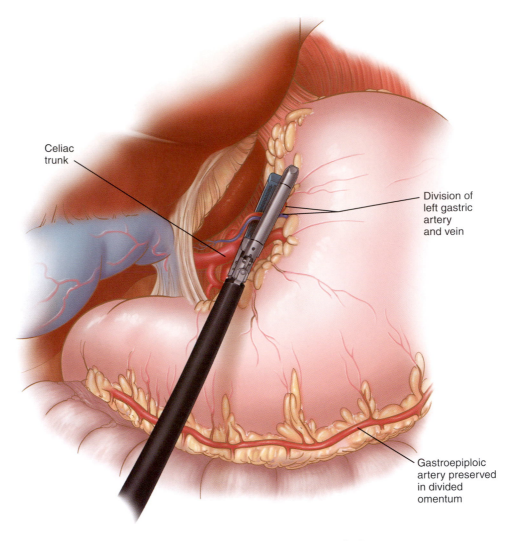

Celiac trunk

Division of left gastric artery and vein

Gastroepiploic artery preserved in divided omentum

FIGURE 1-10 Division of the left gastric artery and vein.

this step. The larger bore needle, which allows passage of the needle catheter (Compat Specialty Feeding Tube, 5 F; Novartis, Minneapolis, MN), is inserted through the abdominal wall percutaneously and enters the jejunum near the tacked site. Under laparoscopic view, the catheter is threaded into the jejunum for a distance of 20 cm. The feeding tube then is injected with 10 mL of air. Distention of the small bowel confirms intraluminal placement of the feeding tube. Two additional sutures then are placed to secure the jejunum to the peritoneal wall. A final stitch is placed several centimeters away from the tacked site to avoid torsion of the bowel around a single point. To complete the laparoscopic dissection, the right and left crura are partially divided to allow passage of the stomach into the mediastinum, and the phrenoesophageal membrane is divided.

A horizontal neck incision then is made to expose the cervical esophagus. We typically leave the Penrose drain around the esophagus during the VATS mobilization and push this drain into the neck at the conclusion of thoracoscopy. This allows quick identification of the correct dissection plane. The specimen then is pulled out of the neck, and the cervical esophagus is divided 1 to 2 cm below the cricopharyngeus. We then perform an extracorporeal end-to-side esophagogastrostomy using a circular 25-mm end-to-end anastomotic (EEA) stapler (Fig. 1-15). A nasogastric tube is passed across the anastomosis

and into the gastric tube. The gastrotomy made for introduction of the stapler head then is amputated with a linear stapler-cutter (Fig. 1-16).

After the neck anastomosis has been completed, we return to the laparoscopic view. Any excess gastric conduit that was pulled into the thoracic cavity is reduced. This can be achieved by gently tugging the antrum downward toward the abdomen; often several centimeters of the gastric conduit will reduce before the anastomosis will move caudad. When this occurs, one can assume the redundant gastric tube is within the abdomen. Failure to perform this step may lead to a slight sigmoid curve of the redundant gastric antrum within the chest; this may lead to poor gastric emptying and the need for subsequent revision.

Three tacking sutures then are placed between the gastric tube and the diaphragm to prevent hiatal herniation. Usually one suture is placed between the left crus and the stomach, just anterior to the greater curve arcade. The second suture is placed on the right side of the gastric tube just above the right gastric vessels, and the third stitch is placed anteriorly between the stomach and the diaphragm. We then close the neck incision very loosely. Tight closure of the platysma may allow a leak to track into the mediastinum rather than out the neck. To prevent this, we usually leave the neck incision open, except for a single staple to oppose the skin edges. The horizontal

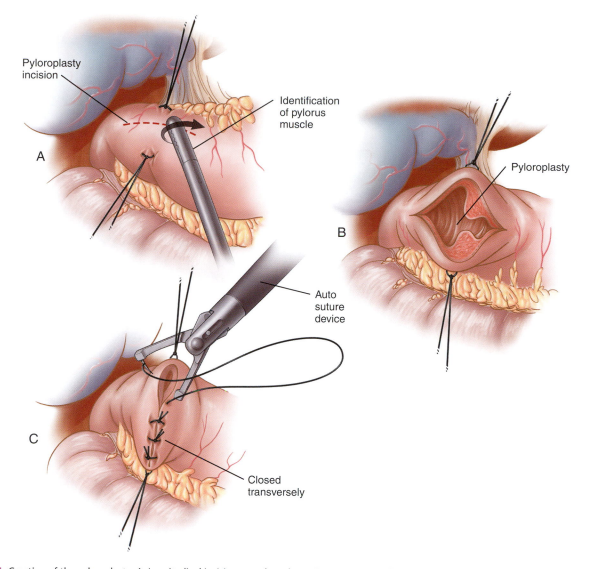

FIGURE 1-11   Creation of the pyloroplasty. **A,** Longitudinal incision over the pylorus. **B,** Stay sutures splaying the incision open. **C,** Incision closed transversely.

incision that we use heals remarkably well with this loose closure. The completed minimally invasive esophagectomy is shown in Figure 1-17.

Minimally Invasive Ivor Lewis Esophagectomy

As described earlier in the chapter, our standard MIE is concluded with a cervical esophagogastric anastomosis. Creation of an intrathoracic anastomosis, however, does carry some benefits. Avoiding dissection in the neck lowers the risk of injury to the recurrent laryngeal nerves. In addition, a small group of patients with intact nerves will develop problems with esophageal transit and aspiration. Although these complications are rarely fatal, they may increase the risk of aspiration pneumonia and decrease clearance of pulmonary secretions and overall quality of life. Furthermore, creation of a lower anastomosis may be necessary in patients with tumor extension onto the cardia. In these cases, more stomach must be resected in order to obtain an adequate margin; the remaining gastric tube may not have sufficient length to reach the neck.

The traditional concern with an Ivor Lewis esophagectomy was the risk of pulmonary complications. It would seem that a minimally invasive Ivor Lewis esophagectomy would combine the advantages of no neck dissection with the benefits of reduced pulmonary morbidity seen with minimally invasive surgery. The conduct of this operation is similar to that for a standard minimally invasive esophagectomy, although we begin the Ivor Lewis esophagectomy with laparoscopy. Once the abdominal phase has been completed, the patient is turned to the left lateral decubitus position. We use the same port sites for thoracoscopy described above. The only modification is to enlarge the posterior inferior eighth intercostal port site to 3 to 4 cm to allow the introduction of circular EEA stapler and for the removal of the specimen. A laparoscopic wound protector is used at this site to minimize the risk of port contamination. Once the esophagus has been mobilized to 4 to 5 cm above the azygos vein, the distal esophagus and stomach are brought through the hiatus into the chest, along with the gastric tube that was sutured to the specimen. The esophagus is elevated and transected 2 to 3 cm above the level of the azygos vein.

The specimen is removed using an endo-catch bag to prevent wound contamination. The anvil of a 28-mm EEA stapler then is placed into the proximal esophagus and secured using two concentric purse-string stitches. A gastrotomy is then made just lateral to the lesser curve staple line to allow introduction of the

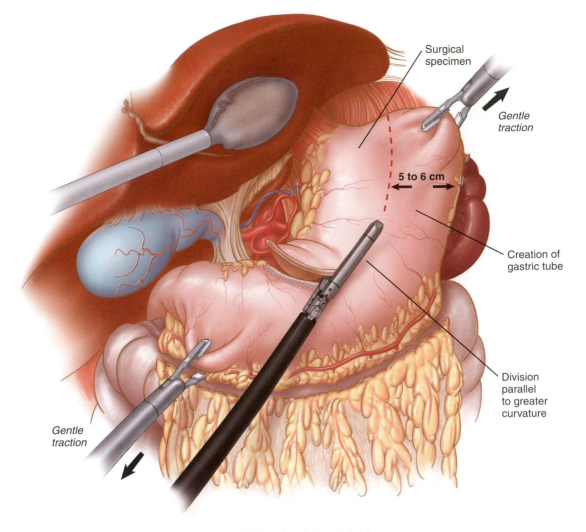

FIGURE 1-12 Creation of the gastric tube.

circular stapler. The stapler is placed through the enlarged posterior port and introduced into the gastrotomy. Prior to creating the anastomosis, we carefully ascertain the amount of conduit that will lie in the chest. It is a common mistake to bring an excess amount of stomach into the chest in an effort to minimize tension on the anastomosis. This excess conduit will often assume a sigmoid curve above the diaphragm and may lead to significant problems with gastric emptying. Once the stapler is introduced into the conduit and we are satisfied with the length of the conduit in the chest, the tip of the stapler is brought out along the greater curve of the stomach. Ensuring proper orientation of the stomach at this point is critical to prevent torsion. The tip of the stapler and the anvil are docked and the stapler fired, creating a circular esophagogastric anastomosis (side of gastric conduit to end of esophagus) at the level of the azygos vein. The excess gastric conduit (that was above the gastrotomy where the stapler was introduced) is trimmed using an articulating linear stapler, and a 28-F chest tube and a Jackson-Pratt drain are placed by the anastomosis. The potential space between the conduit and the right crus of the diaphragm then is closed with a single interrupted stitch to prevent delayed herniation.

POSTOPERATIVE CARE

Patients may be extubated in the operating room and observed overnight in the intensive care unit. The following morning the patient is transferred to the regular floor; ambulation and the use of incentive spirometry are encouraged. Tube feedings are begun on the second postoperative day and gradually are increased to the target rate. The chest tube is removed once the output is below 250 mL over a 24-hour period. We usually keep the chest tube in place until tube feedings are initiated to ensure that there is no evidence of a chylothorax. The nasogastric tube is removed on the third postoperative day and if there is no concern for aspiration, the patient is allowed to take sips of clear liquids. For the patient with a cervical anastomosis, we do not perform a barium swallow unless there is concern for a leak. The patient with an intrathoracic anastomosis undergoes a barium swallow on postoperative day 6 and is discharged if the study is normal. Patients are discharged home on a soft diet and night-time tube feedings. The jejunostomy catheter usually is removed in the clinic after 2 or 3 weeks, if the oral intake is adequate.

MANAGEMENT OF PROCEDURE-SPECIFIC COMPLICATIONS

Esophagectomy carries the potential for severe morbidity, whether performed through an open or minimally invasive approach. In the largest series that reported outcomes following minimally invasive esophagectomy, major complications occurred in 32% of patients. The most common major complication was anastomotic leak (11%). We found that a higher leak

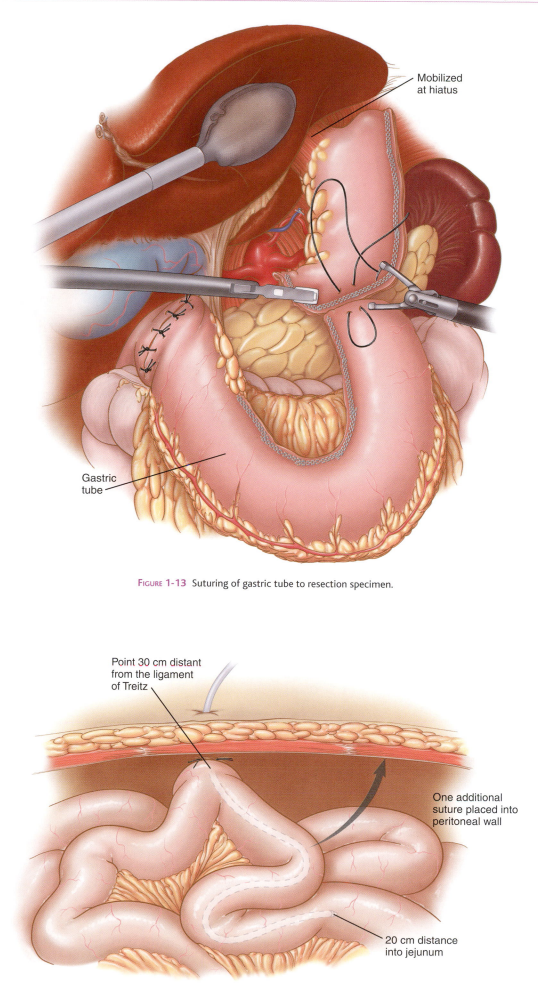

Mobilized
at hiatus

Gastric
tube

FIGURE **1-13** Suturing of gastric tube to resection specimen.

Point 30 cm distant
from the ligament
of Treitz

One additional
suture placed into
peritoneal wall

20 cm distance
into jejunum

FIGURE **1-14** Placement of a feeding jejunostomy.

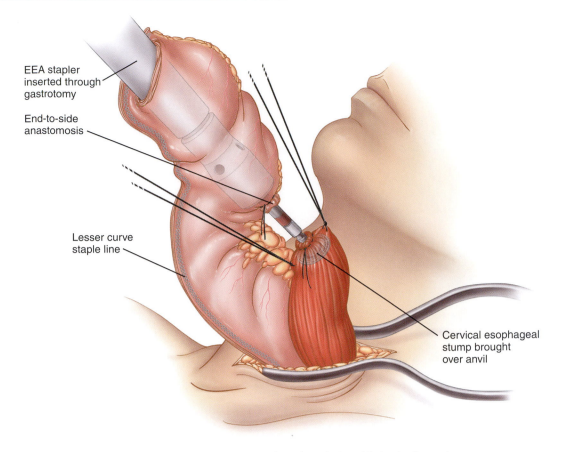

EEA stapler
inserted through
gastrotomy

End-to-side
anastomosis

Lesser curve
staple line

Cervical esophageal
stump brought
over anvil

FIGURE 1-15 Restoration of gastroesophageal continuity with the circular stapler.

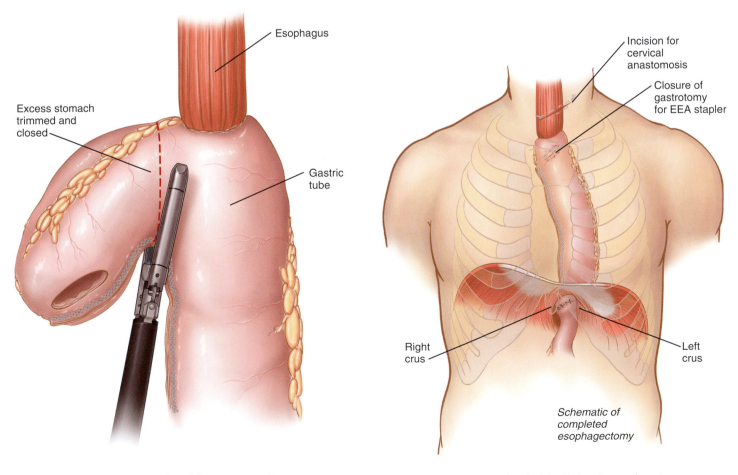

Esophagus

Excess stomach
trimmed and
closed

Gastric
tube

FIGURE 1-16 Amputation of the gastrotomy site.

Incision for
cervical
anastomosis

Closure of
gastrotomy
for EEA stapler

Right
crus

Left
crus

*Schematic of
completed
esophagectomy*

FIGURE 1-17 Completed minimally invasive esophagectomy.

rate occurred when a narrow (3 cm) gastric tube was created. The leak rate was far less with a larger (5 cm) gastric tube. Most anastomotic leaks were localized to the neck and were managed by opening the cervical wound, administration of antibiotics, and enteral nutrition. On occasion a cervical leak will track into the mediastinum. In these cases, a VATS procedure or open thoracotomy and decortication may be necessary. We have found that leaving the mediastinal pleura intact above the level of the azygos vein is important. Should a leak occur, the intact pleura may seal a leak that would otherwise track downward.

Pneumonia was the second most common major complication, occurring in 8% of patients. Vocal cord palsy (4%), chylothorax (3%), and gastric tip necrosis (3%) were uncommon but serious complications. Minor complications included atrial fibrillation and pleural effusion. Anastomotic stricture occurs commonly following esophagectomy, and we take a liberal approach with dilation. Any patient with dysphagia following esophagectomy undergoes endoscopy by the primary surgeon in the operating room, with dilation if needed. We perform all of our dilations under fluoroscopy using a guidewire, in order to minimize the likelihood of perforation. In our experience nearly all patients with an anastomotic leak will develop a stricture, so these patients will need frequent and graded dilations.

RESULTS AND OUTCOME

We published an analysis of 222 consecutive patients who have undergone minimally invasive esophagectomy at the University of Pittsburgh. Although early in the series we selectively performed MIE on patients with smaller tumors and no previous therapy, 35% of the patients in this series had been treated with chemotherapy and 16% with radiation. In addition, 25% of patients had undergone prior open abdominal surgery. MIE was completed as planned in 206 (93%) patients. No emergent conversions to an open procedure were necessary for bleeding. Of the 16 cases who required nonemergent conversion, 11 required a minithoracotomy for adhesions and, in one case, oversewing of bleeding from a persistent intercostal vessel that could not be controlled by VATS.

Overall there were three deaths in the series (1.4% mortality rate): postoperative pneumonia and multisystem organ failure ($n = 1$); a myocardial infarction on postoperative day 5 ($n = 1$); and pericardial tamponade that developed 3 days after MIE ($n = 1$). None of these deaths were in patients who developed an anastomotic leak or gastric tube necrosis. The rate of anastomotic leak in this series was 11.7%. As described above, this

complication was clearly related to the size of the gastric tube. The leak rate associated with a smaller diameter tube (3–4 cm) was 26% in our experience. In those patients who underwent creation of a larger conduit (5–6 cm diameter), the leak rate was only 6%. Stage-specific survival rate in this series was comparable to that in large series of open esophagectomy.

We have also published our early experience with the minimally invasive Ivor Lewis esophagectomy. In our series of 50 patients, 35 underwent a hybrid procedure consisting of laparoscopic preparation of the gastric conduit followed by a minithoracotomy for creation of the anastomosis. The remaining 15 patients had a completely minimally invasive procedure. Among these 50 patients, the rate of anastomotic leak and mortality were both 6%. All of the patients with an anastomotic leak were managed with chest tube drainage alone without the need for reoperation. Importantly, no patient in this small series developed an injury to the recurrent laryngeal nerve. The length of follow-up in this study was insufficient to determine patterns of recurrence and overall survival. However, given the very encouraging results in this series we have continued to offer an Ivor Lewis esophagectomy to patients with cancers of the gastroesophageal junction. At present we have performed over 150 minimally invasive Ivor Lewis esophagectomies at the University of Pittsburgh.

Suggested Reading

Ackroyd R, Watson D, Majeed A, et al: Randomized clinical trial of laparoscopic versus open fundoplication for gastro-oesophageal reflux disease. Br J Surg 2004;91(8):975–982.

Bizekis C, Kent M, Luketich J, et al: Initial experience with minimally-invasive Ivor Lewis esophagectomy. Ann Thorac Surg 2006;82:402–406.

Chiu P, Chan A, Leung S, et al: Multicenter prospective randomized trial comparing standard esophagectomy with chemoradiotherapy for treatment of squamous esophageal cancer: Early results from the Chinese University Research Group for Esophageal Cancer (CURE). J Gastrointest Surg 2005;9(6):794–802.

DePaula AL, Hashiba K, Ferreira EA, et al: Laparoscopic transhiatal esophagectomy with esophagogastroplasty. Surg Laparosc Endosc 1995;5(1):1–5.

Luketich J, Fernando H, Christie N, et al: Outcomes after minimally invasive esophagomyotomy. Ann Thorac Surg 2001;72(6):1909–1912.

Luketich J, Alvelo-Rivera M, Buenaventura P, et al: Minimally invasive esophagectomy: Outcomes in 222 patients. Ann Surg 2003;238:486–495.

Luketich J, Meehan M, Nguyen N, et al: Minimally invasive surgical staging for esophageal cancer. Surg Endosc 2000;14:700–702.

McAnena OJ, Rogers J, Williams NS: Right thoracoscopically assisted oesophagectomy for cancer. Br J Surg 1994;81(2):236–238.

Peracchia A, Rosati R, Fumagalli U, et al: Thoracoscopic esophagectomy: Are there benefits? Semin Surg Oncol 1997;13(4):259–262.

Stahl M, Stuschke M, Lehmann N et al. Chemoradiation with and without surgery in patients with locally advanced squamous cell carcinoma of the esophagus. J Clin Oncol 2005;23(10):2310–2317.

ERIC S. HUNGNESS AND
NATHANIEL J. SOPER

Laparoscopic Esophagomyotomy

Achalasia is a rare primary esophageal motility disorder of unknown etiology that results from degeneration of neurons in the myenteric plexus. Because the lower esophageal sphincter (LES) fails to relax and the esophagus lacks peristalsis, patients with achalasia experience worsening dysphagia, initially with solids and progressing to liquids. Regurgitation, aspiration, chest pain, and weight loss are common, which leads to a medical work-up.

Surgical treatment of achalasia in the past was the open Heller esophagomyotomy, which was performed through a left thoracotomy. This resulted in a high incidence of postoperative reflux, because a fundoplication was not included. It also was difficult to adequately extend the myotomy onto the stomach. With the advent of advanced minimally invasive surgery, laparoscopic Heller esophagomyotomy is now the preferred surgical therapy for patients with achalasia. This chapter will discuss operative indications, pre- and postoperative care, and operative technique of this complex esophageal operation.

OPERATIVE INDICATIONS

Many patients diagnosed with achalasia undergo a trial of medical therapy prior to seeking a surgical consultation. Pharmacologic therapy with calcium channel blockers or nitrates only is transiently effective and may have significant side effects. Endoscopic therapy consists of either pneumatic dilatation or Botox (botulinum toxin type A) injection. For patients undergoing dilatation, the LES is disrupted with progressively larger balloons, up to 40 mm in diameter. This can be performed as an outpatient procedure in the endoscopy suite with conscious sedation. There is a 3% to 5% perforation rate that results in emergency operation in 50% of the cases. Reports suggest that dilatation may be effective in up to 70% of patients at 1 year; the rate of long-term symptom relief, however, is only 50%. Botox therapy may be useful in patients with severe comorbid disease, or in those reluctant to have more invasive treatment. It should be noted that nonsurgical treatments of achalasia, especially Botox injection, can result in scarring of the submucosa, which can make subsequent laparoscopic esophagomyotomy more difficult.

Laparoscopic esophagomyotomy offers patients with achalasia the best chance for long-term symptom resolution with low morbidity in a single therapy session. The esophagomyotomy commonly is combined with a partial fundoplication (Toupet or Dor) or a "floppy" Nissen fundoplication to prevent postoperative pathologic reflux.

PREOPERATIVE EVALUATION, TESTING, AND PREPARATION

Most patients come to their initial surgical evaluation with the diagnosis of achalasia already established. Barium swallow in these patients may show the classic "bird's beak" appearance. Patients with long-standing achalasia also may show a massively dilated esophagus (megaesophagus). Endoscopy should be part of the preoperative evaluation, especially in older patients and in those with long-standing achalasia, in order to rule out pseudoachalasia secondary to tumor. Typically there is minimal resistance to passage of the endoscope into the stomach. Esophageal manometry may confirm the diagnosis by demonstrating failure of LES relaxation and dysmotility or aperistalsis of the esophagus after swallowing.

Patients are counseled that gastric or esophageal perforation, vagal injury, splenic injury, or open conversion are rare but possible outcomes. The typical patient is admitted the day of surgery and might have been limited to clear liquids for 48 hours prior to the operation. The anesthetist should consider rapid sequence induction or awake fiberoptic intubation to reduce the risk of aspiration of retained food in the esophagus.

PATIENT POSITIONING IN THE OPERATING SUITE

The surgeon stands between the patient's abducted legs, facing directly forward during the operation (Fig. 2-1). We prefer flat padded boards that allow the knees to be extended and which minimize the potential for lower extremity neurovascular traction injury. Video monitors are positioned at the head of the operating table. The patient should be secured to the operating table and padded in the appropriate locations because the table is maintained in steep reverse Trendelenburg position during the procedure. To do this, we like to utilize a vacuum beanbag that supports the patient's sides and perineum and minimizes intraoperative movement and displacement of the body.

An angled 30-degree laparoscope allows alternative views of the operative field, including the retrofundic and retroesophageal regions. An atraumatic liver retractor is important for prolonged

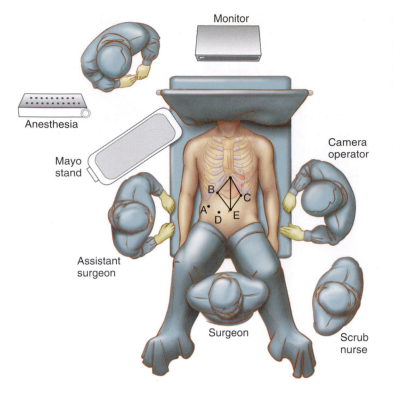

FIGURE 2-1   Room layout and port placement for laparoscopic esophagomyotomy.

on either side of the laparoscope. The surgeon's right-hand port generally is placed 10 cm from the xiphoid and two finger-breadths below the left costal margin. We prefer a 10-mm port in this location, because a curved SH needle can be inserted through the valve. If a 5-mm port is used, then straight or "ski" needles must be used for suturing. Other "automatic" suturing devices also require a 10-mm port. The 5-mm liver retractor port is then placed at least 15 cm from the xiphoid process, two fingerbreadths below the right costal margin. The assistant's 5-mm port is then placed halfway between the camera and liver retractor ports. The left lateral segment of the liver is elevated with a self-retaining liver retractor, and then the surgeon's left-hand 5-mm port is placed. Its precise location depends somewhat on the size and location of the liver lobe and the shape of the retractor itself. A Veress needle may be used to "sound out" potential sites on the abdominal wall for port placement before the port incision is made.

Other surgeons have described alternative operative approaches, such as having the assistant stand to the left of the patient and manipulate tissue through a port placed in the left subcostal region. Some prefer the laparoscopic camera port to be placed in a midline position. Each of these alternatives for port positioning is valid, and the surgeon must decide the optimal positioning for the operating team in his or her own suite.

OPERATIVE TECHNIQUE

Basic Tenets and Techniques

General technical principles of esophageal operations include (1) avoidance of dissection into the esophageal wall; (2) use of atraumatic graspers; (3) dissection under direct vision; (4) plication of the fundus, not the gastric body around the esophagus; and (5) keeping the area tension-free, with respect to axial (tending to pull the repair up into the mediastinum) or rotational (pulling the fundus back to the left) forces.

Initial Dissection

The anterior gastric wall or the gastroesophageal fat pad is then grasped by the assistant and pulled caudally and to the patient's left, placing traction on the gastrohepatic omentum. Using ultrasonic shears, the gastrohepatic omentum is divided, beginning just superior to the hepatic branch of the vagus nerve. The surgeon must be wary of an aberrant left hepatic artery running adjacent to the hepatic branch of the vagus nerve. Although they are encountered in fewer than 5% of patients, such an artery may supply the majority of arterial inflow to the left lateral segment of the liver. The hepatic branch of the vagus nerve generally does not need to be divided for visualization if the angled laparoscope is employed. The gastrohepatic omentum is divided up to the level of the right bundle of the right crus of the diaphragm, and the phrenoesophageal membrane is divided in a transverse direction, taking care to divide only the most anterior portion in order to prevent injury to the underlying esophagus and anterior vagus nerve. The gastric fundus is then pulled inferiorly and to the right. The gastrophrenic ligament is divided to mobilize the gastric cardia.

During the hiatal dissection, the assistant retracts the fat pad inferiorly to place tension on the distal esophagus. Having divided the phrenoesophageal membrane, it is generally easy to insert a blunt-tipped instrument just medial to the right bundle of the right crus of the diaphragm in order to establish a plane between the esophagus and the right crus. The surgeon's left-hand instrument

periods of retraction. We prefer a self-retaining "snake" liver retractor. Atraumatic grasping instruments and hemostatic cutting devices (such as ultrasonic shears or bipolar cutters) also should be available. Also, a flexible endoscope would be helpful to evaluate the esophagus and stomach, as well as to detect mucosal perforation.

PLACEMENT OF TROCARS

We like to place our ports in an arc between 10 and 15 cm inferior to the xiphoid process and costal margin, which are marked prior to pneumoperitoneum (see Fig. 2-1).

An open or closed technique may be used to access the peritoneal cavity. With the open technique, a cut-down is performed through a small incision, and the fascia is incised under direct vision. Sutures are placed at the fascial level, and the peritoneal cavity is entered under direct vision. A Hasson-type trocar and sheath is then placed into the peritoneal cavity, and the pneumoperitoneum is created with the insufflation of carbon dioxide to 12 mm Hg. Alternatively, a Veress needle may be passed directly into the peritoneal cavity.

The esophagus generally enters the abdomen from a slightly right-to-left orientation. We place the laparoscope to the left of the midline in a supraumbilical location approximately 12 cm inferior to the xiphoid process in order to avoid the falciform ligament. An infraumbilical port site generally is too far inferior on the abdominal wall for operations at or around the esophageal hiatus.

The skin incision is made in the appropriate location, and the first trocar is inserted. After laparoscope insertion, a visual exploration of the abdominal cavity is performed, with particular attention paid to the area immediately posterior to the initial trocar insertion site. We prefer the 10-mm diameter laparoscope because it has a wide field of view and brilliant illumination.

The patient is then placed into a *steep* reverse Trendelenburg position, and the rest of the trocars are placed under direct vision. For optimal visual orientation, the working instruments should enter the operative field with a 30- to 60-degree angle

grasps or pushes the right bundle to the patient's right while the right-hand instrument gradually and gently sweeps the esophagus and paraesophageal tissue to the left to mobilize the distal esophagus. The posterior vagus nerve is swept along with the esophagus to the patient's left. This mobilization continues into the chest as far as possible and then distally to the level of the crus. The tissue attached to the medial border of the base of the right bundle is divided so that the origin of the right bundle from the left bundle of the right crus is visualized from the right side of the esophagus.

Once the right side of the esophagus has been mobilized, the surgeon's right-hand instrument sweeps anterior to the esophagus and elevates the anterior crural arch, while gently pushing the esophagus posterior with the left-hand instrument. The postero-medial aspect of the left bundle is visualized, and all the paraesophageal tissue is swept posterior to develop the plane to the left of the esophagus. The anterior vagus nerve and left pleura usually are visualized at this time. The initial dissection of the mediastinum at this point has mobilized the esophagus from the pleura, the aorta, and the lateral crural attachments. The anterior and posterior vagus nerves have been identified to avoid injury. If the parietal pleura is lacerated during the dissection, then the surgeon should communicate this to the anesthetist. Assuming that the lung parenchyma is not injured, the low-tension capnothorax that results usually poses little risk to the patient. The anesthetist can increase the airway pressure while the surgeon slightly decreases the insufflation pressure, and adequate ventilation and perfusion usually can be maintained. Typically, it is not necessary to place a chest tube for these pleural tears.

For the fundal mobilization, the left lateral border of the fundus is grasped, elevated, and retracted to the right while the gastrosplenic ligament is grasped, elevated, and retracted to the left. Division of the short gastric vessels with the ultrasonic shears is started at a point 10 to 15 cm distal to the angle of His. Adequate fundus is mobilized for a tension-free fundoplication. We select a point just superior to the most proximal gastroepiploic vessels, which are identified by their caudal orientation. At this site a "window" is made in the gastrosplenic ligament with the gastric vessel and the entry into the lesser sac, identified by visualizing the space bounded medially by the posterior gastric wall. Once the lesser sac is entered, traction on the stomach and countertraction on the gastrosplenic ligament are maintained to align the greater curvature of the stomach with the visual axis of the laparoscope. The short gastric vessels and all other attachments to the fundus (including any posterior gastric arteries) are then divided sequentially, proceeding from distal to proximal, until the entire fundus has been mobilized. Care must be taken during the division of the most proximal short gastric vessels, as the spleen typically is in close proximity.

After the fundal mobilization, the anterior vagus nerve is dissected from the anterior surface of the esophagus and gastric cardia along the length of the proposed myotomy. Care must be taken not to activate the ultrasonic shears or cautery in proximity to the vagus, as this may lead to injury or paresis. Once the anterior vagus is freed, the retroesophageal space is visualized from the left side of the stomach. The medial border of the left bundle of the right crus of the diaphragm is dissected back to its junction with the right bundle, joining the dissection begun on the right side. A large window is thereby created posterior to the esophagus and proximal stomach and anterior to the left crural bundles. After the retroesophageal window is created, a Penrose drain may be placed around the gastroesophageal junction. This maneuver is helpful if traction is difficult to achieve

by other means. We prefer to use the fundus itself as a retractor, reaching from right to left behind the esophagus to grasp the fundus, and retract it back to the right side behind the esophagus. By placing caudal traction on the wrapped fundus, the gastroesophageal junction and distal esophagus can be brought further into the abdominal cavity.

The distal esophagus then is checked to see if at least 3 cm of esophagus remains in the abdomen when the traction is released. If this is not the case, then further esophageal mobilization should be performed within the mediastinum. In the unlikely event that an adequate length of intra-abdominal esophagus cannot be obtained, the surgeon may consider performing an esophageal-lengthening procedure.

Myotomy

Of note, the myotomy generally is easier to perform on patients who have not had Botox injection or have undergone pneumatic dilatation. With the anterior vagus nerve retracted, the path of the myotomy is scored on the anterior surface of the esophagus and gastric cardia using an L-hook electrocautery device. Atraumatic graspers then grab either side of the scored mark, and then the longitudinal esophageal muscle is separated gently with lateral traction. We prefer to begin this a few centimeters above the gastroesophageal junction. The circular esophageal muscle layer then is carefully divided with hook cautery (Fig. 2-2). Small bites of individual muscle fibers are elevated off the underlying mucosa prior to cautery activation. With a complete myotomy, the underlying mucosa will bulge out. Bleeding during this part of the myotomy is common—the esophageal submucosa has a rich blood supply—but self-limited. Direct pressure usually resolves the bleeding. If used, cautery should be applied sparingly and precisely to avoid mucosal injury. The edges of the myotomy then are grasped with atraumatic graspers to expose more than 120 degrees of the anterior mucosa, ensuring complete division of the circular muscle. The myotomy should continue 6 to 8 cm into the chest and extend 2 to 3 cm onto the

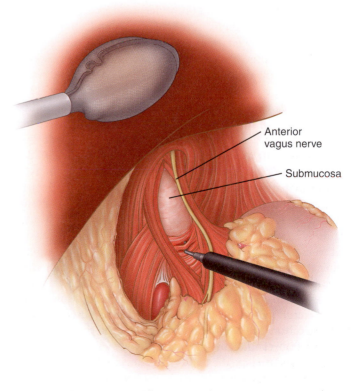

Anterior vagus nerve

Submucosa

FIGURE 2-2 Myotomy with retraction of anterior vagus nerve.

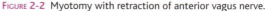

gastric cardia. The latter is identified when the two layers of esophageal muscle become thickened and ill-defined. Once the myotomy is completed an upper endoscope is passed under direct visualization into the lower esophagus in order to detect any mucosal perforation. A perforation is repaired primarily with fine absorbable interrupted sutures, and covered with a Dor fundoplication. After a complete myotomy, it should be possible to view a widely patent gastroesophageal junction with the endoscope several centimeters proximal. If a patent gastroesophageal junction is not visible, then further dissection/myotomy should be considered.

Crural Closure

The crural bundles are then approximated posterior to the esophagus. Inferior traction is maintained on the proximal stomach either by atraumatic graspers placed on the wrapped fundus or with the sling of the Penrose drain. Crural closure is necessary, because even though a hiatal hernia may not have existed preoperatively, an iatrogenic one potentially was created by the paraesophageal dissection. We use 2-0 nonabsorbable braided polyester sutures on a curved (SH) needle for this purpose. The crural fascia should be incorporated in the sutures along with the muscular fibers. The crura are closed until they lightly touch the empty esophagus; it should be possible to pass an instrument between the esophagus and the closed crura. Esophageal dilators can stiffen the esophagus, making it difficult to retract the esophagus anteriorly for the posterior crural closure. We therefore prefer not to use these dilators during crural closure.

Fundoplication

One purpose of a partial fundoplication is to prevent reflux with minimal esophageal outflow resistance. We prefer to perform a partial fundoplication with laparoscopic esophagomyotomy, since some recent studies have suggested that the addition of a partial fundoplication reduces the incidence of postoperative gastroesophageal reflux without increasing dysphagia. A partial fundoplication may be more difficult to conceptualize and perform for the nonspecialist surgeon compared to a total fundoplication, which can limit the widespread application of partial fundoplication. We prefer the Toupet fundoplication (Fig. 2-3), since it "holds" the edges of the myotomy open and is easier to construct. For this procedure, the fundus is pulled posterior to the esophagus with suture of the leading edge of the wrapped fundus to the right edge of the esophageal myotomy. The left (medial) side of the fundus is sutured to the left edge aspect of the esophageal myotomy. Varying numbers of sutures may be placed between the fundus and the crura for further stabilization. The Dor fundoplication (Figs. 2-4 and 2-5) is a 180- to 200-degree anterior fundoplication that has been used primarily in association with laparoscopic esophagomyotomy.

Although it may be possible to construct a partial fundoplication without fundic mobilization or division of the short gastric vessels, we prefer a complete fundic mobilization regardless of the fundoplication. The technical details of the Toupet fundoplication vary considerably among different surgeons. Some describe fixation of the fundoplication to the crura, whereas others have omitted this step. Most individuals use multiple interrupted sutures of heavy-gauge nonabsorbable sutures to fix the fundoplication 200 to 270 degrees around the posterior circumference of the esophagus.

Prior to suturing, the fundus is checked for rotational tension and torsion by first observing the wrapped fundus after it

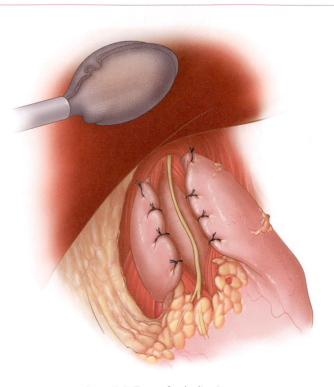

FIGURE 2-3 Toupet fundoplication.

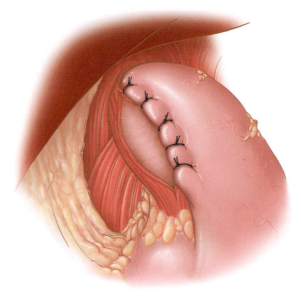

FIGURE 2-4 Dor fundoplication—initial sutures.

is released. If it retracts back around the esophagus to the left, then there is tension that should be eliminated by dividing more fundic attachments. Next, we check for a twist or entrapment of the wrapped fundus in the posterior window by performing a "shoeshine" maneuver. The leading edge of the fundus that has been passed behind and to the right of the esophagus is grasped, along with the fundus to the left of the esophagus. The fundus is then retracted back and forth to make sure that it slides easily, that the tissues on both sides are in continuity, and that the fundus is not twisted.

The wrapped fundus is pulled well to the patient's left to expose the posterior aspect of the wrapped fundus and the crural bundles. We use 2-0 nonabsorbable braided polyester sutures on a curved needle for the fundoplication. Several interrupted sutures are placed between both the posterior left aspect of the

tron intravenously for the first 12 to 18 hours after the operation. The intent of this regimen is to minimize the risk of postoperative nausea and vomiting. Since edema narrows the esophagus in the early postoperative interval, the patient is kept on a soft diet for 2 to 4 weeks. Most patients, however, notice a dramatic resolution of the dysphagia immediately. If a patient experiences severe chest or abdominal pain, or if the patient vomits in the early postoperative period, then a water-soluble contrast swallow radiograph is obtained to evaluate for perforation or disruption, or displacement of the wrap. Each patient is seen in the outpatient office 2 to 4 weeks after the operation. Rapid resumption of full activity is encouraged, with the exception of any activity requiring a Valsalva maneuver. This is discouraged for at least 6 weeks after the operation.

MANAGEMENT OF PROCEDURE-SPECIFIC COMPLICATIONS

Mucosal Perforation

The risk for mucosal perforation may be minimized by careful and meticulous surgical technique, especially in patients who have had previous endoscopic therapy. Lateral traction to the muscularis should be applied slowly. Individual circular muscle bundles should be dissected free and elevated from the underlying mucosa, which is thinner in the stomach. Electrocautery should be used sparingly and accurately. The endoscope should be advanced under direct visualization by a skilled endoscopist.

If the surgeon suspects a mucosa perforation during the operation, then an oral gastric tube should be used for a diagnostic instillation of methylene blue. Another option includes the passage of an endoscope with insufflation of the esophagus and stomach. Most esophageal and gastric perforations discovered during esophagomyotomy may be closed laparoscopically with fine sutures. The adequacy of the repair can be checked by flooding the area with saline solution and then insufflating air or carbon dioxide into the esophagus. We perform a Dor fundoplication if a mucosal perforation has occurred to help buttress the mucosal repair.

Capnothorax

The risk for capnothorax can be minimized with careful dissection of the pleura away from the esophagus. If the pleura is lacerated during hiatal dissection, then a capnothorax will usually be discovered when the diaphragm is seen bulging caudad. This generally does not have deleterious effects; however, the anesthesia team should be made aware (see Chapter 32). In the event of respiratory compromise, the airway and insufflation pressures should be increased and decreased, respectively. Rarely, if ever, does a chest tube need to be placed. Routine postoperative chest x-ray is not performed. A capnothorax will almost always resolve on its own. Supplemental O_2 may be given to facilitate absorption of CO_2. Only in the setting of respiratory compromise is tube thoracostomy performed.

Vagus Nerve Injury

Vagus nerve injury is best avoided by early identification of the nerve during the hiatal dissection. Only superficial bites of the phrenoesophageal membrane should be taken. Blunt dissection should be used liberally during hiatal dissection in order to identify the nerves prior to dividing any structures with scissors or

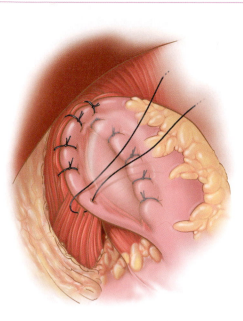

FIGURE 2-5 Dor fundoplication—final appearance.

fundus and the left bundle and between the posterior right aspect of the fundus and the right bundle of the diaphragm to stabilize the wrap. We generally place three sutures between the right edge of the esophageal myotomy and the leading edge of the wrapped portion of fundus to create a wrap that is 2 to 3 cm in length. The fundus to the left of the esophagus is then approximated to the left edge of the esophageal myotomy with three interrupted sutures. Care is taken to avoid the underlying mucosa while these sutures are being placed. The completed fundoplication has been described as a "hot dog in a bun" (see Fig. 2-3).

We construct a Dor fundoplication if mucosal perforation has occurred, or when there is too much anterior angulation of the esophagus as the fundus is brought through the retroesophageal window. The medial posterior fundus is sutured to the left edge of the myotomy with three interrupted 2-0 braided permanent sutures (see Fig. 2-4). The superior suture incorporates the left bundle, anchoring the fundoplication. The "floppy" superior lateral fundus is then brought 180 degrees anteromedially and sutured to the right edge of the myotomy and right bundle. Two additional sutures approximate the fundus to the myotomy, completing the fundoplication (see Fig. 2-5).

Upon completion of the fundoplication, the liver retractor is removed and the undersurface of the liver is examined for capsular tears or bleeding. The upper abdomen is aspirated and checked for hemostasis. The ports are then removed under direct vision. Any port larger than 5 mm diameter and located below the costal margin on exsufflation should have fascial closure with heavy-gauge suture. We perform this approximation using a fascial closure device with laparoscopic visualization. The abdomen is exsufflated, the ports are removed, and each incision is infiltrated with bupivacaine.

POSTOPERATIVE CARE

Our protocol specifies that, prior to leaving the operating room, the patient is administered intravenous ketorolac and ondansetron. A nasogastric tube is rarely used. We admit all patients to the hospital after the operation and give them ice chips that evening. The patients are allowed clear liquids the morning after the operation; if this is tolerated, then a soft diet is ordered for lunch. The patient receives scheduled ketorolac and ondanse-

ultrasonic shears. If one or both of the vagus nerves are suspected of being injured, no immediate therapy is mandatory. Even in the setting of complete vagotomy, most patients will not develop symptoms of delayed gastric emptying.

RESULTS AND OUTCOME

Most studies have demonstrated good to excellent results in patients undergoing laparoscopic esophagomyotomy for achalasia, with greater than 90% of patients experiencing relief of dysphagia at 1 year. Longer follow-up has also yielded good to excellent results, depending on the criteria used. Relief of preoperative symptoms must be weighed against postoperative gastroesophageal reflux, which has been reported to occur in nearly 50% of patients if a fundoplication is not added to the myotomy. A recent randomized controlled trial showed that the incidence of pathologic gastroesophageal reflux as measured with 24-hour pH monitoring is significantly reduced with the addition of a partial fundoplication. Other studies have shown that the incidence of symptomatic reflux is much less than that measured by 24-hour pH monitoring. Overall, quality of life studies have shown a dramatic improvement in the majority of patients, even taking into account postoperative gastroesophageal reflux. An alternative to partial fundoplication in conjunction with esophagomyotomy is to employ a floppy 360-degree fundoplication after the myotomy. No prospective randomized studies which compare antireflux procedures in this setting are available at this point in time.

Certain factors have been shown to be predictors of good outcome following laparoscopic esophagomyotomy. Multiple studies have suggested that endoscopic therapy, whether dilatation or Botox injection, prior to surgical myotomy results in a worse outcome compared to results with myotomy as the initial treatment. Endoscopic therapy results in scarred tissue planes that can lead to insufficient myotomy or mucosal perforation.

Laparoscopic esophagomyotomy offers patients with achalasia the best chance for long-term resolution of symptoms with low morbidity. This complex operation should be performed by surgeons skilled in advanced laparoscopic surgery. Although there is little controlled data to support this statement, it is our contention that this complex operation is best performed by surgeons with experience in its execution and who also are skilled in advanced laparoscopic surgery.

Suggested Reading

Frantzides CT, Moore RE, Carlson MA, et al: Minimally invasive surgery for achalasia: A 10-year experience. J Gastrointest Surg 2004;8(1):18–23.

Oelschlager BK, Chang L, Pellegrini CA: Improved outcome after extended gastric myotomy for achalasia. Arch Surg 2003;138:490–497.

Perrone JM, Frisella MM, Desai KN, et al: Results of laparoscopic Heller-Toupet operation for achalasia. Surg Endosc 2004;18:1565–1571.

Richards WO, Torquati A, Holzman MD, et al: Heller myotomy versus Heller myotomy with Dor fundoplication for achalasia: A prospective randomized double-blind clinical trial. Ann Surg 2004;240:405–412.

Rosetti G, Brusciano L, Amato G, et al: A total fundoplication is not an obstacle to esophageal emptying after Heller myotomy for achalasia: Results of a long-term follow-up. Ann Surg 2005;241:614–621.

Smith CD, Stival A, Howell DL, et al: Endoscopic therapy for achalasia before Heller myotomy results in worse outcomes than Heller myotomy alone. Ann Surg 2006;243:579–586.

CONSTANTINE T. FRANTZIDES AND
MARK A. CARLSON

Laparoscopic Nissen Fundoplication

The Nissen fundoplication has been and remains one of the most popular, if not the most popular, procedures performed for gastroesophageal reflux disease (GERD). The efficacy of this operation has been demonstrated in controlled clinical trials and, though not in complete concordance, the available data support the use of this procedure for the treatment of complicated gastroesophageal reflux disease. The popularity of the Nissen fundoplication surged with the advent of laparoscopy in the mid-1990s, and the annual number of these procedures performed in the United States subsequently underwent several doublings. Since this period, however, the enthusiasm of referring physicians for the Nissen fundoplication seems to have waned somewhat; it may have been that this procedure was overutilized in the quest to "stamp out" gastroesophageal reflux disease. Nevertheless, a well-performed Nissen procedure in the selected patient for the appropriate indication remains a proven therapy.

Since its introduction in the 1950s, the Nissen operation has undergone a number of technical modifications and refinements. The current "best approach" for the performance of a Nissen operation is somewhat controversial, and the literature is full of opinions with very little good-quality, controlled data to support them. Having said this, we will describe in this chapter what we believe to be the important technical aspects of this procedure, based on our experience and that of others. In brief, these technical features include (1) complete mobilization of the fundus of the stomach with division of the short gastric vessels; (2) extensive mobilization of the esophagus in the lower mediastinum such that 3 to 5 cm of the distal esophagus will lay below the diaphragm without tension; (3) preservation of the vagal nerves; (4) suture closure of the esophageal hiatus, with prosthetic reinforcement of the crural repair for large hiatal defects; and (5) creation of a short (2–3 cm), floppy, 360-degree wrap using the fundus only.

OPERATIVE INDICATIONS

The first-line treatment for gastroesophageal reflux disease is, of course, medical therapy, and not surgery. The indication for surgical correction of gastroesophageal reflux disease is relative, meaning that the decision to operate typically is worked out between the patient and his/her physician. In general, a Nissen fundoplication is performed in the patient in whom medical therapy for gastroesophageal reflux disease has failed. The definition of "medical failure" is intentionally left loose; examples would

include (1) a patient who is noncompliant with medication, (2) a patient who has persistent regurgitation while on maximal medical therapy, (3) a patient with reflux-induced asthma while on maximal medical therapy, and (4) a patient who simply chooses to have operative treatment of his/her gastroesophageal reflux disease. Stronger relative indications for an antireflux procedure include severe erosive esophagitis which has not responded adequately to medical therapy and esophageal metaplasia (Barrett's esophagus) complicated by dysplasia. To reiterate, there are few if any absolute indications for a Nissen fundoplication; the point in time at which surgical therapy is chosen over medical therapy is patient- and physician-dependent.

Fundoplication, and in particular Nissen fundoplication, has been the most popular procedure employed when surgical treatment has been elected to correct gastroesophageal reflux disease. Recently, several endoscopic therapies have emerged for gastroesophageal reflux disease, including endoscopic plication of the gastroesophageal junction or application of radiofrequency energy to the gastroesophageal junction. These therapies appear to have limited utility in the patient with uncomplicated gastroesophageal reflux disease who do not have a concomitant hiatal hernia. The long-term (e.g., 10-year) follow-up to these endoluminal therapies is incomplete, so it is difficult to make a firm recommendation regarding laparoscopic versus endoscopic treatment of gastroesophageal reflux disease. The endoscopic therapies may be useful in the patient who is at high risk for general anesthesia or pneumoperitoneum, or who simply does not want to have any external surgical incisions. Patient education would be paramount in these situations.

Other antireflux procedures have been used to treat gastroesophageal reflux disease, including the partial (Toupet) fundoplication. One of the rationales for this procedure has been to decrease the incidence of postoperative dysphagia, especially in patients with esophageal dysmotility. For instance, the Toupet procedure commonly is employed in conjunction with an esophagomyotomy for achalasia. In our own experience, however, we have utilized the floppy Nissen fundoplication for this clinical scenario, and postoperative dysphagia has not been a problem (see Suggested Reading). In general, we do not believe that the presence of esophageal dysmotility is a contraindication to a floppy 360-degree wrap. Absence of motility is a different issue, but such a patient would be better served by esophageal replacement rather than an antireflux procedure.

PREOPERATIVE EVALUATION

The goals of the preoperative evaluation for the patient being considered for laparoscopic Nissen fundoplication are (1) to confirm the diagnosis of gastroesophageal reflux disease; (2) to characterize the extent of the disease, including the status of the esophageal mucosa; (3) to evaluate for hiatal hernia; (4) to evaluate for any confounding diagnoses, such as neoplasm, dysmotility, or gastric outlet obstruction; and (5) to determine the patient's suitability for the operation, including consideration of the patient's comorbid conditions and whether the patient has failed medical therapy. In addition to a directed history and physical and routine blood tests, it may be helpful to have information derived from the following tests:

Chest x-ray. A chest film may demonstrate a hiatal hernia and provide information about its size and associated contents. Concomitant chest disease also can be identified.

Upper gastrointestinal (GI) contrast study. Also known as a barium esophagogram, this study will provide information on the anatomy of the esophagus and stomach, which would be especially relevant if there is an associated hiatal hernia or volvulus. In addition, an upper GI study can provide direct evidence of gastroesophageal reflux, although the absence thereof does not rule out the diagnosis. In the hands of an experienced gastrointestinal radiologist, the upper GI study also can provide qualitative information on the patient's esophageal motility and can identify concomitant gastric emptying problems.

Upper endoscopy. Also known as esophagogastroduodenoscopy (EGD), this study permits direct evaluation of the esophagogastric mucosa, allowing for the diagnosis and grading of the esophagitis. The EGD also can verify the presence of a hiatal hernia and is important to identify patients with Barrett's esophagus and those who (rarely) might have an esophageal neoplasm.

Ambulatory pH monitoring with manometry. If the patient has equivocal evidence of gastroesophageal reflux disease (e.g., symptoms of reflux but no esophagitis on endoscopy), then pH monitoring and manometry may be useful to demonstrate or exclude the diagnosis. In addition, if the patient has signs or symptoms of esophageal dysmotility, then manometric information may be helpful in determining whether or not to perform a fundoplication.

Chest computed tomography (CT) scan. If the patient has a large hiatal hernia, then a CT scan of the chest is helpful in delineating the anatomy and contents of the hernia sac, including the presence of organs other than the stomach, the presence of gastric volvulus, and so on.

Pulmonary function tests, ENT (ear, nose, throat) evaluation. These findings are helpful if the patient is having manifestations of supraglottic gastroesophageal reflux disease.

It is not necessary to obtain all the foregoing tests on every patient. We obtain a chest x-ray, upper GI study, and EGD routinely, and the other tests are employed selectively (see Suggested Reading). Ambulatory pH monitoring with manometry is expensive and difficult for the patient. Furthermore, although the information obtained from pH monitoring/manometry may be scientifically interesting, it typically does not influence subsequent management unless the routine testing (patient history, EGD, and upper GI study) has produced equivocal or conflicting results. In addition, all patients have preoperative liver function tests (transaminases, bilirubin, alkaline phosphatase, etc.) in case an aberrant left hepatic artery is encountered during the procedure (see later discussion). The algorithm describing our typical preoperative evaluation is shown in Figure 3-1.

PATIENT POSITIONING

The patient is positioned supine on the operating table with split-leg support; this is our preferred position, although others may prefer supine, with legs straight. Alternatively, the patient may be placed in stirrups (the "French," or modified low-lithotomy, position), but this may predispose the patient to deep vein thrombosis. The patient may have security straps across the chest and legs to allow for extreme positioning (rotation, tilt) of the operating table. Routine positioning for many procedures, including the

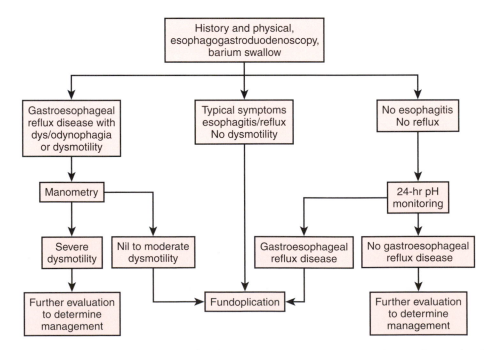

FIGURE 3-1 Algorithm for the selective use of esophageal manometry and 24-hour pH monitoring in the patient under consideration for a laparoscopic Nissen fundoplication. (From Frantzides CT, Carlson MA, Madan AK, et al: Selective use of esophageal manometry and 24-hour pH monitoring before laparoscopic fundoplication. J Am Coll Surg 2003;197:358.)

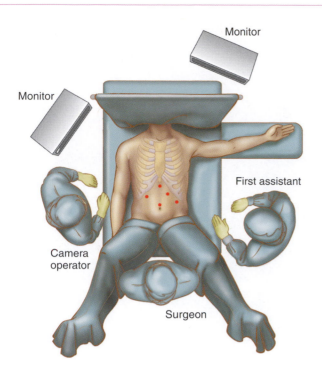

FIGURE 3-2 Positioning in the operating room. The patient is in the supine split-leg position.

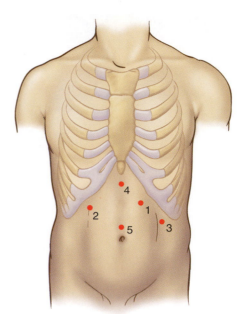

FIGURE 3-3 Trocar positions for a laparoscopic Nissen fundoplication. The trocars (all 10 mm) typically are placed in the numerical order as shown, starting with an optical bladeless trocar at position 1.

Nissen, includes calf sequential compression devices and forced-air patient warmer. The monitors are placed on either side of the patient's head, whether on towers or hung from the ceiling (Fig. 3-2). With the patient's legs split, the surgeon should stand between the patient's legs; the first assistant should be on the left, and the camera operator should be on the patient's right.

POSITIONING AND PLACEMENT OF TROCARS

Pneumoperitoneum most often is established with a Veress needle, a Hasson cannula, or an optical bladeless trocar. The authors prefer the optical bladeless trocar, although there is insufficient controlled data to demonstrate the superiority of one entry technique over the others. Each port site is infiltrated with a long-acting local anesthetic. The optical bladeless trocar is inserted in the left subcostal region in the midclavicular line (Fig. 3-3), and a 15-mm Hg pneumoperitoneum with CO_2 is established. The remaining four trocars are depicted in Figure 3-3; a total of five 10-mm trocars are inserted. Other authors have described a combination of 5- and 10-mm trocars for this procedure; we prefer all to be 10-mm trocars for maximal instrument versatility. Furthermore, the jaws of a 10-mm grasping instrument have a relatively broad surface, thus making tissue trauma less likely compared to the use of a 5-mm grasping instrument.

A crucial component of most laparoscopic operations, including the Nissen, is the placement of trocars. The arrangement of the trocars can strongly influence degree of difficulty of the subsequent laparoscopic procedure. The trocar positioning illustrated in Figure 3-3 is only a suggestion; adjustments to the actual positioning may be needed based on the patient's body habitus. It is a good idea to fully insufflate the abdomen and then decide on port positioning; the surgeon then can make a visual estimate to determine if the instruments will reach the targeted intra-abdominal region through the planned trocar sites, prior to inserting the trocars. In addition, we like to transilluminate the abdominal wall with the intra-abdominal laparoscope; if the abdominal wall is not too thick, then this transillumination can demonstrate abdominal wall vasculature which the surgeon then can avoid.

OPERATIVE TECHNIQUE

The surgeon operates through ports 1 and 2 (see Fig. 3-3); the first assistant utilizes port 3 and 4 for retraction, and the camera is manipulated through port 5. A 30-degree angled 10-mm laparoscope is preferable for this operation and is placed through port 5. The operating table is placed in steep reverse Trendelenburg position. The left lobe of the liver is retracted with an atraumatic retractor through port 4; our preference has been to use an inflatable balloon retractor (Soft-Wand, Gyrus-ACMI, Southborough, MA) for this step. This can be held in place with a self-retaining device, or manually by the first assistant. The first assistant grasps the gastric body and retracts this caudad; the surgeon introduces a grasper through port 2 and the gastrohepatic ligament and phrenoesophageal ligament are incised with a hook electrocautery or with an ultrasonic scalpel through port 1 (Fig. 3-4).

The dissection proceeds in the avascular plane of the gastrohepatic omentum anterior to the caudate lobe of the liver. The division of the gastrohepatic omentum allows entry into the lesser sac.

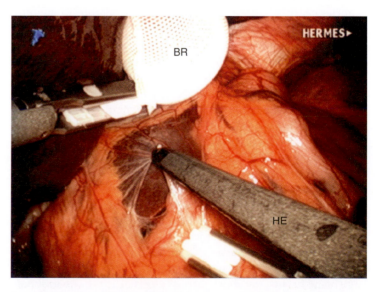

FIGURE 3-4 Incision of the gastrohepatic ligament with a hook electrocautery (HE). An inflatable balloon retractor (BR) is retracting the left lateral lobe of the liver. The other two instruments visible are both 10-mm atraumatic graspers.

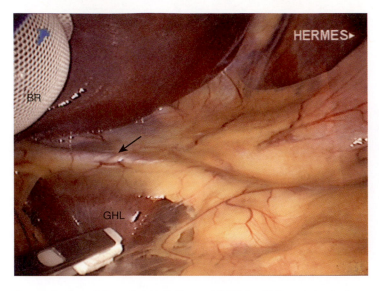

FIGURE 3-5 View of the gastrohepatic ligament (GHL) in which an anatomically variant blood vessel is seen transversely crossing the field *(arrow)*. A balloon retractor (BR) is retracting the liver, and an atraumatic grasper is seen at the lower left.

An aberrant or replaced left hepatic artery may be encountered traveling through the gastrohepatic ligament (i.e., lesser omentum), as shown in Figure 3-5. Division of this vessel usually would have no consequences to a patient with a normal liver; however, liver necrosis may occur in patients with underlying liver disease. Thus, preoperative knowledge of liver function would be crucial in this scenario. If the patient does have abnormal preoperative liver function tests, then preservation of an aberrant left hepatic artery would be advisable.

With the gastrohepatic omentum incised, the right bundle of the right diaphragmatic crus can be visualized. The peritoneum overlying the surface of the right bundle is scored and opened with hook electrocautery. Using a blunt dissection probe introduced through port 1 and a laparoscopic Babcock forceps through port 2, the retroesophageal space then is opened up with gentle blunt dissection. At this point in the procedure, we like to have the anesthetist insert a lighted bougie into the esophagus to aid in the subsequent dissection (Fig. 3-6A). Other authors believe that such a maneuver is not necessary and perhaps risks esophageal perforation. In our experience, this lighted dissection aid has been quite helpful, especially with a large hiatal hernia (see Chapter 4). Sharp dissection is not required to develop the retroesophageal space. It is our preference to leave the posterior vagus nerve attached to the esophagus (Fig. 3-6B). It usually is not necessary to complete this retroesophageal dissection/mobilization until after the short gastric vessels have been divided and the left side of the esophagus has been mobilized. This practice should minimize injury to the superior pole of the spleen.

After the initial mediastinal dissection has been accomplished, the surgeon grasps the gastric fundus through port 2 with an atraumatic grasper, the first assistant similarly grasps the gastrosplenic omentum through port 3, and the short gastric vessels are placed on modest stretch for division using the ultrasonic scalpel or the LigaSure device (Fig. 3-7). Once the lesser sac has been entered through the gastrosplenic omentum, the division of the short gastrics proceeds cephalad to the angle of His. Other than with a large hiatal hernia, the short gastric vessels near the superior pole of the spleen can be quite short, and care should be taken to avoid splenic injury at this location. Once the short gastric vessels have

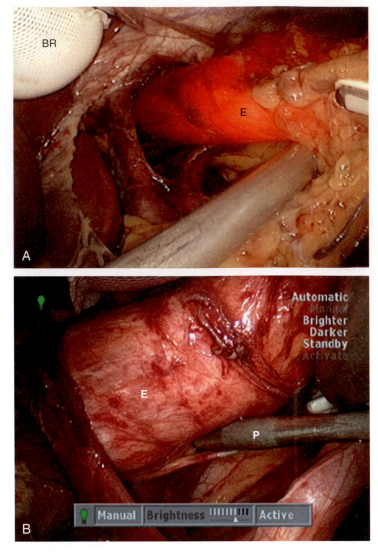

FIGURE 3-6 **A,** Creation of a "window" posterior to the gastroesophageal junction. A lighted bougie is illuminating the esophagus (E). An atraumatic grasper has been placed into the window and is levering the gastroesophageal junction anteriorly. A balloon retractor (BR) is retracting the liver. **B,** The posterior vagus has been left attached to the esophagus (E), but has been pulled inferiorly by a palpation probe (P) for demonstration purposes.

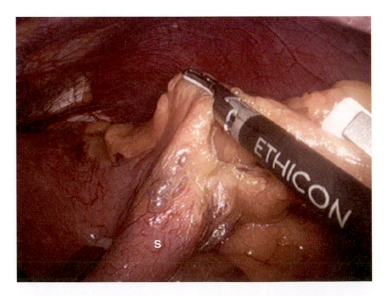

FIGURE 3-7 Ligation of the short gastric vessels with ultrasonic scalpel (instrument with the Ethicon label). Two atraumatic graspers are providing tension/countertension on the stomach (S) and the gastrosplenic omentum.

been divided, the posterior gastric fundus should be inspected for adhesions and vessels, which should be ligated to ensure a completely mobile fundus.

After the fundus has been mobilized, the left side of the esophagus is mobilized from the left bundle of the right crus using blunt dissection. The assistant then retracts the stomach caudad, and the surgeon creates a "window" posterior to the gastroesophageal junction, from right to left, using a Babcock grasper through port 2 and a blunt probe through port 1 (see Fig. 3-6A). This can be done by placing the Babcock grasper posterior to the gastroesophageal junction, levering anteriorly, and then bluntly dissecting with the probe until the superior pole of the spleen is visualized. A sutured cruroplasty then is performed in all patients with the lighted bougie (typically 50–60 F) advanced into the stomach; we feel that reduces the risk of an overly tight crural closure. The bundles are approximated with interrupted sutures of 2-0 braided polyester or other similar nonabsorbable material; the surgeon should take wide, ample bites of the crural bundles, and use a stitch interval of about 5 mm (Fig. 3-8). For large hiatal defects (generally greater than 5 cm) or weak crural tissue, the surgeon can consider cruroplasty reinforcement with prosthetic mesh (see Chapter 4).

To create the fundoplication, a Babcock grasper is introduced through port 2 and passed posterior the gastroesophageal junction through the above-described window, and the superior portion of the fundus is delivered into the jaws of this Babcock forceps. In order to prevent wrapping the fundus to the gastric body (a common mistake in creating a fundoplication), the inferolateral portion of the fundus should be stabilized by the assistant's Babcock forceps in port 3. The surgeon then carefully draws the superior portion of the fundus from the left side of the esophagus back through the window to the right side of the esophagus. Using a back-and-forth motion ("shoe-shine" maneuver) on the fundus around the esophagus, the laxity of the fundoplication can be assessed. These maneuvers help assure that a fundus-to-fundus (rather than a fundus-to-corpus) wrap will be created.

The Endo Stitch (U.S. Surgical, Norwalk, CT) device or other suturing instrument then is introduced through port 1, and the fundus from the right side of the esophagus is sutured to the fundus from the left side of the esophagus using interrupted sutures of braided 2-0 polyester. Generous fundal bites should be utilized;

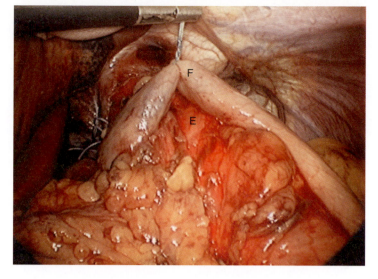

FIGURE 3-9 Placement of the first stitch of the fundoplication (F). The wrap is intentionally loose around the esophagus (E). The tails of this first stitch are left long, so the surgeon may use this stitch as a retraction aid.

typically three sutures are placed to create a wrap that is 2 to 3 cm in length. This is done with the esophageal bougie in place. The middle stitch is placed first; the wrap then is elevated by grasping the stitch tails in order to evaluate the laxity of the fundoplication before the placement of the cephalad stitch (Fig. 3-9). Ideally, one should easily be able to place a Babcock forceps alongside the esophagus (with the bougie in place) under the wrap, as an indicator of proper laxity.

The cephalad stitch is the most crucial, as improper placement may result in an excessively tight or nonsecured wrap. This stitch also is placed with the Endo Stitch device through port 1, using the tails of the previously placed stitch as a retraction aid. The left portion of the fundal wrap is taken first with the cephalad stitch, then a bite of the anterior arch of the esophageal hiatus, and then the right portion of the fundal wrap (Fig. 3-10). This cephalad stitch anchors the fundoplication to the diaphragm, reducing the risk of postoperative wrap herniation into the thorax. The final caudad stitch is placed 1 cm distal to the middle stitch. The completed wrap is shown in Figure 3-11.

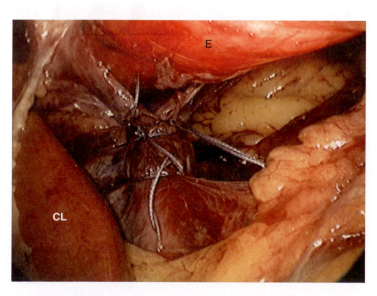

FIGURE 3-8 A completed posterior cruroplasty. E, esophagus (illuminated with the bougie); CL, caudate lobe of the liver.

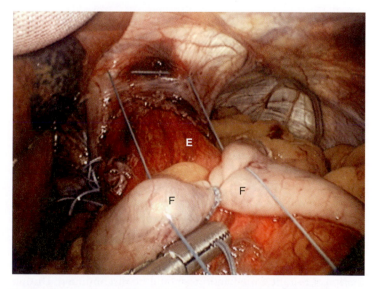

FIGURE 3-10 Placement of the cephalad stitch of the fundoplication (F). This stitch takes a bite of the fundus on either side of the esophagus (E) and also incorporates the crura anterior to the esophagus. This stitch anchors the wrap to the diaphragm.

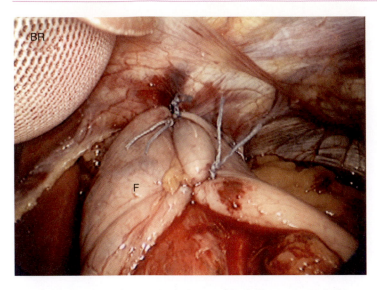

FIGURE 3-11 A completed Nissen fundoplication (F). A balloon retractor (BR) is retracting the liver.

Suturing with the Endo Stitch device with extracorporeal knot tying permits tissue approximation under mild tension with greater ease compared to suturing with intracorporeal knotting. As with other operations (open or laparoscopic), a suture should be tied such that the tissue within the knot is approximated rather than strangulated. Another advantage to the Endo Stitch device is that the rigidity of its jaws makes suturing of the crura and the fundoplication (especially with the cephalad stitch) less cumbersome than with a conventional needle and driver.

After completion of the wrap, it is checked one more time for appropriate laxity. The field is irrigated with saline. The pneumoperitoneum is evacuated, the fascia of all ports is closed using a fascial closure device (e.g., Carter Thomason CloseSure System, Inlet Medical, Trumbull, CT) and 1-0 absorbable suture, the skin of the incisions is closed with a 4-0 polyglactin intracuticular stitch, and the procedure is terminated.

POSTOPERATIVE CARE

Upon completion of the operation, the Foley catheter is removed, and the patient is given a dose of ketorolac tromethamine for analgesia. Most patients will not require narcotics for analgesia. Within 2 hours after the procedure has been completed, we expect that the patient will be up and walking. Coughing, deep breathing, and incentive inspirometry are encouraged. While same-day discharge has been feasible, we prefer to observe the patient for 23 hours before discharging home. A Gastrografin swallow (Bracco Diagnostics, Princeton, NJ) is not performed unless there is a question of the wrap's integrity. Severe bloating requiring nasogastric decompression is rare after a laparoscopic fundoplication; therefore, routine nasogastric tube utilization is not needed.

On postoperative day 1, the patient is given clear liquids in the morning. The patient is discharged home by noon on postoperative day 1 with instructions to begin a soft diet and to refrain from lifting anything heavier than 15 pounds (7 kg). Small and more frequent meals should be the rule in order to avoid gastric distention. Antireflux medications should be discontinued. During the first 2 weeks, the patient should avoid red meat; in the first 3 months, the patient should avoid carbonated beverages and gas-producing foods such as beans, peas, broccoli, and cauliflower.

Chewing gum also should be avoided because of the associated aerophagia. Based on a 16-year observation study, most patients will have temporary dysphagia that will resolve within the first 3 months. Alteration of bowel habits is common after fundoplication, but this also resolves after 3 months in virtually all patients. In addition, most patients will lose some weight during the initial few months, but this invariably is followed by a period of weight gain. Follow-up visits may be performed at 1 week and at 1, 3, 6, and 12 months.

PROCEDURE-SPECIFIC COMPLICATIONS

Intraoperative complications of laparoscopic Nissen fundoplication include perforation, pneumothorax (for management of these first two incidents, see Chapter 4, on hiatal hernia repair), bleeding, and vagal injury. If bleeding occurs, it typically arises from the short gastric vessels and was more common when clips were used for short gastric ligation. The incidence of splenic injury has been reduced drastically by the minimally invasive approach. Splenectomy is quite rare during laparoscopic Nissen fundoplication. Tears in the splenic capsule can be managed with compression from an inflatable balloon retractor or similar device or with local hemostatic agents. In order to avoid bleeding, hemostatic scalpels which employ ultrasonic or bipolar energy are recommended; in order to avoid splenic injury, the surgeon should always employ gentle traction during the fundal mobilization or if the omentum is adherent to the spleen. Vagal injury/transection is best avoided with careful identification of the vagal trunks.

Complications in the postoperative period include perforation/abscess (to be discussed in Chapter 4), esophageal stenosis, recurrent herniation, wrap slippage, and valve malfunction. Esophageal stenosis may be the result of a tight cruroplasty or a tight fundoplication. This may be avoided by hiatal closure and floppy fundoplication over a 50- to 60-F bougie. Dysphagia that lasts beyond 3 months should be evaluated with a barium swallow; if there is a stenosis, then pneumatic dilatations may be performed. If this is not successful, then reoperation may be required to either remove 1 or 2 cruroplasty sutures or redo the fundoplication. Recurrent herniation is discussed in Chapter 4. A slipped wrap typically manifests with recurrent pyrosis and is diagnosed with a barium swallow or an EGD. A redo fundoplication typically is necessary to correct a slipped wrap. A slipped wrap may be avoided by anchoring to the anterior arch of the crura (rather than the esophagus). Valve malfunction usually is secondary to a malpositioned or disrupted wrap. This also may be diagnosed with a barium swallow or an EGD. Wrap disruption may be avoided by large tissue bites during the fundoplication with nonabsorbable sutures, and tying the sutures without strangulating tension. Proper wrap positioning requires exact identification of the fundus, with subsequent wrap creation utilizing the fundus and not the gastric corpus. A malpositioned wrap typically requires a redo fundoplication.

RESULTS AND OUTCOME

Fundoplication is one of the few nonamputative procedures performed in general surgery. The objective of this procedure is to create a functional valve at the gastroesophageal junction; therefore, the technical aspects of this procedure are especially crucial for a successful outcome. In a review of over 10,000 published procedures in 2001, the overall success rate for laparoscopic

Nissen fundoplication in the hands of experienced surgeons was 90%; if patients with large hiatal hernia are excluded, then this success rate is even higher. While the failure rate of laparoscopic Nissen fundoplication is quite low in the hands of experienced/specialized surgeons, the results in the general community of surgeons is not known. It has been our impression as medicolegal experts that a patient who has a poor outcome after fundoplication will have a greater propensity to pursue legal action than a patient who has a poor outcome after an operation for a life-threatening condition.

Laparoscopic Nissen fundoplication began in 1991 and quickly became the gold standard for the surgical management of GERD. From a physiologic standpoint, the best method to "cure" GERD is to create a new antireflux valve. A disparity exists between surgeons and gastroenterologists regarding the "cure" for GERD. Medical management consists of symptomatic relief with proton pump inhibitors, but this does little to prevent the actual episodes of reflux. An interesting observation in the treatment of GERD has been the development of several endoscopic methods to create an antireflux valve; this suggests that at least some gastroenterologists have not been completely satisfied with pure medical management of GERD. It has been our impression that the number of patients referred for Nissen fundoplication peaked in the mid-latter 1990s, but subsequently has been declining. This decline may be secondary to the perceived poor outcome of patients operated on in the general community. In actuality, there has been no direct comparison of modern surgical treatment (i.e., laparoscopic Nissen fundoplication) and modern medical treatment (i.e., proton pump inhibitors) with long-term follow-up (10 years or more); and, to our knowledge, such a study has not been initiated. Furthermore, the long-term risks of proton pump inhibitor treatment (such as adenocarcinoma) have not been defined. So currently, many of these issues regarding the treatment of GERD are unresolved.

Suggested Reading

Anvari M, Allen C: Five-year comprehensive outcomes evaluation in 181 patients after laparoscopic Nissen fundoplication. J Am Coll Surg 2003;196:51–57; discussion 57–58; author reply 58–59.

Booth MI, Jones L, Stratford J, Dehn TC: Results of laparoscopic Nissen fundoplication at 2–8 years after surgery. Br J Surg 2002;89:476–481.

Carlson MA, Frantzides CT: Complications and results of primary minimally invasive antireflux procedures: A review of 10,735 reported cases. J Am Coll Surg 2001;193:428–439.

Donahue PE, Samelson S, Nyhus LM, Bombeck CT: The floppy Nissen fundoplication: Effective long-term control of pathologic reflux. Arch Surg 1985;120:663–668.

Frantzides CT, Carlson MA, Zografakis JG, et al: Postoperative gastrointestinal complaints after laparoscopic Nissen fundoplication. J Soc Laparoendosc Surg 2006;10:39–42.

Frantzides CT, Carlson MA, Madan AK, et al: Selective use of esophageal manometry and 24-hour pH monitoring before laparoscopic fundoplication. J Am Coll Surg 2003;197:358–363; discussion 363–364.

Frantzides CT, Richards C: A study of 362 consecutive laparoscopic Nissen fundoplications. Surgery 1998;124:651–654; discussion 654–655.

Hinder RA, Filipi CJ, Wetscher G, et al: Laparoscopic Nissen fundoplication is an effective treatment for gastroesophageal reflux disease. Ann Surg 1994;220:472–481; discussion 481–483.

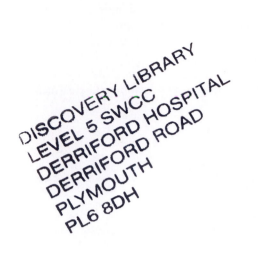

CONSTANTINE T. FRANTZIDES, FRANK A. GRANDERATH,
URSULA M. GRANDERATH, AND MARK A. CARLSON

Laparoscopic Hiatal Herniorrhaphy

The diaphragm is perforated with three major openings through which pass the vena cava, the aorta, and the esophagus (Fig. 4-1). The opening for the esophagus, or esophageal hiatus, is bounded by the right and left crura of the diaphragm, which are musculotendinous structures that originate from the central tendon of the diaphragm and insert into the vertebral bodies. A hiatal hernia is the protrusion of abdominal organs through the esophageal hiatus. Although the anatomic relationships can vary, the typical arrangement of the crura is shown in Figure 4-1. Note that (in most cases) the actual structures that the surgeon sutures together when performing a posterior cruroplasty are the right and left bundles (columns) of the right crus; the left crus per se is not involved in a posterior cruroplasty.

Sliding (type I) hiatal hernia occurs in the majority of patients with gastroesophageal reflux disease (Fig. 4-2A). The presence of such a hiatal hernia generally inhibits the integrity and function of the gastroesophageal antireflux barrier. It follows that reduction of a hiatal hernia and closure of the esophageal hiatus have been considered essential for the success of an antireflux procedure. Not surprisingly, one of the most common reasons for anatomic failure of a laparoscopic antireflux operation is the recurrence of hiatal hernia, with resultant intrathoracic migration of the fundoplication. Therefore, the importance of a secure hiatal closure during laparoscopic fundoplication has received increasing emphasis in the surgical literature.

Although the type I hiatal hernia is by far the most common type of hiatal hernia (85% to 95%, depending on the series), the other types of hiatal hernia also may require surgical correction. Paraesophageal (types II and III hiatal) hernias represent approximately 5% to 15% of all hiatal hernias. In a type II hernia (classic paraesophageal; see Fig. 4-2B), the gastroesophageal junction remains subdiaphragmatic, in its normal anatomic position. Characteristically, the phrenoesophageal ligament with the gastric fundus migrates anteriorly or laterally alongside the esophagus into the mediastinum. In a type III hernia (mixed paraesophageal; see Fig. 4-2C), the gastroesophageal junction has herniated through the diaphragm, and the gastric fundus has migrated alongside the esophagus. In addition, a type IV (giant) hiatal hernia has been described (see Fig. 4-2D), characterized by the migration of other intra-abdominal organs (e.g., omentum, colon, small bowel, spleen) in addition to the stomach into the mediastinum.

Similar to gastroesophageal reflux disease, laparoscopic management of large hiatal hernia has become standard in most centers. A considerable amount of retrospective data suggests that laparoscopic repair of hiatal hernia is associated with a lower morbidity rate, a shorter hospitalization, and a quicker recovery compared to the open approach. Whether performed open or laparoscopically, however, hiatal hernia repair with primary closure of the crural bundles has a high recurrence rate, in some series ranging up to 40%. Since the late 1990s a body of literature has accumulated which indicates that crural closure supplemented with prosthetic mesh results in a lower rate of recurrence compared to simple sutured cruroplasty.

Currently there is no agreement regarding a standardized technique for mesh-reinforced hiatoplasty. Debate exists regarding the type of mesh to employ, the shape and size of mesh in relation to the defect, the method of mesh fixation, and so forth. In addition, controversy still exists regarding the rationale and safety of placing prosthetic material at the esophageal hiatus. In this chapter we will describe several alternatives for mesh-reinforced hiatoplasty which we have used with salutary outcome; we also will address safety concerns with a summary of the world's literature on the controversial subject of mesh at the esophageal hiatus.

OPERATIVE INDICATIONS

The indication for repair of a hiatal hernia depends on the hernia type. For a sliding (type I) hiatal hernia, repair generally is indicated if the hernia is associated with gastroesophageal reflux disease that is, for one reason or another, not satisfactorily treated with medication; this is probably the most common indication for repair of a hiatal hernia. In this case the hernia is repaired in conjunction with an antireflux procedure (e.g., Nissen wrap). A small, asymptomatic sliding hiatal hernia does not need to be repaired. In between these two extremes are moderate-sized sliding hiatal hernias that produce mild or modest symptoms; the indication for repair in these patients is more relative and should be left to discussion between the physician and the patient.

For an uncomplicated type II to IV (paraesophageal) hernia, elective operation may be pursued after appropriate preoperative evaluation and optimization of patient. Traditional dogma stated that the mere presence of a type II to IV hernia was an indication for repair; however, that may not be necessary, as literature contains some series in which observation of asymptomatic paraesophageal hernias has been done safely. In general, we still feel inclined to offer surgery for these hernias, especially

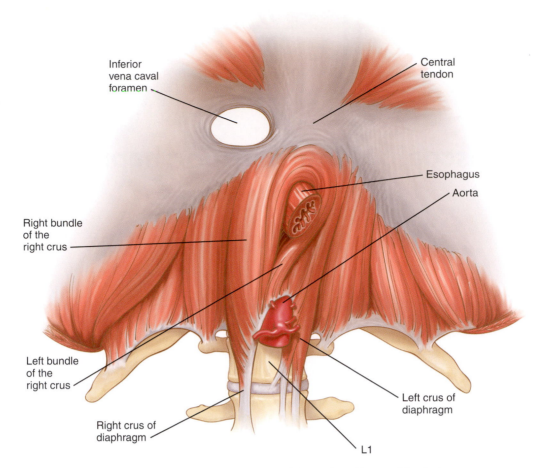

Inferior
vena caval
foramen

Central
tendon

Esophagus

Aorta

Right bundle
of the
right crus

Left bundle
of the
right crus

Left crus of
diaphragm

Right crus of
diaphragm

L1

FIGURE 4-1 Typical anatomic arrangement of the esophageal hiatus of the diaphragm.

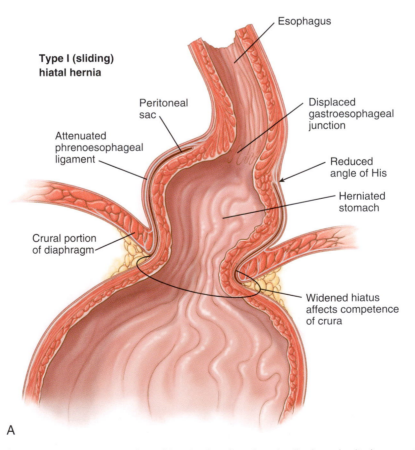

**Type I (sliding)
hiatal hernia**

Esophagus

Peritoneal
sac

Displaced
gastroesophageal
junction

Attenuated
phrenoesophageal
ligament

Reduced
angle of His

Herniated
stomach

Crural portion
of diaphragm

Widened hiatus
affects competence
of crura

A

FIGURE 4-2 A, Type I (sliding) hiatal hernia. The gastroesophageal junction has slipped proximally above the diaphragm and into the mediastinum.

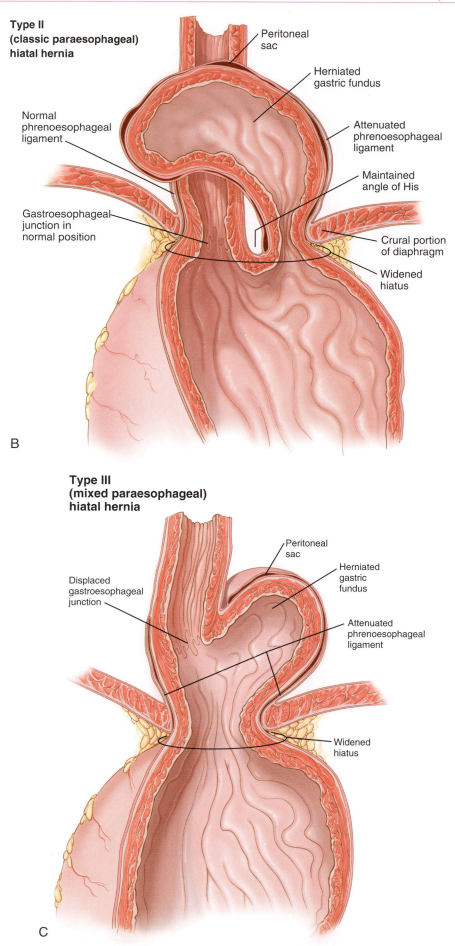

**Type II
(classic paraesophageal)
hiatal hernia**

Peritoneal
sac

Herniated
gastric fundus

Normal
phrenoesophageal
ligament

Attenuated
phrenoesophageal
ligament

Maintained
angle of His

Gastroesophageal
junction in
normal position

Crural portion
of diaphragm

Widened
hiatus

B

**Type III
(mixed paraesophageal)
hiatal hernia**

Peritoneal
sac

Herniated
gastric
fundus

Displaced
gastroesophageal
junction

Attenuated
phrenoesophageal
ligament

Widened
hiatus

C

FIGURE 4-2 CONT'D **B,** Type II (classic paraesophageal) hiatal hernia. The gastroesophageal junction remains at or below the diaphragm. The gastric fundus/body has migrated into the mediastinum alongside the esophagus, thereby disrupting the normal relationship between the fundus and the gastroesophageal junction. **C,** Type III (mixed paraesophageal) hiatal hernia. The gastroesophageal junction has slipped proximally above the diaphragm and into the mediastinum. The gastric fundus/body has migrated into the mediastinum alongside the esophagus, which again disrupts the normal relationship between the fundus and the gastroesophageal junction.

Continued

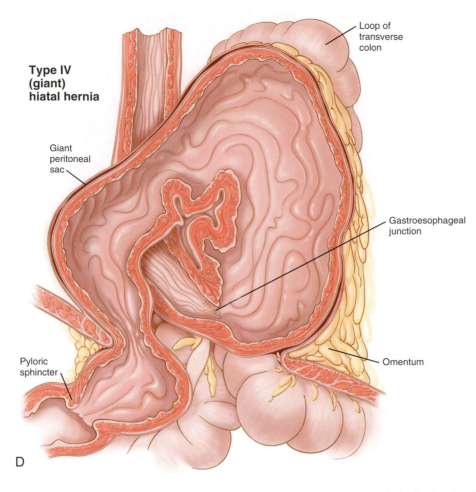

Type IV (giant) hiatal hernia

Loop of transverse colon

Giant peritoneal sac

Gastroesophageal junction

Omentum

Pyloric sphincter

D

FIGURE 4-2 CONT'D   **D,** Type IV (giant) hiatal hernia containing stomach, colon, and omentum. The portion of the stomach that has herniated into the chest has twisted (volvulized) along the long axis of the stomach. This can cause gastric ischemia and necrosis.

if the patient is a good operative risk. Incidentally, a truly asymptomatic paraesophageal hernia is not common. If the patient is symptomatic, then the indication for repair is much stronger.

If the patient has symptoms of gastric ischemia/necrosis secondary to volvulus of a paraesophageal hernia (see Fig. 4-2C and D), then this is a surgical emergency, and urgent operative intervention is indicated. The patient with an upper gastrointestinal hemorrhage should undergo a standard algorithm for GI bleeding and, after stabilization, undergo operative repair. The obstructed patient should undergo resuscitation, optimization, and semiurgent repair. In summary, a patient with a complicated type II to IV hiatal hernia who can tolerate general anesthesia should undergo urgent operative repair; otherwise, there is a high risk of death.

PREOPERATIVE EVALUATION

The preoperative evaluation for a patient with hiatal hernia is similar to that for a preoperative Nissen patient (please refer to Chapter 3). The findings on the upper GI radiograph and computed tomography (CT) scan will provide information on the hernia contents and give the surgeon an idea of how large the hiatal defect is. This latter dimension is relevant in that the surgeon should have a strategy prepared to deal with a defect that cannot be closed primarily, or for which the closure is under excessive tension. In addition to obtaining anatomic information on the hernia, the surgeon should ensure that the patient

will be able to tolerate a prolonged period of pneumoperitoneum; many patients with paraesophageal hernia are elderly or frail.

PATIENT POSITIONING AND TROCAR PLACEMENT

The positioning of the patient and the placement of the trocars is similar to that of a Nissen fundoplication (see Chapter 3). During repair of a large hiatal hernia, it may be helpful to have the upper trocars placed as close to the costal margin as possible in order to have better access to the mediastinum. Alternatively, bariatric-length instruments may be used (but these may not be universally available). In order to optimize the locations for trocar insertion, the mapping of these sites is best done after the abdomen has been fully insufflated.

OPERATIVE TECHNIQUE

With the patient in steep reverse Trendelenburg position, the contents of the hiatal hernia sac are reduced into the abdomen with three atraumatic graspers (two manipulated by the surgeon, one by the first assistant; Fig. 4-3). In the vast majority of cases, the anterior contents of the sac, whether stomach, colon, or small bowel, are freely mobile and can be reduced with modest traction; adhesions that tether the contents inside the sac usually indicate that there may be another process involved. Once the anterior hernia contents are reduced, the gastrohepatic omentum

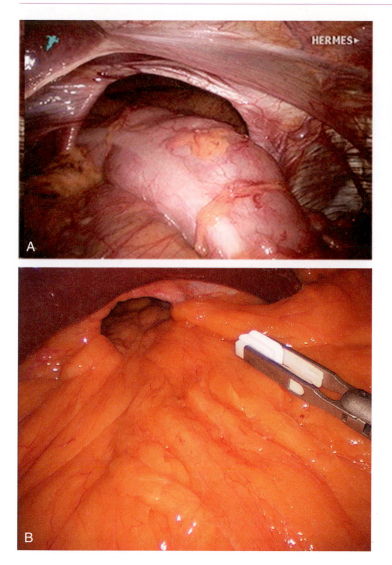

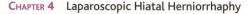

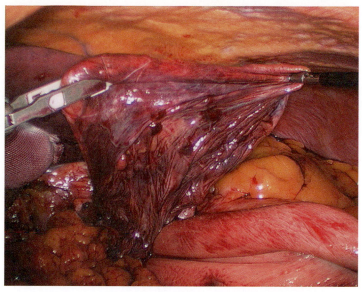

FIGURE 4-4 Reduction of the hiatal hernia sac into the abdomen in preparation for excision.

FIGURE 4-3 **A** and **B**, Laparoscopic views of a large type IV hiatal hernia with hernia sac contents consisting of the stomach, omentum, and colon. The atraumatic grasper shown will reduce the contents of the hernia sac.

(also known as the lesser omentum or pars flaccida) is placed on stretch and incised in its thin area over the caudate lobe of the liver. This incision is carried superiorly to the anterior arch of the esophageal hiatus. The hernia sac then is grasped anteriorly and pulled slowly but with persistence out of the mediastinum and into the abdomen (Fig. 4-4). The hernia sac typically is quite thin and can tear easily. Of note, the hernia sac on the left side usually is in contact with the parietal pleura. A tear in the parietal pleura will result in pneumothorax; the surgeon should endeavor to avoid this complication (see "Complications").

After the anterior hernia sac has been reduced, the sac is entered just over the crural arch with an ultrasonic scalpel or similar device. This incision into the sac is carried from right to left over the top of the hiatus to the left crural bundle. The anterior portion of the sac is kept under constant tension as it is dissected out of the mediastinum. Once reduced, the anterior sac typically is amputated from the anterior surface of the stomach with the ultrasonic scalpel. Although the sac can be an excellent handle on which to provide traction, more often than not the sac is so large that it impedes the progress of the dissection, so the sac should be removed.

The right crural bundle then is swept away from the body of the stomach with blunt technique. At this point the posterior hiatus usually is still occupied by gastric body, which means that the

left gastric artery has been drawn into the posterior mediastinum and will be at risk for injury during subsequent dissection. After dissecting the right bundle free, the surgeon should be able to see into the mediastinum, with the medial side of the esophagus and stomach in view. At this point an illuminated esophageal bougie may be inserted per os and advanced into the distal esophagus with the surgeon monitoring the advancement of the lighted bougie with the laparoscope.

Aided by the esophageal illumination, the surgeon mobilizes the esophagus medially and anteriorly along the distal portion. This mobilization mostly is done with blunt technique; it is somewhat risky to use an electrical or other power source in the confined workspace of the mediastinum. After this anteriomedial dissection has been accomplished, the surgeon can reduce the posterior portion of the stomach which, in a mixed paraesophageal hernia (see Fig. 4-2C), typically is situated behind the gastroesophageal junction. As mentioned above, care should be taken in this location to identify the left gastric artery, as its normal anatomic arrangements likely will be distorted. This vascular supply to the lesser curvature should be preserved, since the short gastric vessels on the fundus are ligated later on; thus, compromise of the left gastric artery in this situation might render the fundus ischemic. The trunk of the left gastric artery may be adherent to the posterior fornix created by the right and left crural bundles and in this case will require meticulous, sharp dissection for mobilization. In addition, the posterior vagal trunk should be kept apposed to the esophagus. Separation of the posterior vagus from the esophagus may expose this nerve to injury or entrapment during the subsequent cruroplasty.

Upon reduction of the posterior stomach and the left gastric artery, the surgeon may pass a 10-mm grasper (from medial to lateral, through the right lateral trocar) behind the gastroesophageal junction and retract in an anterocaudad direction. This elevates the esophagus and stomach, exposing the retrogastric space such that the surgeon can identify and clear off the right and left crural bundles. At this point the surgeon also may be able to create a "window" posterior to the stomach, that is, a continuous space between the lesser curvature, passing beneath the fundus, and exiting laterally near the angle of His by the upper pole of the spleen. Creating a window at this point is not crucial, but the surgeon should ensure that the crural bundles have been well

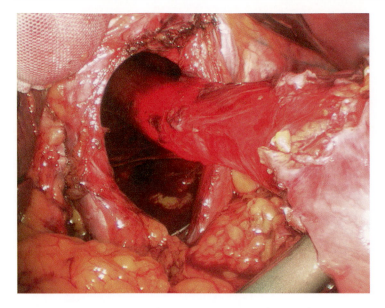

FIGURE 4-5 Circumferential mobilization of the lower esophagus and upper stomach; the esophagus is illuminated with the lighted bougie.

delineated. It is easier and safer to complete the window after the fundus has been mobilized.

After the anterior, medial, and posterior dissections have been accomplished, the short gastric vessels that supply the fundus of the stomach can be transected with the ultrasonic scalpel. It is helpful to identify the angle of His first, so that the transection of the short gastric vessels does not begin too distally on the greater curve. In a patient with a large hiatal hernia the short gastric vessels often become elongated, which makes their transection relatively easy. Once the fundus has been mobilized, the remaining lateral attachments of the distal esophagus in the mediastinum may be taken by retracting the stomach and esophagus inferomedially. Any remaining hernia sac that was situated posteriorly is placed on stretch and amputated.

The goal of the mediastinal dissection is a circumferential mobilization of the lower esophagus and upper stomach, so that upon completion of this dissection the gastroesophageal junction and all of the stomach will lie below the diaphragm without tension (Fig. 4-5). Some authors have described the syndrome of "short esophagus" in paraesophageal hernia, meaning that it was not possible to obtain adequate esophageal length during the mediastinal mobilization. The advice that has been given for this situation is to perform an esophageal-lengthening maneuver (e.g., Collis procedure). In contrast, we have not come across the short esophagus syndrome in our cases of paraesophageal hernia; that is, we have been able to obtain adequate esophageal length without performing a Collis procedure.

The next step after the circumferential mobilization of the lower esophagus and upper stomach is the cruroplasty (hiatoplasty). The surgeon should first manipulate the crural bundles, and determine if a primary hiatal closure without tension may be performed. After this determination, a posterior cruroplasty is performed with (our preference) interrupted sutures of 2-0 braided polyester (Fig. 4-6A and B). Anterior leverage of the gastroesophageal junction with a 10-mm instrument (as described earlier) facilitates crural exposure during this step; in addition, the esophageal bougie (50–60 F) should be in place so that the closure is not made too tight. The tissue bites should be as large as the surgeon can manage; care should be exercised when taking a deep bite into the crural bundles because of the proximity of the

aorta and vena cava. We begin suturing at the level of the posterior fornix/commissure and progress anteriorly, placing stitches about every 5 mm. This posterior primary cruroplasty is performed to the extent that the tissue permits; if the sutures begin tearing through the tissue, or the crural columns become taut, then the surgeon should not force further sutures. An anterior cruroplasty may be added as long as there is not excessive tension in the arch above the esophagus.

If a sutured (i.e., primary) cruroplasty results in tension across the suture line, then the surgeon may consider bolstering the repair with a sheet of prosthetic mesh. Our indication for mesh utilization in a previous clinical trial was a hiatal defect diameter of 8 cm or larger. We have liberalized this indication somewhat, because in defects down to 5 cm the primary cruroplasty still may be under too much tension. As mentioned above, tissue tearing or taut columns should alert the surgeon to this problem. In addition, there are other "risk factors" for breakdown of a primary cruroplasty and the surgeon should consider them (including advanced age, obesity, and chronic straining/lifting) when deciding whether to use mesh. It should be acknowledged that the indications for mesh utilization at the esophageal hiatus are controversial (see "Results and Outcome").

As indicated earlier, we will use mesh at the hiatus if the cruroplasty appears at risk; prior to any mesh hiatoplasty, however, the surgeon should perform a careful inspection of the proximal stomach and fundus in order to ensure that no full-thickness injury has been incurred. If there is a question of a leak, then the surgeon may have the anesthesiologist insufflate the organ while it is submerged in saline. Placement of a permanent prosthesis in the presence of a full-thickness esophageal or gastric injury is risky and, generally speaking, is not recommended (see the section, Procedure-Specific Complications).

The precise technique of mesh repair varies among the authors of this chapter. One technique is to place a circumferential sheet of PTFE (double-surfaced; e.g., DualMesh, W.L. Gore and Associates, Flagstaff, AZ) around the gastroesophageal junction and against the diaphragm. A circular sheet of PTFE is cut 15 cm in diameter, and a 3-cm "keyhole" with slot is cut from the center (refer to the accompanying DVD for visual details). The mesh is inked with an indelible marker at 3 and 9 o'clock (the

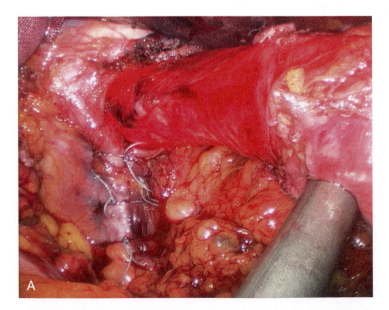

FIGURE 4-6 Posterior cruroplasty with interrupted permanent sutures. A, Intraoperative image.

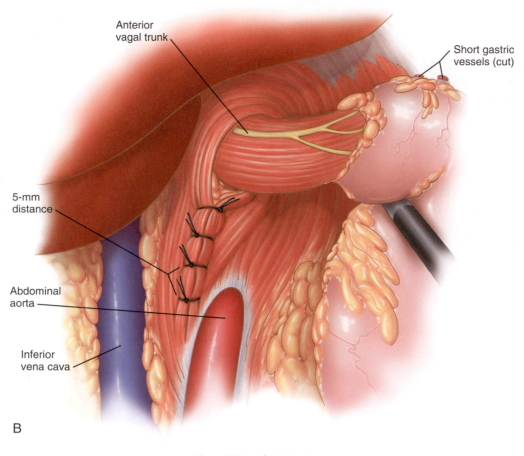

Anterior
vagal trunk

Short gastric
vessels (cut)

5-mm
distance

Abdominal
aorta

Inferior
vena cava

B

FIGURE 4-6 CONT'D B, Drawing.

"equator"), and also at 12 o'clock (medial leaf only). Three poly-glactin sutures are placed for orientation and grasping, one at the upper corner of each leaf of the keyhole, and one at 6 o'clock. The mesh then is rolled up and passed through a trocar into the abdomen. Mesh contact with the patient's skin should be avoided. Alternatively, the surgeon may use a lightweight coated polyester mesh (Parietex, U.S. Surgical, Norwalk, CT), which generally is easier to manipulate than PTFE and has a "see-through" advantage because of its macroporous construction.

Once inside the abdomen, the mesh is unfolded and the medial leaf of the keyhole is passed underneath the esophagus from right to left; care should be taken to avoid introducing a twist in the mesh as it passes underneath the gastroesophageal junction. Using the ink marks and polyglactin sutures for orientation, the mesh is positioned with the keyhole slot oriented vertically. For anchorage of the mesh, the surgeon can employ a multifeed 10-mm hernia stapler which fires conventional staples (e.g., Ethicon EMS, Ethicon Endo-Surgery, Cincinnati, OH). The first staple is fired at the superior corner of the medial leaf of the keyhole and, progressing in a counterclockwise fashion, the medial mesh perimeter is secure down to the 6 o'clock position. The stapler head is oriented radially so that one end of each staple catches the mesh, while the other end gets a bite of the diaphragm. Firing staples (or tacks) into the diaphragm should be done with prudence, as there have been case reports of cardiac injury secondary to this technique.

After the medial perimeter of the mesh has been secured, the medial margin of the keyhole is secured to the underlying right crural bundle, again progressing from 12 to 6 o'clock. The mesh should not be applied to the esophagus by this inner row of staples; in addition, the bougie should be kept in place in order to avoid mesh constriction of the esophagus. The lateral leaf of the keyhole then is secured to the diaphragm/left crural bundle with the stapler in a similar fashion, but this time going in a clockwise fashion from 12 to 6 o'clock. The two leaflets of the keyhole then are secured to each other along the vertically oriented slot; see Figure 4-7 for the appearance of the completed mesh hiatoplasty. During the stapling of the mesh, the surgeon frequently should check its position with respect to the ink marks to ensure continued proper placement of the mesh. In the posterolateral region, care should be taken to avoid applying the mesh to the spleen or the gastrosplenic omentum.

An alternative method of mesh hiatoplasty involves the use of a V-shaped, U-shaped, or rectangular polypropylene or PTFE mesh, which is slipped underneath the gastroesophageal junction and applied to the primary cruroplasty as a buttress (Fig. 4-8). These repairs also have been shown to have excellent efficacy and durability. A potential advantage to a noncircumferential mesh configuration as shown in Figure 4-8 is that the theoretical risk of constriction or strangulation of the esophagus by mesh contraction or "shrinkage" would be decreased compared to the circumferential mesh configuration shown in Figure 4-7. Although mesh constriction of the gastroesophageal junction probably is a real concern if a heavyweight polypropylene mesh is used for hiatoplasty, clinical experience has not demonstrated constriction to be a problem with the mesh repair shown in Figure 4-7.

Upon completion of the hiatoplasty, the surgeon then has the option of performing an antireflux procedure. We prefer to

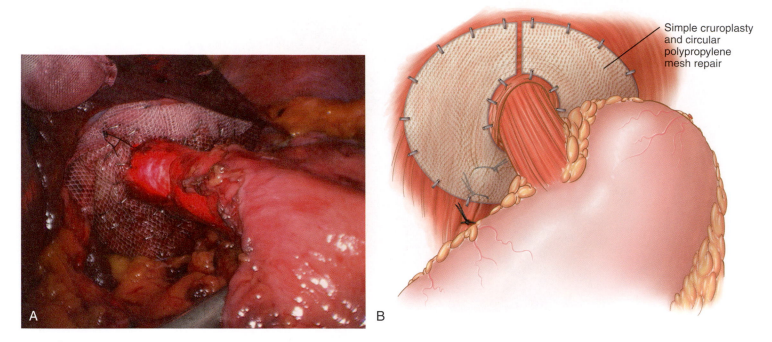

A   Simple cruroplasty
                                                                                   and circular
                                                                                   polypropylene
                                                                                   mesh repair

B

FIGURE 4-7   The completed circumferential mesh hiatoplasty. **A,** Intraoperative image. **B,** Drawing.

create a Nissen wrap in most of our patients (Fig. 4-9); in the presence of the circumferential mesh hiatoplasty shown in Figure 4-7, concomitant Nissen construction has not produced long-term dysphagia in our patients. We feel that some sort of antireflux procedure is necessary in these patients because any remnant of the natural antireflux mechanism was destroyed by the dissection. The details of this wrap construction are the same as described for Nissen fundoplication in Chapter 3. In addition, we will anchor the fundoplication to the mesh with most cephalad stitch of the wrap. After completion of the wrap, the operation is concluded by closing the fascia of the ports and evacuating the pneumoperitoneum.

POSTOPERATIVE CARE

Compared to a simple Nissen fundoplication with repair of a small hiatal hernia, a procedure on a large hiatal hernia is more prone to gastric or esophageal perforation. Therefore, a routine Gastrografin swallow (Bracco Diagnostics, Princeton, NJ) is obtained in the morning of postoperative day 1. If this study does not demonstrate extravasation, then the patient is given a clear liquid diet. Because the typical patient is older, several days of hospitalization may be necessary. At the time of discharge the patient may be placed on a soft diet, as described in Chapter 3 for Nissen fundoplication. Activity restrictions and follow-up also

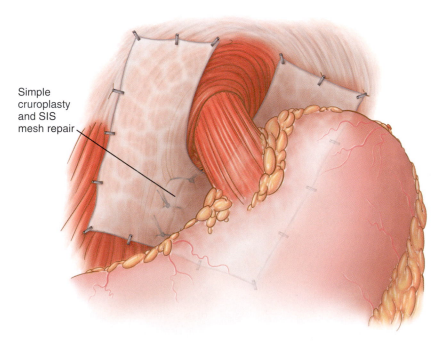

Simple
cruroplasty
and SIS
mesh repair

FIGURE 4-8   Posterior mesh (U-shaped) hiatoplasty.

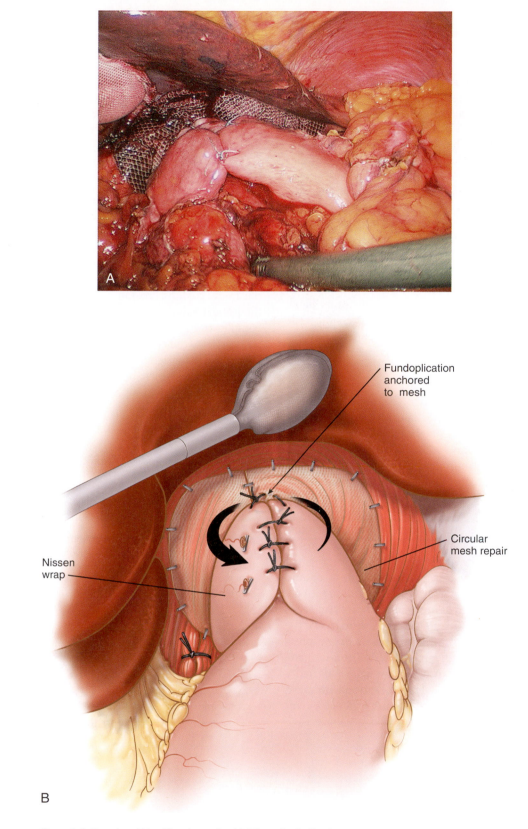

Fundoplication
anchored
to mesh

Circular
mesh repair

Nissen
wrap

FIGURE 4-9 Completed hiatal hernia repair with Nissen fundoplication. **A**, Intraoperative image. **B**, Drawing.

are similar to that described in Chapter 3, except that a barium swallow is obtained at the 6-month visit.

PROCEDURE-SPECIFIC COMPLICATIONS

The complications described in Chapter 3 also can occur after repair of a large hiatal hernia; in addition, the latter procedure is more prone to vagal injury, pneumothorax, perforation, and abscess/leak. In addition, there are other, rarer complications of large hiatal hernia repair including cardiac tamponade (from overvigorous application of diaphragmatic tacks) and aortic injury (during the cruroplasty). If not recognized immediately and treated, these latter complications can be quickly fatal. A more common and benign complication is pneumomediastinum with subsequent subcutaneous emphysema in the chest, neck, and head regions. Although this complication can produce a temporary yet distressing cosmetic appearance, the complication is self-limiting and rarely has physiologic consequences. Another common and benign postoperative finding is a mediastinal seroma. This may appear on a chest x-ray as an air-fluid level. In the absence of signs and symptoms, such a seroma requires no specific intervention.

The occurrence of a pneumothorax may be recognized intra-operatively by eventration of the diaphragm into the left upper abdomen; in addition, there also may be tachycardia, oxygen desaturation, hypercarbia, hypotension, and other well-known physical signs of pneumothorax. This complication may not necessitate open conversion; the surgeon may address the situation by decreasing the pressure of the pneumoperitoneum and having the anesthesiologist hyperventilate the patient. These maneuvers often will correct the derangements in vital signs. Tube thoracostomy usually will require conversion because of the inability to maintain pneumoperitoneum; on the other hand, needle thoracostomy may provide enough decompression while allowing ongoing pneumoperitoneum. If the patient remains unstable despite the above interventions, then conversion to open surgery may be necessary.

The primary mechanism of perforation is traction from grasping forceps. In order to minimize this risk, we like to use 10-mm graspers with atraumatic jaw inserts (Atraugrip, Specialty Surgical Instrumentation, Nashville, TN). In large hiatal hernia, the esophagus may be displaced posteriorly and "accordioned" in the mediastinum. A lighted bougie carefully inserted into the esophagus after reduction of the hernia will aid in the identification and mobilization of the esophagus. Some surgeons feel that the use of the bougie risks esophageal perforation; however, it is our opinion that benefits of this dissection aid outweigh its risks. If a perforation is diagnosed intraoperatively, then primary closure should be performed with interrupted sutures. Whether permanent mesh should be utilized in the presence of a perforation is a judgment call; confounding factors like spillage of luminal contents and security of the repair will influence this decision. Alternatively, the surgeon may consider the use of a bioprosthesis in the presence of a perforation. If the diagnosis of perforation is made during the postoperative period in a patient who has had a mesh-reinforced cruroplasty, then early reoperation with mesh explantation will be likely. If the patient has not had placement of mesh, then a postoperative leak might be successfully managed with nonoperative care consisting of antibiotics, parenteral nutrition, and percutaneous drainage.

A rare complication of mesh-reinforced hiatal hernia repair is mesh erosion or mesh-induced stenosis. In the event that one of these complications occurs, we presume that mesh explantation will be necessary; however, we have never had to do this in our 16 years of experience with laparoscopic hiatal hernia repair.

RESULTS AND OUTCOME

It has been documented that primary hiatal herniorrhaphy (laparoscopic or open) has a high recurrence rate. Since the 1990s a number of studies have demonstrated that mesh-reinforced hiatal hernia repair has a much lower recurrence rate compared to primary repair. The opponents of mesh repair have argued that prosthetic utilization at the esophageal hiatus is prone to complications such as erosion and stenosis. While these risks have theoretical validity, there is little documented evidence of such complications with the use of modern mesh material. We do acknowledge the criticisms of the opponents to mesh utilization, but in our experience (which includes a randomized trial) we have found no discernable adverse effects with the use of modern mesh material at the esophageal hiatus.

Suggested Reading

Carlson MA, Condon RE, Ludwig KA, Schulte WJ: Management of intrathoracic stomach with polypropylene mesh prosthesis reinforced transabdominal hiatus hernia repair. J Am Coll Surg 1998;187:227–230.

Carlson MA, Frantzides CT: Prosthetic reinforcement of posterior cruroplasty during laparoscopic hiatal herniorrhaphy. Surg Endosc 1997;11:769–771.

Frantzides CT, Carlson MA: Paraesophageal herniation. In Baker RJ, Fischer JE (eds): Mastery of Surgery, 4th ed. Philadelphia, Lippincott Williams & Wilkins, 2001.

Frantzides CT, Madan AK, Carlson MA, Stavropoulos GP: A prospective, randomized trial of laparoscopic polytetrafluoroethylene (PTFE) patch repair vs. simple cruroplasty for large hiatal hernia. Arch Surg 2002;137:649–652.

Granderath FA, Carlson MA, Champion JK, et al: Prosthetic closure of the esophageal hiatus in large hiatal hernia repair and laparoscopic antireflux surgery. Surg Endosc 2006;20:367–379.

Granderath FA, Schweiger UM, Kamolz T, et al: Laparoscopic Nissen fundoplication with prosthetic hiatal closure reduces postoperative intrathoracic wrap herniation: Preliminary results of a prospective randomized functional and clinical study. Arch Surg 2005;140:40–48.

Oelschlager BK, Pellegrini CA, Hunter J, et al: Biologic prosthesis reduces recurrence after laparoscopic paraesophageal hernia repair: A multicenter, prospective, randomized trial. Ann Surg 2006;244:481–490.

Stomach

MANISH PARIKH AND
ALFONS POMP

Laparoscopic Total Gastrectomy for Malignancy

5

Laparoscopic total gastrectomy is a recent minimally invasive modality used for early proximal gastric cancers. Although there is a paucity of data compared to laparoscopic colorectal resection for malignancy, international data are now emerging demonstrating that laparoscopic gastrectomy is safe and feasible and can satisfy all oncologic principles in experienced hands. The most common reconstruction after laparoscopic total gastrectomy is Roux-en-Y esophagojejunostomy. This operation is one of the most difficult laparoscopic procedures currently performed and should be done only by a surgeon skilled in laparoscopy and familiar with the oncologic principles of gastric cancer.

OPERATIVE INDICATIONS

Surgical resection is the primary therapeutic modality for potentially resectable (stages I–III) gastric cancer. A T1 tumor of the stomach (limited to the submucosa) may be treated with radical gastrectomy; T2 and higher lesions may receive preoperative chemotherapy followed by radical gastrectomy. If the tumor is located in the body or antrum, then a subtotal gastrectomy may be performed; if the tumor is in the cardia, then a total gastrectomy may be performed (although proximal gastrectomy also has been described for this indication). Longitudinal margins of more than 5 cm are preferable. If the patient has M1 disease (including peritoneal seeding) or encasement of a major vascular structure (e.g., celiac axis), or a complete (R0) resection cannot otherwise be obtained, then a resection for cure is not indicated. A minimum of 15 nodes should be removed with the specimen for staging purposes. Of note, the extent of resection and lymphadenectomy for gastric cancer have been issues of debate. In the United States and Europe, a D1 resection (removal of the stomach and the greater and lesser omenta) generally is preferred. In Japan, more extensive D2 resections have found favor. Total gastrectomy also may be indicated for palliation of M1 gastric tumors that are bleeding or causing obstruction. Other forms of surgical therapy for gastric cancer include endoscopic mucosal resection and laparoscopic wedge resection; both of these modalities are utilized for the treatment of early gastric cancer. Experience in the West with these minimalistic procedures has been nominal, and further study is needed before recommendations can be given.

PREOPERATIVE EVALUATION, TESTING, AND PREPARATION

Preoperative history and physical examination in a patient with known gastric cancer should focus on detecting occult metastatic disease (e.g., supraclavicular lymph nodes, umbilical nodes, pouch of Douglas). The patient should undergo esophagogastroduodenoscopy with biopsy to confirm malignancy. Endoscopic ultrasound may be useful to determine the depth and extension of the malignancy. Computed tomography (CT) scan of the chest and abdomen is important to stage the tumor. Some centers frequently utilize positron emission tomography (PET) combined with CT scan as an adjunctive modality to identify metastasis. The patient should undergo thorough nutritional evaluation, and preoperative total parenteral nutrition may be used when indicated.

PATIENT POSITIONING AND PLACEMENT OF TROCARS

We prefer the Alphastar table (Maquet, Rastatt, Germany) with footplate attachments. The patient is placed in the "French" split-leg position with the legs abducted, but not flexed, and properly secured (Fig. 5-1). The surgeon stands between the patient's legs, the first assistant (liver retractor and camera holder) stands on the patient's right, and the second assistant stands on the patient's left. A total of six trocars are used in our standard approach (Fig. 5-2). A 10-mm trocar is used at the umbilicus (we prefer the open technique to enter the peritoneal cavity). Two additional 10-mm trocars are placed: one in the left epigastric paramedian position (optics) and one in the right subcostal position in the midclavicular line (liver retraction). Two 5-12–mm trocars (Versaport, U.S. Surgical, Norwalk, CT) are used: one in the subxiphoid position and one in the left midclavicular line, four fingerbreadths inferior to the costal margin. Finally, a 5-mm port in the left anterior axillary line lateral to the 5-12–mm trocar is placed for additional gastric retraction. A second insufflator is attached to optimize pneumoperitoneum (15 mm Hg carbon dioxide) in case frequent aspiration is necessary.

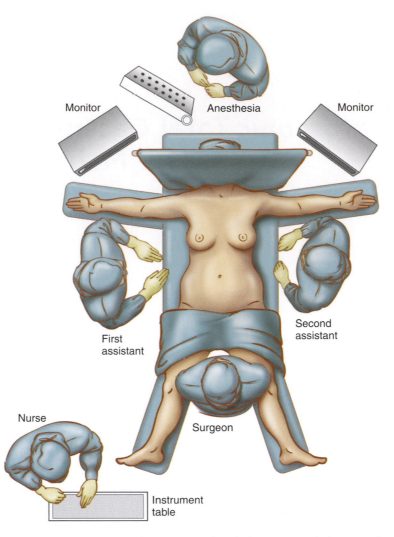

FIGURE 5-1 Operating room setup for a laparoscopic total gastrectomy. The patient is in the split-leg position with the surgeon between the patient's legs, the first assistant (camera operator/liver retractor) on the patient's right, and the second assistant on the patient's left.

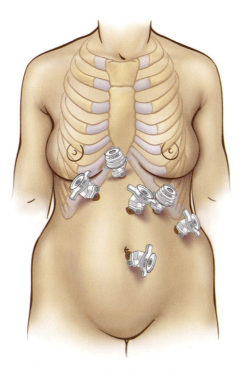

FIGURE 5-2 Trocar positions for a total gastrectomy.

OPERATIVE TECHNIQUE

The 10-mm 30-degree laparoscope is introduced and general exploration is performed. The surgeon determines resectability of the tumor. A careful inspection of the peritoneal surfaces, liver, pancreas, and base of the mesocolon is performed. If ascites is present, then cytologic examination is performed. Malignant ascites does not render the tumor unresectable, but this finding does portend a worse prognosis. If the surgeon cannot identify the gastric tumor, then endoscopy should be performed to confirm the location of the malignancy.

Mobilization of Omentum and Short Gastric Vessels

The patient is placed in steep reverse Trendelenburg position. If the stomach is distended, then the anesthesiologist should place an orogastric tube for decompression; this tube must be removed as soon as possible in order to avoid any problems during subsequent stapling. With the camera in the midabdominal port and the surgeon's hands utilizing the subxiphoid and left subcostal 5-12–mm trocars, the entire greater omentum is mobilized off the transverse colon (from the duodenum to the spleen; Fig. 5-3). The left lateral liver segment is retracted anteriorly and superiorly with a hand-held retractor. Troublesome bleeding can be avoided by keeping the appropriate plane of dissection between the appendices of the

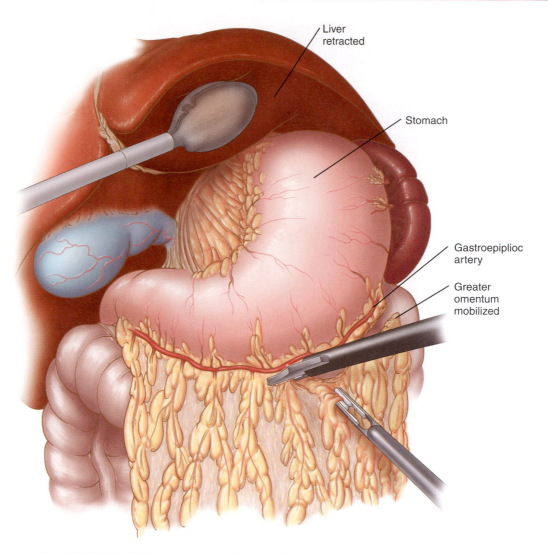

FIGURE 5-3 Division of the greater omentum between the greater curve of the stomach and the colon.

colon and the omentum. The second assistant may use an atraumatic bowel grasper (left lateral 5-mm port) to maintain caudad traction on the transverse colon. As the dissection continues, it is important to elevate the omentum away from the transverse mesocolon in order to avoid injury to the middle colic vessels.

The lesser sac is entered, and the short gastric vessels are divided with the ultrasonic scalpel (Fig. 5-4). This continues superiorly to the level of the left crus. Exposure while dividing the short gastric vessels and dissecting near the left crus often is difficult. Helpful maneuvers include the following:

- Place the second assistant's grasper on the lateral fold of the omentum (in the midgastrosplenic ligament) and retract this laterally toward the spleen.
- Temporarily increase the pneumoperitoneum to 20 mm Hg.
- Place the patient in maximal reverse Trendelenburg position.
- Tilt the patient laterally with the right side down.
- Maintain an adequate level of paralysis during anesthesia.
- Position the second assistant's grasper on the posterior fundus and retract (push) this toward the patient's right side.
- A 5-mm trocar in a higher, more medial left upper quadrant position occasionally is required to retract the perigastric fat in order to expose the gastroesophageal junction.

All posterior attachments to the pancreas must be lysed, taking care not to injure the splenic artery. This is best performed with laparoscopic scissors. Placing the second assistant's graspers

on the posterior fundus and retracting this toward the patient's right shoulder facilitates exposure of these attachments. If these attachments are not divided prior to stapling, then tearing and troublesome bleeding can occur.

Duodenal Dissection/Transection

The second assistant retracts the greater curvature anteriorly and laterally toward the patient's right shoulder. The surgeon's left hand grasps the fat of the gastrocolic ligament (via the right midclavicular 5-12–mm trocar) and retracts it caudad. The surgeon's right hand manipulates the ultrasonic scalpel. The remainder of the gastrocolic ligament between the antrum and gastroepiploic arcade is divided with the ultrasonic scalpel. The right gastroepiploic vessels are divided either with a 2.5-mm Endo GIA linear stapler with a 60-mm cartridge length (U.S. Surgical) or between 10-mm titanium clips.

The pylorus and first portion of duodenum are palpated with the laparoscopic graspers in order to confirm/delineate the anatomy. Any remaining branches between the gastroepiploic arcade and the antrum/pylorus are divided with the ultrasonic scalpel, proceeding toward the inferior aspect of the first portion of the duodenum. Typically, the dissection extends to just beyond the vascular complex inferior to the pylorus. Superiorly, the right gastric artery is dissected and ligated. It is important to avoid hemostatic clips in this area (especially on the duodenal side)

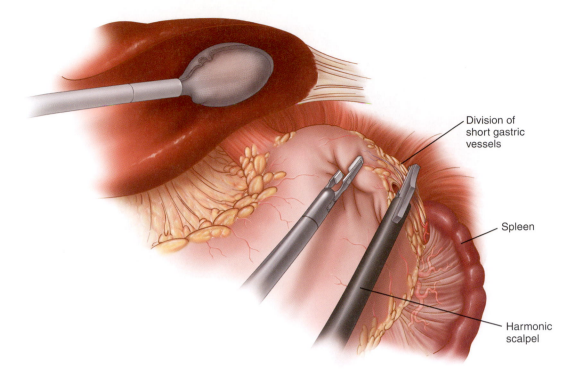

Division of
short gastric
vessels

Spleen

Harmonic
scalpel

FIGURE 5-4 Division of the short gastric vessels.

to prevent clip interference with the staple line. The retroduo-denal and supraduodenal tissue are dissected with the ultrasonic scalpel, taking care not to cause thermal injury to the duodenum. The second assistant retracts the stomach laterally and anteriorly so the surgeon can see both the greater curvature and the posterior stomach for the retroduodenal dissection. The gastroduodenal artery, which lies posteriorly between the first and second portion of duodenum, marks the distal aspect of dissection.

Using a 10-mm right-angle dissector, a 1-cm window (wide enough to accommodate a linear stapler) is made posterior and superior to the first portion of the duodenum, medial to the common bile duct (Fig. 5-5). Ideally, the supraduodenal window is between the serosa of the duodenum and the pyloric branches of the right gastric artery. The duodenum is transected with a 3.5-mm Endo GIA linear stapler (60-mm cartridge length), buttressed with Bioabsorbable Seamguard (W.L. Gore and Associates, Flagstaff, AZ); a 2- to 5-cm duodenal cuff should be left (Fig. 5-6). The stapler usually is applied via the left midclavicular 5-12–mm port. The second assistant retracts the antrum toward the patient's left side in order to facilitate this. The Seamguard buttressing material obviates the need to oversew the duodenal stump. If the surgeon is unable to complete the supraduodenal window, an alternate method is to transect the most inferior two thirds of the duodenum with the linear stapler, complete the supraduodenal window, and then transect the remaining duodenum with another application of the stapler.

Hiatal Dissection, Celiac Axis Dissection, and Division of Left Gastric Vessels

The second assistant grasps the pylorus and retracts this inferiorly to slightly stretch the lesser omentum. The transparent lesser omentum is incised to expose (from right to left) the caudate lobe, right crural bundle, esophageal hiatus, and if present, a hiatal hernia. The second assistant's grasper is repositioned to retract the cardia of the stomach toward the patient's left side. An aberrant left hepatic artery, which can be found in up to 20%

of patients, will need to be divided if present. The peritoneum over the right crural bundle is incised with the hook electrocautery or ultrasonic scalpel, and mobilization of the medial edge of the crus is carried out superiorly to the apex of the hiatus and inferiorly to the confluence of the right and left crural bundles (Fig. 5-7). The phrenoesophageal membrane is divided. The posterior vagus is identified (typically 2–3 cm lateral and posterior to the right esophageal wall) and then transected. The anterior vagus (running anteriorly on the esophagus) is also divided.

The dissection of the posterior window behind the distal esophagus and proximal stomach is completed by dividing all attachments between the esophagus and the inferior crural confluence. Any remaining attachments between the stomach and left crus and not divided during transection of the short gastrics should now be divided. With the stomach retracted toward the left and inferiorly, the surgeon places a 7-inch long 0.25-inch wide Penrose drain through the posterior window (Fig. 5-8). Both ends of the Penrose drain are grasped and a clip is applied. The second assistant then holds the Penrose drain to provide better esophageal retraction while the posterior window is widened.

The esophagus is mobilized in order to increase its intra-abdominal length. Esophageal attachments in the posterior mediastinum are divided as cranially as possible. Traction on the Penrose drain is used to optimize exposure posteriorly and laterally. The esophagus is mobilized in this manner from the pleura, aorta, and lateral crural attachments. The surgeon should be cautious with lateral dissection in this location because of the risk of breaching the pleura. If the pleural space is inadvertently entered, then the surgeon must communicate with the anesthesiologist in order to monitor airway pressures and ventilation. Generally, chest tubes are not necessary in this scenario.

The second assistant elevates the fundus of the stomach and retracts it anteriorly and toward the patient's right shoulder. The left gastric vessels now should be visible extending to the lesser curvature. The artery should be dissected toward the celiac axis, sweeping the lymph nodes along the left gastric artery toward the

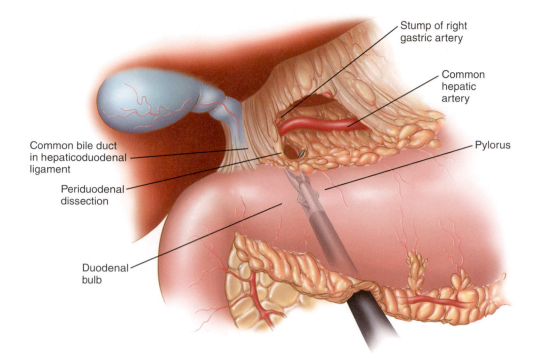

FIGURE 5-5 Creation of a window posterior to the first portion of the duodenum.

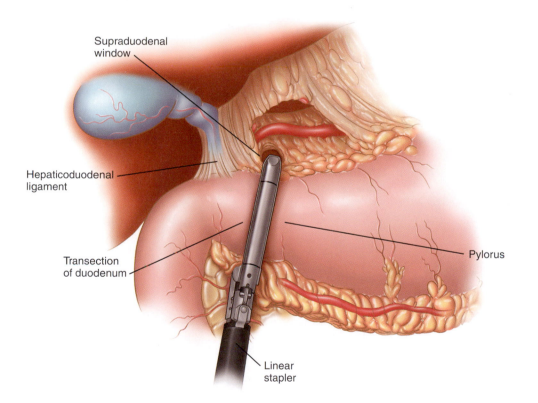

FIGURE 5-6 Duodenal transection with linear stapler.

lesser curvature. The left gastric pedicle then may be transected using the 2.5-mm Endo GIA stapler. The coronary vein (which lies caudal to the left gastric artery) often can be transected with the artery.

If a D1 (perigastric) lymph node dissection is planned, at least 15 nodes are required for adequate staging. Some centers (especially in Japan) routinely perform a more extensive D2 lymph node dissection, although the Western data have not completely substantiated the benefits of a D2 dissection. If a D2 dissection is desired, then all lymphatic tissue along the common hepatic artery, left gastric artery, celiac axis, and splenic artery (in addition to perigastric lymph nodes) should be retrieved. The peritoneum along the common hepatic artery extending distally to the gastroduodenal artery and proximally to the celiac axis is incised. The artery is carefully dissected, sweeping the lymphatic tissue toward the lesser curve. In a similar fashion, the surgeon should sweep the lymph nodes along the splenic artery toward the lesser curve.

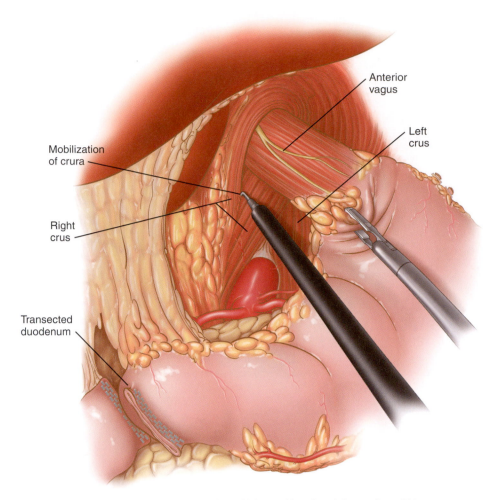

Anterior
vagus

Left
crus

Mobilization
of crura

Right
crus

Transected
duodenum

FIGURE 5-7 Exposure of the right and left crural bundles of the esophageal hiatus.

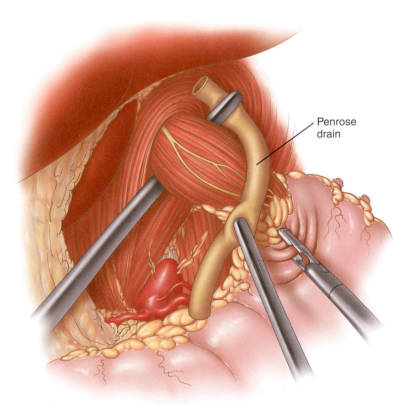

Penrose
drain

FIGURE 5-8 Placement of a Penrose drain through the window posterior to the gastroesophageal junction.

Esophageal Transection and Esophagojejunostomy with Circular Stapler

Intraoperative endoscopy may help verify the exact location of the esophagogastric junction. An Endo GIA stapler (3.5 mm) is placed through the subxiphoid 5-12–mm port, and the esophagus is divided just above the junction. The left subcostal 5-12–mm trocar is removed and this incision is enlarged (the circular stapler will be placed through here later). An impermeable bag is placed through this incision, and the specimen is removed. To facilitate removal of the specimen, the bag may need to be exteriorized and the duodenal stump may need to be delivered first. The rest of the stomach and omentum can then be delivered in a spiral twisting motion. It may facilitate the operation (especially with more bulky specimens) to remove the surgical specimen at the end of the case, so that the surgeon does not have a larger incision to close in order to maintain pneumoperitoneum. A disadvantage of this latter approach is that the pathologist cannot confirm the surgical margins prior to completion of the anastomosis.

We prefer the CEEA 25-mm circular stapler (OrVil, U.S. Surgical) to construct the esophagojejunostomy. A 2-0 Prolene suture is passed through the spike of the stapler and an air knot is tied to facilitate subsequent removal from the abdomen. This spike then is retracted completely into the stapler. In addition, camera drape is cut and attached with an adhesive strip around the shaft of the stapler (for wound protection during removal). The anesthesiologist then passes this nasogastric tube apparatus through the mouth until the tip abuts the esophageal staple line. The surgeon's left instrument and the second assistant gently grasp the corners of the staple line and retract inferomedially to facilitate passage of the tube. An esophagotomy is made using ultrasonic energy dissection, and the tip of the tube is pulled out through the left subcostal port. A jaw thrust maneuver by the anesthesiologist facilitates passage of the anvil through the upper esophageal sphincter. On occasion, the balloon of the endotracheal tube needs to be temporarily deflated in order to deliver the anvil. The excess tubing is pulled through the trocar until the metal tip of the anvil exits the esophagus. The tubing is removed after cutting the suture between the anvil and the tube, thus freeing the anvil from the tube.

The laparoscope is moved to the umbilical port. A V-shaped rent can be made in the omentum to facilitate antecolic passage of the Roux limb. With the assistants retracting the transverse colon superiorly, the ligament of Treitz is located and the proximal jejunum is run about 50 cm (usually sufficient to provide enough mesentery) in preparation for the esophagojejunostomy. Flat 5-mm forceps (Dorsey, Karl Storz, Tutlingen, Germany) are used to avoid serosal tears. The jejunum is elevated to inspect the mesentery and ascertain whether it will reach the hiatus in a tension-free manner. If the jejunal mesentery is short, it may be necessary to make mesenteric relaxing incisions. A 10-mm right-angle forceps is used to make a window between the jejunal mesentery and the bowel wall. The jejunum is transected with a 2.5-mm Endo GIA stapler (45-mm cartridge length), buttressed with Bioabsorbable Seamguard. The distal staple line then is excised with the ultrasonic scalpel.

After the jejunal transection, the left subcostal trocar is removed and the circular stapler is passed transabdominally into the enterotomy of the distal jejunum. The circular stapler is advanced into the opened end of the distal jejunal limb for several centimeters, and then advanced cephalad toward the hiatus. The stapler head must reach the esophagus (containing the anvil) without tension. If this is not possible, then a retrocolic route may be necessary

or additional esophageal mobilization should be done. The white plastic perforator is advanced through the antimesenteric wall of jejunum approximately 6 to 7 cm distal to the opened jejunum. The spike then is removed from the abdominal cavity by grasping the suture attached to the spike. The laparoscope is returned to the midabdominal port. The anvil (in the esophagus) then is united with the stapler (Fig. 5-9). It is important that no tissue is caught between the esophagus and jejunum within the stapler, and that there is no pinching of the bowel wall (which can create an obstruction). The stapler is fired, and then backed out of the enterotomy with a gentle, rocking motion. The adhesive strip holding the wound protector is removed, and the stapler is removed from the trocar site while advancing the wound protector over the tip of the stapler, in order to prevent the stapler from contacting the wound.

Reinforcement sutures of 3-0 Vicryl may be placed at the anastomosis as needed. The opened Roux limb is inspected for bleeding; any oozing emanating from the enterotomy may indicate bleeding from the esophagojejunostomy and should be evaluated. If necessary, the laparoscope can be placed through the enterotomy to directly visualize the anastomosis. If there is no bleeding from the opened limb, then a 2.5-mm linear stapler buttressed with Seamguard is used to close the open end of jejunal limb through the port site which the circular stapler had passed. The tip of the stapler must be in the jejunal mesentery to ensure that the opened jejunum has been completely closed; otherwise, a leak may occur into the mesentery. The small stump of jejunum is extracted from the right midclavicular trocar site. Finally, the anesthesiologist inserts an orogastric tube (or nasogastric tube if it is to remain in place postoperatively), the Roux limb is clamped, and a methylene blue test is instilled to evaluate

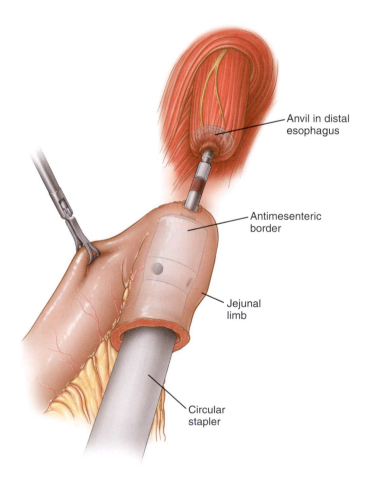

Anvil in distal esophagus

Antimesenteric border

Jejunal limb

Circular stapler

FIGURE 5-9   Creation of esophagojejunostomy with a 25-mm circular stapler.

for leak. Alternatively, an endoscope can be used to inspect the esophagojejunostomy and to perform an air leak test. The disadvantage of the latter approach is that air may distend the small bowel and make the distal anastomosis more difficult.

Alternate Techniques for Construction of Esophagojejunostomy

Some surgeons prefer retrocolic passage of the Roux limb. The second assistant's graspers are placed on the epiploic appendages of the transverse colon and retracted superiorly. The ultrasonic scalpel is used to make a window between the ligament of Treitz and the middle colic vessels. The Roux limb is then passed through this window toward the esophageal hiatus. In addition, the esophagojejunostomy can be constructed with the linear stapler or with hand-sewn technique. In order to use the linear stapler, an enterotomy is made in the antimesenteric border of the Roux limb, and the midpoint of the esophageal staple line is opened. The jaws of a 3.5-mm Endo GIA stapler (45-mm length) are placed into these openings and the stapler is fired, creating a posterior anastomosis. The anterior aspect then is closed with sutures. A completely hand-sewn technique can be done in two layers over a nasogastric tube or an endoscope (to ensure patency). Using this technique may prolong operative time. Irrespective of the technique used for construction of the esophagojejunostomy, it is critical that this is done in a tension-free manner and that the anastomosis is tested in order to rule out a leak.

Jejunojejunostomy and Closure

The laparoscope is brought back to the umbilical port. The surgeon moves to the patient's right side. The Roux limb is run for at least 40 to 50 cm (in order to minimize bile reflux), and an enterotomy is made at this point with the ultrasonic scalpel on the antimesenteric side of the jejunum. Another enterotomy is made approximately 1 to 2 cm away from the stapled end of the proximal jejunum. The stapled proximal jejunum (biliopancreatic limb) should be on the patient's left and cephalad; the Roux limb should be on the patient's right side and caudad. The surgeon should take care that there has been no twisting of the mesentery and that both staplers are fired on the antimesenteric border in order to avoid creating an ischemic anastomosis. The 2.5-mm linear stapler (60-mm cartridge length) is introduced through the subxiphoid trocar, aiming toward the pelvis. A standard side-to-side anastomosis is created between the biliopancreatic limb and the Roux limb. The enterotomy is closed in two layers with 2-0 silk.

It is important to close all mesenteric defects in order to avoid internal hernias and their associated complications. With the same position (surgeon and first assistant on the patient's right side), the jejunojejunostomy mesenteric defect is closed with a running 2-0 silk suture (24-cm length). We prefer to incorporate the serosa of the jejunum in the last stitch of this closure. The surgeon then returns between the patient's legs in order to close Petersen's defect (between the jejunal mesentery and transverse mesocolon). The patient is placed in slight reverse Trendelenburg position. Sometimes it is necessary to insert an additional 5-mm trocar in the left lower quadrant to optimize suturing angles. The assistants grasp the epiploic appendages of the transverse colon and retract this superiorly. The space between the transverse colon mesentery and the jejunal mesentery is closed with a running 2-0 silk suture. The last stitch should incorporate the serosa of jejunum and tenaie of the transverse colon.

A feeding jejunostomy (Witzel-type) can be placed 30 to 40 cm distal to the jejunojejunostomy, though this is not universally performed. We no longer place suction drains near the duodenal stump nor near the esophagojejunostomy. All fascial defects larger than 5 mm are closed with a suture-passing device with 0-Vicryl sutures. The skin incisions are closed with subcuticular absorbable monofilament sutures.

POSTOPERATIVE CARE

Patients are closely monitored for at least 6 hours. Maintenance intravenous fluids are continued to ensure urine output of at least 0.5 to 1 mL/kg/hour. Early ambulation is critical; the majority of our patients ambulate the very evening of surgery. Patients usually require an intravenous patient-controlled analgesic pump for the first 2 days. An upper GI contrast study is performed on the second or third postoperative day, depending on the clinical scenario. If this study is satisfactory, then the patient can receive clear liquids for 24 hours followed by a pureed diet. Once the patient is tolerating pureed foods, he or she may be discharged home (usually by the fifth or sixth postoperative day).

PROCEDURE-SPECIFIC COMPLICATIONS

A leak at the esophagojejunostomy is the most severe complication of this procedure. The critical factor in determining anastomotic leak is tension at the anastomosis. Thus, it is important to do everything possible to construct a tension-free anastomosis. Management of a leak depends on the clinical scenario. If the leak is minor (seen on contrast study only) and the patient is stable, then percutaneous drainage, nasogastric tube decompression, and antibiotic therapy may be adequate. If a leak is diagnosed early, then the patient may be explored laparoscopically and additional suture, biologic glue, large-bore drains, and a feeding jejunostomy can be placed. The anastomosis should not be completely redone because this almost inevitably will result in another leak or complete anastomotic breakdown. In some circumstances, thoracoscopy or thoracotomy may be necessary to establish adequate drainage. In the most dire circumstances, an end cervical esophagostomy may be required. Bleeding can be avoided by meticulous hemostasis intraoperatively. The ultrasonic scalpel may be used for 1- to 2-mm vessels; however, major vessels such as the right gastric, right gastroepiploic, and left gastric should be divided with a linear stapler or 10-mm metal clips. If immediate hemostasis is needed for heavy intraoperative bleeding, then conversion to hand-assist still may maintain some of the benefits of laparoscopic surgery.

RESULTS AND OUTCOME

Although laparoscopic gastric surgery for benign disease is well established, the role of laparoscopic gastric resection for malignancy has not been well defined. Originally, laparoscopy was described mainly for staging purposes prior to gastrectomy for malignant disease. Now, laparoscopic gastrectomy is being performed with increasing frequency, primarily for benign indications. A few specialized centers (especially in Japan) are performing laparoscopic gastrectomy for malignant disease in large numbers. The main advantages of laparoscopic gastrectomy over the equivalent open procedure are similar to those for other laparoscopic procedures: shorter hospital stay and convalescence, less surgical trauma (as evidenced by biologic markers), less pain, and earlier recovery of gastrointestinal function. In parallel to the growing body of data supporting the use of laparoscopic surgery for colorectal malignancies, recent reports also have shown that minimally invasive gastrectomy for malignancy can satisfy the oncologic criteria for an R0 resection. A recent randomized trial reported similar 5-year overall and disease-free survival rates in the laparoscopic versus the open gastrectomy groups. Thus, in experienced hands, laparoscopic gastrectomy appears to be oncologically adequate in terms of margins and lymph node retrievals. The performance of a formal D2 lymphadenectomy (as defined in the *Japanese Classification of Gastric Carcinoma*) still is a technical challenge laparoscopically, but this too can be accomplished by the experienced surgeon. As more follow-up data emerge, we anticipate that laparoscopic gastrectomy for malignancy will be as common as laparoscopic colon resection for malignancy.

Suggested Reading

Dulucq J, Wintringer P, Perissat J, Mahajna A: Completely laparoscopic total and partial gastrectomy for benign and malignant diseases: A single institute's prospective analysis. J Am Coll Surg 2005;200:191–197.

Dulucq J, Wintringer P, Stabilini C, et al: Laparoscopic and open gastric resections for malignant lesions: A prospective comparative study. Surg Endosc 2005;19:933–938.

Goh PM, Alponat A, Mak K, Kum CK: Early international results of laparoscopic gastrectomies. Surg Endosc 1997;11:650–652.

Goh P, Khan A, So J, et al: Early experience with laparoscopic radical gastrectomy for advanced gastric cancer. Surg Laparosc Endosc Percutan Tech 2001;11:83–87.

Huscher C, Mingoli A, Sgarzini G, et al: Laparoscopic versus open subtotal gastrectomy for distal gastric cancer: Five-year results of a randomized prospective trial. Ann Surg 2005;241:232–237.

Japanese Gastric Cancer Center: Japanese classification of gastric carcinoma, 2nd English edition. Gastric Cancer 1998;1:10–24.

Kitano S, Shiraishi N, Uyama I: A multicenter study on oncologic outcome of laparoscopic gastrectomy for early cancer in Japan. Ann Surg 2007;245:68–72.

Miura S, Kodera Y, Fujiwara M, et al: Laparoscopy-assisted distal gastrectomy with systemic lymph node dissection: A critical reappraisal from the viewpoint of lymph node retrieval. J Am Coll Surg 2004;198:933–938.

National Comprehensive Cancer Network: Clinical Practice Guidelines in Oncology: Gastric Cancer. Version 1, 2007. Available at www.nccn.org.

Pugliese R, Maggioni D, Sansonna F, et al: Total and subtotal laparoscopic gastrectomy for adenocarcinoma. Surg Endosc 2007;21:21–27.

Tanimura S, Higashino M, Fukunaga Y, et al: Laparoscopic gastrectomy with regional lymph node dissection for upper gastric cancer. Br J Surg 2007;94:204–207.

Ueda K, Matteotti R, Assalia A, Gagner M: Comparative evaluation of gastrointestinal transit and immune response between laparoscopic and open gastrectomy in a porcine model. J Gastrointest Surg 2006;10:39–45.

Weber K, Reyes C, Gagner M, Divino C: Comparison of laparoscopic and open gastrectomy for malignant disease. Surg Endosc 2003;17:968–971.

CONSTANTINE T. FRANTZIDES AND
JOHN G. ZOGRAFAKIS

Laparoscopic Gastric Bypass with Roux-en-Y Gastrojejunostomy

6

The surgical management of obesity has evolved dramatically since its inception in the early 1960s. Completely malabsorptive procedures including the jejunoileal intestinal bypass (JIB) were succeeded by purely restrictive procedures such as the vertical banded gastroplasty (VBG). Although the weight loss from the JIB was satisfactory, severe protein-calorie malnutrition, hepatic failure, and other malabsorptive complications led to the abandonment of this procedure. The VBG has fallen out of favor because of inadequate long-term sustained weight loss and many technical failures. In the mid- to late 1980s, open Roux-en-Y gastric bypass (ORYGB) evolved as the gold standard for weight-loss surgery. This is considered a hybrid operation because both restrictive and malabsorptive components are combined in order to maximize safe and sustained weight loss. With the advent of minimally invasive surgery and the availability of advanced laparoscopic instrumentation, the laparoscopic Roux-en-Y gastric bypass (LRYGB) has experienced exponential growth. The safety, efficacy, and popularity of the LRYGB has attracted more patients to consider surgical treatment who otherwise might not have sought such intervention.

The surgeon performing laparoscopic weight reductive procedures should have a background in bariatric surgery and advanced laparoscopic surgical skills. In order to advance an individual's laparoscopic surgical skills, surgeons may choose year-long surgical fellowships, week-long mini-fellowships, or a variety of intensive continuing medical education (CME) courses available at national meetings. Without question, a significant time investment is necessary in order to master the advanced laparoscopic surgical techniques required to complete these procedures.

OPERATIVE INDICATIONS

The surgical treatment of morbid obesity evolved secondary to the unsatisfactory outcome of medical therapies for weight loss. Untreated morbid obesity places the patient at risk for multiple comorbid conditions and ultimately a shortened life span. Risk stratification is done with the body mass index (BMI); increasing BMI is associated with increasing medical risk and surgical complications. In March 1991, the National Institutes of Health Consensus Conference on Obesity concluded that (1) surgery is the only way to obtain consistent and permanent weight loss for patients with morbid obesity, and that (2) weight reductive surgery is indicated for those patients with a BMI of greater than $40\,kg/m^2$, as well as for those patients with a BMI of 35 to $39.9\,kg/m^2$ with associated medical comorbidities, including hypertension, diabetes, and obstructive sleep apnea. Patients should have documentation of failed efforts to lose weight. It is important for patients who seek weight-loss surgery to be educated regarding the risks and benefits of the bariatric procedure, as well as the postoperative dietary requirements that are essential for long-term success. Finally, neither surgery nor a dietary program alone will be successful without dedicated exercise by the patient.

Relative contraindications to a laparoscopic weight-loss procedure would include previous intra-abdominal open surgery, especially that of the foregut, and previous abdominal wall herniorrhaphy (with mesh). These relative contraindications are dependent upon the laparoscopic experience of the surgeon. In fact, laparoscopic gastric bypass may be performed safely after almost any laparoscopic or open surgery.

PREOPERATIVE EVALUATION, TESTING, AND PREPARATION

Patients are often well informed prior to a surgical consultation, since a vast amount of educational information is available on the Internet. Patient education is paramount to a good outcome. Attendance at a preoperative weight-loss surgery seminar is encouraged, as well as completion of preoperative education classes. Other components of the preoperative work-up may include nutritional and psychological assessments. These tests may serve to identify those patients who may suffer from untreated psychiatric conditions such as major depressive disorder, binge eating, or drug abuse/alcoholism. Appropriate psychotherapy or counseling may be necessary before surgery. A thorough physical examination ultimately is performed by the primary surgeon, and then the decision to proceed with an open or laparoscopic procedure can be made. The risks and benefits specific to the procedure should be explained to the patient and family in detail so that informed consent can be obtained.

Many health insurance companies require the completion of a physician-supervised weight-loss program that includes a dietary and exercise regimen. Sometimes these requirements result in a lengthy waiting period (3 to 18 months) prior to allowing for insurance preauthorization. There has been no controlled trial that has documented long-term benefits for patients who have completed such a program.

Preoperative laboratory testing may include a chest x-ray, blood chemistries, hemogram, ultrasound of the gallbladder, electrocardiogram (ECG), cardiac stress testing, pulmonary function testing (including an overnight polysomnogram), upper gastrointestinal (UGI) endoscopy, and a UGI contrast study. If the patient has a personal or family history of pulmonary embolism (PE) or deep venous thrombosis (DVT), further work-up for hypercoagulability may be required (see Chapter 10). For patients found to have cholelithiasis on preoperative ultrasound, the gallbladder may safely be removed concurrently with the LRYGB. For patients without stones, 3 months of ursodiol (Actigall) therapy has been shown to reduce the risk of developing symptomatic gallstones. Nausea and abdominal pain are the most frequent side effects of ursodiol therapy. If a hiatal hernia is identified intraoperatively (or by preoperative UGI contrast study or endoscopy), then it may safely be repaired at the time of the LRYGB. After reduction of the hiatal hernia and appropriate esophageal mobilization, the diaphragmatic defect should be closed with an anterior and posterior cruroplasty over a fixed-diameter bougie, placed per os by an anesthesiologist. It is important to completely reduce the hiatal hernia in order to avoid creating too large a pouch. Once the crural repair is complete, the bougie is removed and the gastric pouch is then created. The goal of preoperative testing is to identify and optimize the patient's medical comorbid conditions prior to surgery and general anesthesia.

Effective preoperative diets include a high-protein, low-calorie diet, or physician-prescribed programs including Optifast (a meal replacement program). Preoperative dietary restrictions may decrease the size of the liver (especially the left lobe) and decrease intra-abdominal mesenteric adipose tissue, allowing for easier laparoscopic manipulation of the stomach and bowel. Prescribed meal replacement programs such as Optifast may be cost-prohibitive for a number of patients. Of note, it is important to monitor electrolytes and diuretic therapy while on a restricted preoperative diet plan.

Some surgeons have adopted the routine use of mechanical bowel preparation and antimicrobial prophylaxis prior to an elective weight-loss operation. Preoperative preparation of the patient may include standard mechanical bowel cleansing in addition to oral antibiotics. If desired, a mechanical bowel preparation with polyethylene glycol electrolyte (PEG) matrix, as well as neomycin and erythromycin base oral antibiotics, may be utilized (also known as the modified Condon-Nichols bowel preparation). In addition to mechanical and antibiotic bowel preparations, the patient can shower/bathe the evening before surgery with a chlorhexidine-based topical antiseptic (e.g., Hibiclens). Perioperative intravenous antibiotics (such as a second-generation cephalosporin) should be initiated prior to skin incision. Two doses can be administered postoperatively and then antibiotic therapy should be discontinued. Alternative antibiotic prophylaxis is described in Chapter 31.

In addition to the utilization of size-appropriate lower extremity intermittent pneumatic compression garments, it is recommended that venous thromboembolism (VTE) prophylaxis be instituted prior to surgical intervention. There have been no studies that have demonstrated a difference between unfractionated heparin and low-molecular-weight heparin. Some surgeons have suggested subcutaneous administration of 5000 units of heparin 2 hours prior to surgery, and then every 8 hours until hospital discharge. There have been many successful alternative therapies documented in the medical literature. The risks of a VTE event versus hemorrhage (the primary complication of VTE prophylaxis) must be weighed by the surgeon. Other options to consider include preoperatively placed temporary IVC filters, or long-term patient anticoagulation. The surgeon should be well versed on VTE prophylaxis and treatment, so that patient therapy can be optimized. Further discussion of VTE appears in Chapter 10.

PATIENT POSITIONING

An operating room table should be utilized that can support patients with morbid obesity (at least up to 800 pounds), that can be positioned low to the floor and in steep reverse Trendelenburg position, and that has appropriate attachments to allow for safe patient positioning. Split-leg attachments as well as right-angle footboards are helpful in supporting the weight of a patient who has been placed in steep reverse Trendelenburg position.

Two monitors are positioned, one over the right shoulder and another over the left shoulder of the patient. Two 40-L, high-flow CO_2 insufflators are helpful in maintaining pneumoperitoneum in the obese patient. In addition to high-resolution camera equipment, a variety of bariatric-length laparoscopes, including 5-mm and 10-mm diameter 0- and 30-degree angulation scopes are helpful. Because standard 33-cm laparoscopic equipment often is not long enough to complete the procedure, typically bariatric length (45 cm) instrumentation is required. Trocars also come in extended lengths, and although not always necessary, they may be needed for the patient with a very thick anterior abdominal wall. Finally, atraumatic bowel graspers (5 mm and 10 mm) and atraumatic liver retractors complete the tray. A photograph of the positioning and placement of operating room personnel and equipment is shown in Figure 6-1.

Airway maintenance in a morbidly obese patient is critical. Prior to induction of anesthesia, the head of the patient may be positioned in a "sniffing" position. Placing blankets or pillows under the patient's back and head will elevate the ear of the patient parallel to the sternum. This will facilitate vocal cord visualization and endotracheal intubation. Should anatomic considerations preclude rapid sequence intubation, fiberoptic intubation is an option (see Chapter 32).

After induction of anesthesia, care must be taken to pad the exposed bony prominences. The arms of the patient should be in the extended position and should be padded and secured to the arm boards in order to prevent tension on the shoulder and brachial plexus. Pulse oximetry monitoring is done with a soft finger probe. Invasive hemodynamic monitoring (i.e., arterial or central venous access) is left to the discretion of the surgeon/anesthesiologist. The patient is placed in a supine position, and split-leg table attachments are utilized. Right-angle footboards are necessary after splitting the legs in order to accommodate steep reverse Trendelenburg position. A slight flexion is placed in the operating room table in order to open up the upper abdomen and costal margins. Straps should secure the upper thighs to the split-leg attachments and operating room table. Foley catheter and orogastric tubes are placed to decompress the bladder and the stomach, respectively. Standard operative abdominal skin preparation is completed prior to draping.

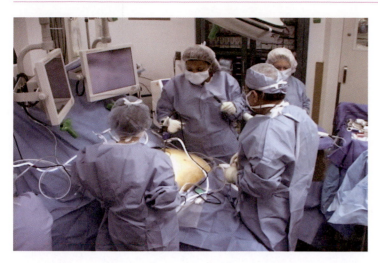

FIGURE 6-1 Operating room equipment and personnel setup.

The surgeon stands between the patient's legs (see Fig. 6-1), and the first assistant stands on the patient's left side. A dedicated camera operator stands on the right side of the patient. The scrub nurse is positioned at the right side of the surgeon, at the left lower side of the patient. A self-retaining retractor can be secured to the operating room table under the right arm of the patient. The patient should be padded against contact with the retractor. The arm of the self-retaining retractor is brought over the right side of the patient, secured to the Soft-Wand Balloon Retractor (Gyrus ACMI, Southborough, MA), and is utilized to elevate the left lobe of the liver.

PLACEMENT OF TROCARS

Access to the abdominal cavity in patients with morbid obesity can be challenging. There are a variety of techniques, including the use of optical bladed trocars (Visiport Plus RPF, U.S. Surgical, Norwalk, CT), bladeless trocars, open access technique (Hasson cannula), and the Veress needle. A safe and reproducible technique for initiating pneumoperitoneum is the bladeless optical trocar. A 0-degree 10-mm laparoscope is inserted into a handled 12-mm Endopath Bladeless Trocar (Ethicon Endo-Surgery, Cincinnati, OH) and is placed in the left subcostal position in the midclavicular line (Fig. 6-2). The handled version offers excellent control of the trocar during abdominal cavity access, reducing the chances of "plunging" into the abdomen. Pneumoperitoneum then is established at 15 to 18 mm Hg. After evaluation of the abdominal contents from this trocar position (trocar 1, see Fig. 6-2), five other 12-mm ports are placed under direct visualization. Trocar 2 is inserted in the right midclavicular line, at the level half the distance between the right subcostal margin and the umbilicus; trocar 3 is placed in the left anterior axillary line, subcostally; trocar 4 is inserted in the subxiphoid area to the left of the falciform ligament (ligamentum teres); trocar 5 is placed in the midline at mid-distance between the xiphoid and the umbilicus; and trocar 6 is inserted at the umbilicus. A solution of 0.5% bupivicaine (Marcaine) is infiltrated into the subcutaneous tissues prior to trocar placement.

OPERATIVE TECHNIQUE

Prior to beginning the procedure, the anvil and Autosuture EEA stapler (U.S. Surgical) should be prepared. The spring on the

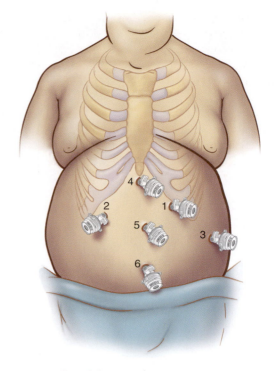

FIGURE 6-2 Trocar placement.

anvil is removed using a hemostat, carefully preventing injury to the blade on the anvil. After removing the spring, a hemostat is placed on the platform of the base (drum), and it is "loosened" in order to allow the anvil to toggle freely. The anvil then can be secured to an 18-F orogastric tube using 2-0 monofilament suture. See Chapter 33 for figures.

In order to prevent contamination of the anterior abdominal wall when the EEA stapler is removed after creation of the gastrojejunostomy, a "wound protection device" is fashioned to the EEA stapler. A standard laparoscopic camera drape is cut approximately 8 to 10 cm from its end and is secured to the head of the EEA stapler using either Steri-Strips or the tape provided with the drape. After firing the stapler, the drape can be everted over the head of the stapler and used to protect the anterior abdominal wall.

Dissection of the Angle of His

The 10-mm atraumatic balloon liver retractor is inserted through trocar 4, and the left lobe of the liver is retracted, exposing the stomach and the gastroesophageal junction (Fig. 6-3). After decompression of the stomach with an orogastric tube, the orogastric tube and any esophageal probes are removed from the patient. The stomach is grasped using two atraumatic Babcock forceps (Atraugrip Atraumatic Grasper, Specialty Surgical Instrumentation, Nashville, TN) introduced through trocars 2 and 3, and the stomach is retracted caudally to expose the phrenoesophageal ligament. The ligament and the peritoneal reflection at the angle of His are divided with the hook electrocautery through trocar 1 (Fig. 6-4). The dissection should continue until the left crus of the diaphragm and the esophagus are identified. Often there is a fat pad overlying this area, but it is not necessary to excise this pad. Sufficient mobilization should occur so that the fat pad is not trapped in the stapler during pouch formation. Care

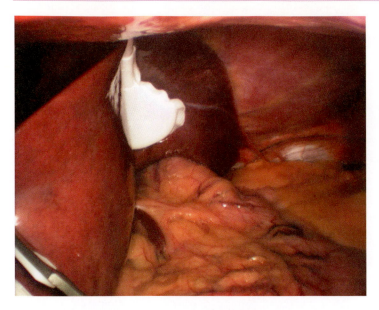

FIGURE 6-3   Retraction of the left lobe of the liver with the Soft-Wand balloon retractor.

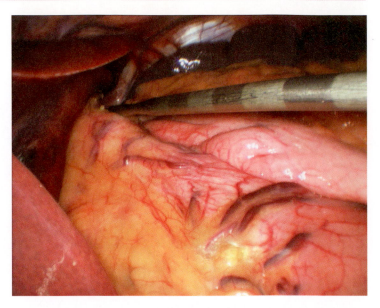

FIGURE 6-5   A calibrated palpation probe is used to measure 5 cm distal to the gastroesophageal junction.

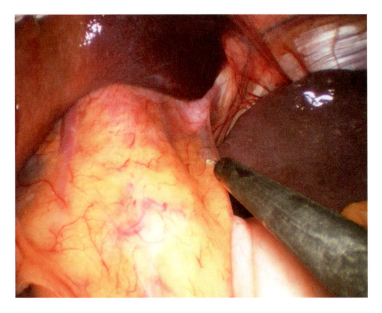

FIGURE 6-4   Identification of the angle of His; division of the peritoneal reflection with hook electrocautery.

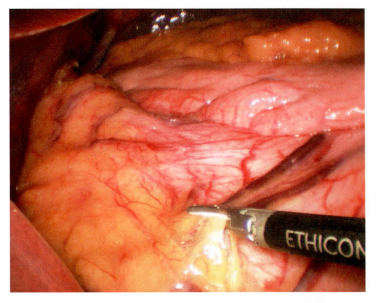

FIGURE 6-6   Division of neurovascular bundle along the lesser curvature of the stomach using the Harmonic ACE scalpel, sparing the nerve of Latarjet.

should be taken not to injure the spleen or the esophagus. Creation of this space will allow the stapler to exit this region safely when the pouch is created. A blunt palpation probe is used to expose the esophagus at the angle of His and the left bundle of the right crus of the diaphragm.

Creation of Gastric Pouch

After releasing the caudal retraction of the stomach, a Babcock grasper placed through trocar 3 is repositioned on the body of the stomach. A blunt palpation probe (with defined 1-cm increment calibrations) is used to measure approximately 5 cm from the gastroesophageal junction (Fig. 6-5). Two of the neurovascular bundles at the lesser curvature are divided with the ultrasonically activated scalpel (Fig. 6-6). This dissection is carried down to the posterior leaflet of the lesser omentum. Once the lesser sac is entered, the opening is enlarged by passing a blunt grasper into the lesser sac from trocar 2 (Fig. 6-7). During this dissection, caution should be exercised to avoid thermal injury or transection of the anterior or posterior nerves of Latarjet. Once a 2- to 3-cm

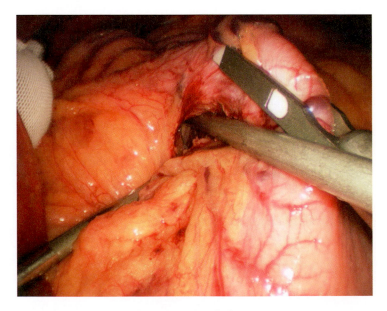

FIGURE 6-7   Entry into the lesser sac.

opening into the lesser sac has been made, the stomach is divided horizontally, 5 cm below the gastroesophageal junction, with a laparoscopic linear stapler containing a blue 45-mm × 3.5-mm staple load (Fig. 6-8), introduced through trocar 2. Prior to firing the stapler the surgeon should confirm that the orogastric tube and any other esophageal or gastric monitoring equipment has been removed from the stomach.

At this point, the blunt palpation probe may be used to divide any adhesions noted in the lesser sac. The probe then may be used to "even out" the posterior wall of the stomach (Fig. 6-9). If care is not taken to smooth out the redundant posterior wall of the stomach, too large of a pouch may be created. After the horizontal gastric transection, the stapler is reinserted through trocar 1, and blue 60-mm × 3.5-mm staple loads are fired to complete the pouch, progressing cephalad toward the angle of His (Fig. 6-10). After firing the first vertical staple load, a right-angle esophageal retractor (placed through trocar 1) is passed posterior to the pouch toward the angle of His. Once deflected, the tip of the esophageal retractor should be visible in the previously prepared space between the esophagus and the fundus of the stomach (Fig. 6-11). This opening is created to the right of the first short gastric bundle. If this vascular pedicle is left attached to the pouch, too large a pouch will be created. Once the thin tissue is divided with the esophageal retractor, the tip may be deflected superiorly to create a window large enough for the stapler. This last firing should transect the gastric remnant from the pouch (Figs. 6-12 and 6-13). An approximated 30-mL gastric pouch thus is created. It may be necessary to use a 4.8-mm staple load (green) for very thick gastric tissue, which is seen primarily in males with central obesity. It may be necessary to use additional sutures to reinforce the perpendicular staple lines on the gastric remnant.

Transoral Anvil Placement

The gastric pouch is grasped using two atraumatic graspers through trocars 2 and 3. The anesthesiologist then advances the orogastric tube through the mouth until the first black line on the tube reaches the patient's front teeth. At this point the tube should be in the distal esophagus, and then can be slowly advanced until it enters the pouch. Under direct visualization, the tip of the orogastric tube is positioned against the staple line of the gastric pouch and held in place by both atraumatic graspers.

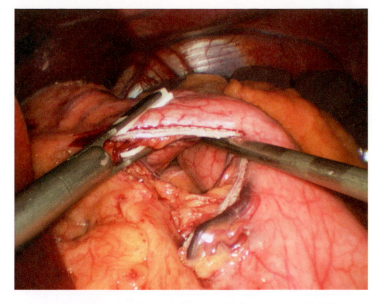

FIGURE 6-9 The palpation probe is used to even out the posterior wall of the stomach in preparation for linear stapler placement.

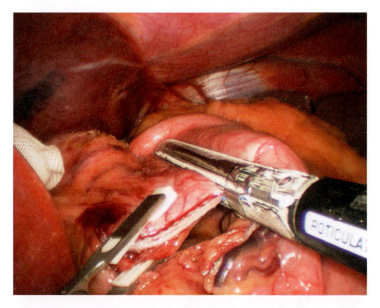

FIGURE 6-10 Vertical transection of the stomach with the stapler aiming at the angle of His.

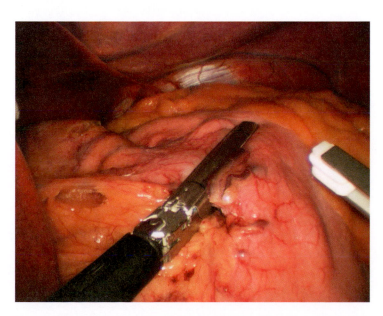

FIGURE 6-8 Horizontal transection of the stomach using a blue 3.5-mm staple load.

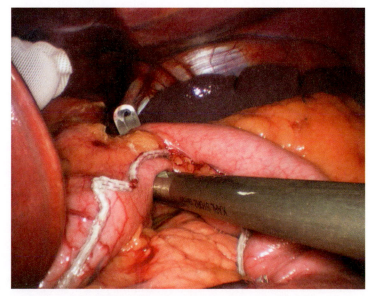

FIGURE 6-11 The esophageal retractor is deflected above the angle of His, lateral to the left bundle of the right crus of the diaphragm.

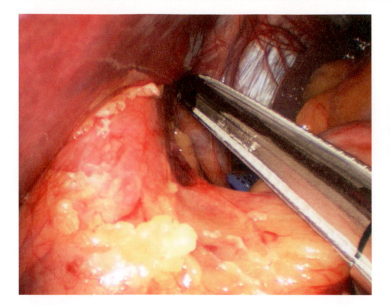

FIGURE 6-12 Positioning the final stapler; note the blue cartridge visible at the angle of His.

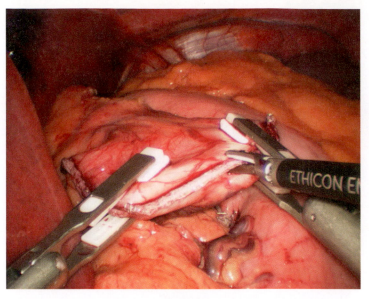

FIGURE 6-14 A small gastrotomy is performed on the gastric pouch using the Harmonic ACE scalpel to allow passage of the orogastric tube.

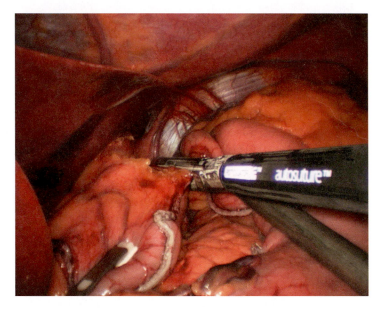

FIGURE 6-13 Final vertical stapler placed, completing pouch formation and separation of gastric remnant.

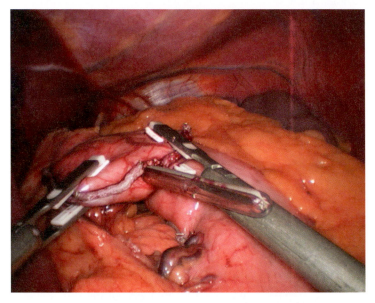

FIGURE 6-15 Orogastric tube passed into the abdomen.

If there are posterior vessels identified on the pouch, then the pouch will need to be rotated clockwise so that the anvil can be positioned to avoid these vessels. The ultrasonic scalpel is used to make a small gastrotomy (Fig. 6-14), allowing a snug exit of the orogastric tube, which then is pulled out of the gastric pouch (Fig. 6-15). Care is taken by the anesthesiologist to orient the smooth part of the anvil toward the hard palate of the patient.

Once the anvil is in position, the assistant surgeon pulls the orogastric tube out of the abdomen (through trocar 3), thereby pulling the anvil through the esophagus and into the pouch. Minimal force should be used to pull the anvil through the esophagus. The monofilament suture then is cut and the anvil is separated from the orogastric tube (Fig. 6-16). The orogastric tube then can be discarded, leaving the anvil in the gastric pouch. While stabilizing the post of the anvil with a Babcock grasper placed through trocar 2, a second grasper placed through trocar 1 deflects the platform of the anvil (within the pouch) back to its original position, perpendicular to the post (Fig. 6-17). Recently, Autosuture released a prefabricated anvil attached to an orogastric

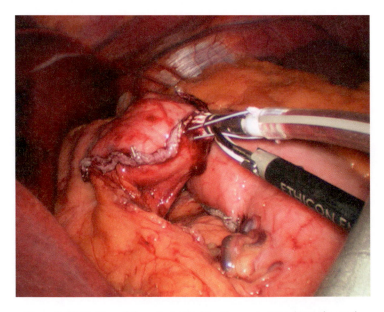

FIGURE 6-16 Division of the suture attaching the orogastric tube to the anvil.

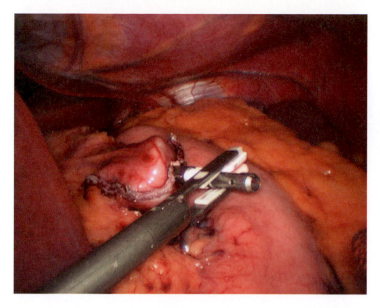

Figure 6-17 A grasper is used to deflect the platform of the anvil in the pouch.

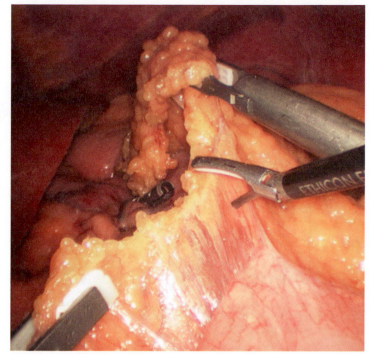

Figure 6-18 Division of the greater omentum.

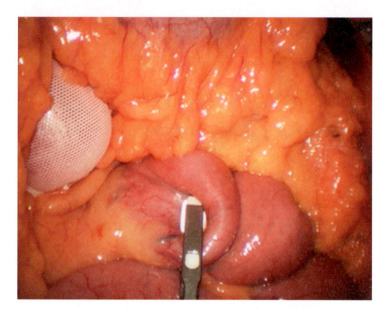

Figure 6-19 Identification of the ligament of Treitz.

tube (OrVil, U.S. Surgical), which eliminates the need for the surgeon to fashion the anvil-orogastric tube conduit. When using the newly designed OrVil, the orogastric tube should be advanced into the esophagus until the third black line reaches the front teeth. Positioning of the anvil into the pouch then may continue as described above. Once the orogastric tube is pulled through into the pouch, the suture can be cut, and the orogastric tube is disconnected from the anvil.

Alternatives to Anvil Placement

As an alternative to the transoral staple placement, a gastrotomy can be created prior to pouch formation, and the anvil can be introduced into the pouch. Most frequently, the post of the anvil is passed into position through the pouch, and then after placement of the anvil, sizing and stapling of the pouch can be performed. Another alternative is to create a linear stapled gastrojejunostomy. After formation of the small gastric pouch, the Roux limb is brought up to the pouch. Both ante-colic/ante-gastric (AC-AG) and retro-colic/retro-gastric (RC-RG) techniques have been described. After securing the two pieces of bowel together using absorbable suture, an enterotomy is made in the small bowel and a gastrotomy is made in the pouch. A linear stapler then can be introduced and fired to create the anastomosis. Once the stapler is removed, the remaining defect can be closed with sutures in one or two layers.

Division of Omentum

Division of the greater omentum frequently is necessary in the AC-AG technique. Using an atraumatic grasper through trocar 3, the left side of the omentum is grasped and retracted cephalad. Using graspers through trocars 2 and 3, and the ultrasonic scalpel (through trocar 1), the omentum is divided to the level of the transverse colon (Fig. 6-18). Care must be taken to avoid injuring the gastric remnant which lies below the divided omentum. After the omental division, the post of the anvil is centered on the divided omentum. The balloon retractor is then repositioned and utilized to retract the transverse colon cephalad, thus exposing the root of the small bowel mesentery and facilitating the identification of the ligament of Treitz (Fig. 6-19).

Creation of the Biliopancreatic Limb

After identification of the ligament of Treitz, atraumatic graspers (trocars 2 and 6) are utilized to measure the appropriate length for the biliopancreatic limb (BPL). A 3-0 permanent (silk) suture is placed 50 to 60 cm distal to the ligament of Treitz. The jejunum then is divided with a linear stapler (placed through trocar 6) just distal to the silk suture, using a white 45-mm × 2.5-mm staple load (Fig. 6-20). The small bowel mesentery is next fanned open using graspers positioned through trocars 2 and 3, and the mesentery is transected using a gray 45-mm × 2.0-mm staple load through the umbilical port (Fig. 6-21). An alternative method of mesenteric hemostasis utilizes SeamGuard, a bioabsorbable staple line reinforcement product (W.L. Gore & Associates, Flagstaff, AZ), which is loaded onto a white 45-mm × 2.5-mm staple load prior to firing. Once in position, this buttress material can be used to

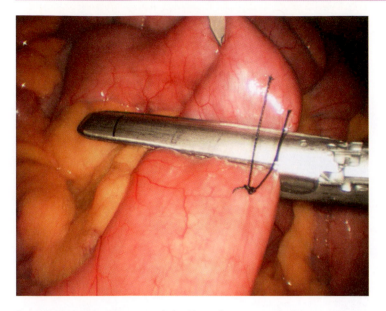

FIGURE 6-20 A white 2.5-mm staple load is used to transect the jejunum 50 cm distal to the ligament of Treitz. Note the permanent suture marking the distal end of the biliopancreatic limb.

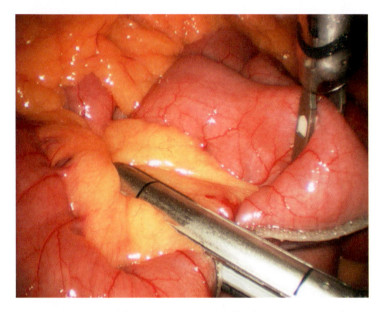

FIGURE 6-21 Division of the mesentery, completed with a gray 2-mm staple load.

position the small bowel without damaging the mesentery. There are other techniques for mesenteric division, including the use of ultrasonic or bipolar shears. We prefer the stapled technique because we believe that it provides more consistent hemostasis. The small bowel then can be measured with graspers through trocars 2 and 6 in order to create a Roux limb measuring 150 cm distal to the jejunal staple line.

Triple-Stapling Technique for the Jejunojejunostomy

The creation of a traditional side-to-side jejunojejunostomy can be complicated by stricture formation. Because of frequent complications at this anastomosis, we devised an alternative triple-stapling technique (Frantzides-Madan triple-stapling technique), which can decrease the risk for stricture/obstruction at the jejunojejunostomy. After measuring an appropriate length for the Roux limb, the BPL and the distal end of the Roux limb are positioned parallel to each other, with the antimesenteric walls opposed. A small enterotomy is created on the antimesenteric border of the distal Roux limb (Fig. 6-22) with the ultrasonic scalpel. Another

enterotomy is created on the antimesenteric border of the biliopancreatic limb about 5 cm from the silk suture (Fig. 6-23). The bowel is positioned so that the enterotomies are adjacent. Using a Babcock grasper through trocar 2, the bowel is stabilized so that the linear stapler can be introduced (Fig. 6-24). The Roux limb and BPL are joined together with a white 45-mm × 2.5-mm staple load through trocar 6 (Fig. 6-25). The stapler is removed (Fig. 6-26) and the anastomosis, instrumentation, and camera are rotated in a counterclockwise position and elevated to the upper abdomen, just to the left of the falciform ligament. This permits the assistant surgeon to introduce the linear stapler through trocar 3 and fire another white 45-mm × 2.5-mm staple load in the opposite direction from the first. This completes two of the three firings of the triple-stapling technique (Fig. 6-27).

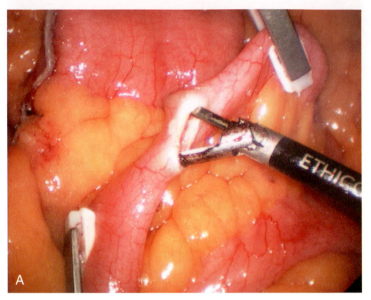

A

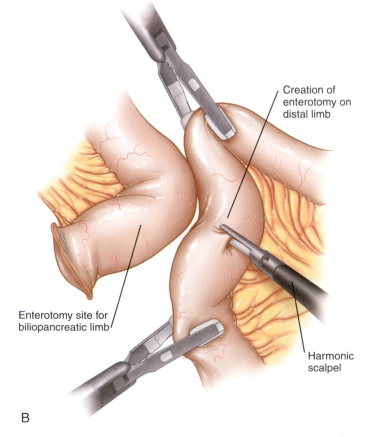

B

FIGURE 6-22 The Harmonic ACE scalpel is used to create an enterotomy on the antimesenteric border of the distal Roux limb. A, Surgical site. B, Schematic representation.

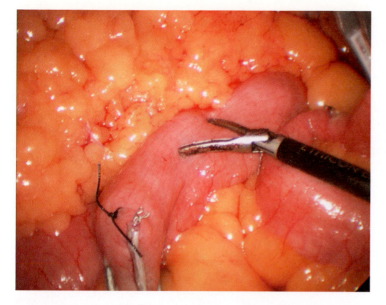

FIGURE 6-23 The enterotomy on the biliopancreatic limb is created three jaw widths proximal to the silk suture.

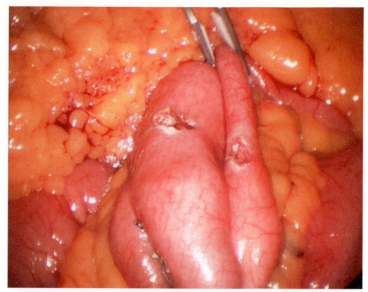

FIGURE 6-24 A Babcock grasper is used to stabilize and align the two loops of bowel in a parallel orientation.

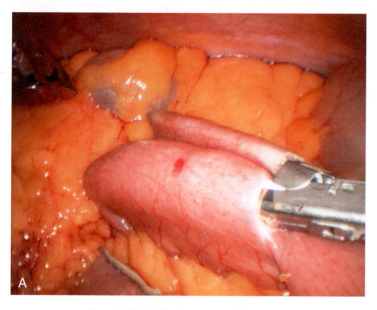

A

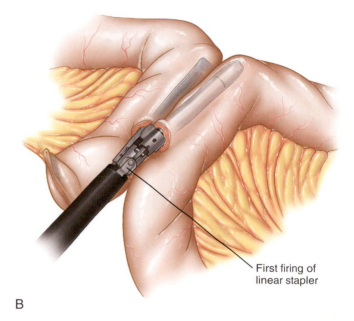

B

First firing of linear stapler

FIGURE 6-25 A white 2.5-mm staple load is used to join together the two loops of bowel. **A,** Surgical site. **B,** Schematic representation.

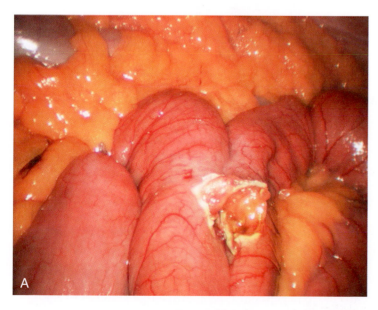

A

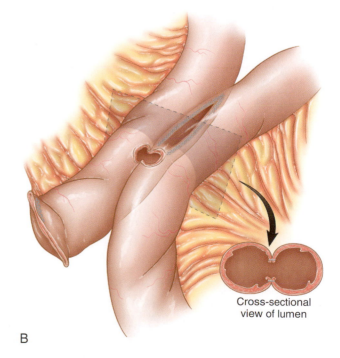

B

Cross-sectional view of lumen

FIGURE 6-26 Defect created after stapler removal. **A,** Surgical site. **B,** Schematic representation.

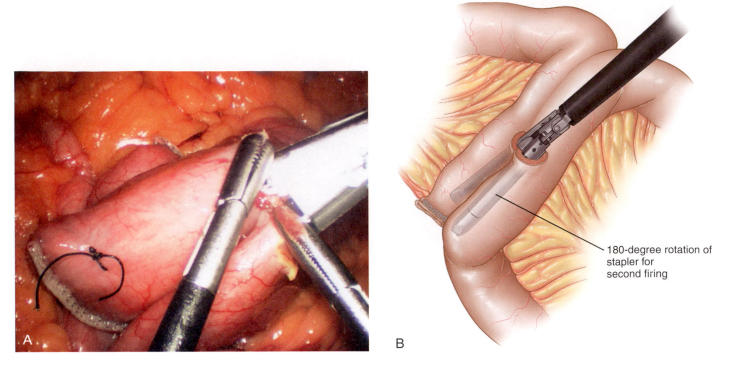

FIGURE 6-27 Second 2.5-mm white staple load is used to create the opposing staple line for the triple-stapling technique. **A,** Surgical site. **B,** Schematic representation.

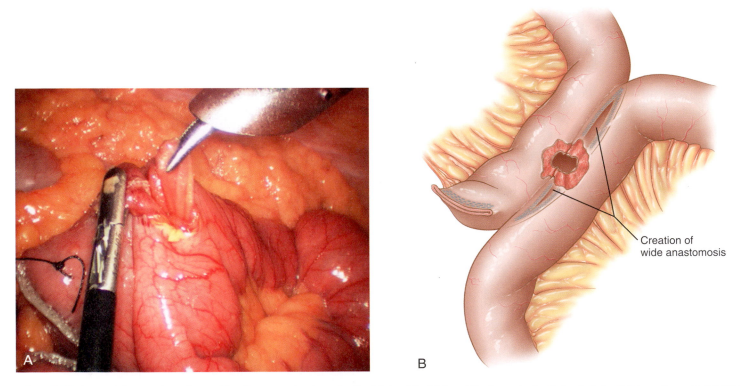

FIGURE 6-28 A curved dissector is used to position the open enterotomy for the third and final firing of the linear stapler. **A,** Surgical site. **B,** Schematic representation.

The opening of the anastomosis is evaluated for hemostasis, and the posterior wall of the anastomosis is inspected to ensure patency. A curved dissector through trocar 3 is used to position the open enterotomy for the third firing of the linear stapler (Fig. 6-28). One or two white 45-mm × 2.5-mm staple loads are fired in a perpendicular fashion to complete the jejunojejunostomy (Figs. 6-29 and 6-30). Metallic clips may be placed on the remnant of the silk suture marking the end of the BPL; these clips can be used to identify the jejunojejunostomy during postoperative contrast studies. In addition, internal herniation of small bowel through the mesenteric defect of the jejunojejunostomy after LRYGB has been described. It therefore is advisable to close this defect by placing interrupted sutures (Fig. 6-31).

Gastrojejunostomy

The Roux limb is brought up toward the gastric pouch in an antecolic fashion between the previously created defect in the greater omentum, carefully avoiding rotation of the bowel and its mesentery. The jejunal staple line is opened with the ultrasonic scalpel. Trocar 3 is removed, and the skin and fascial incision is enlarged to accommodate the EEA stapler, which is introduced into the abdomen and then into the open jejunum. The EEA

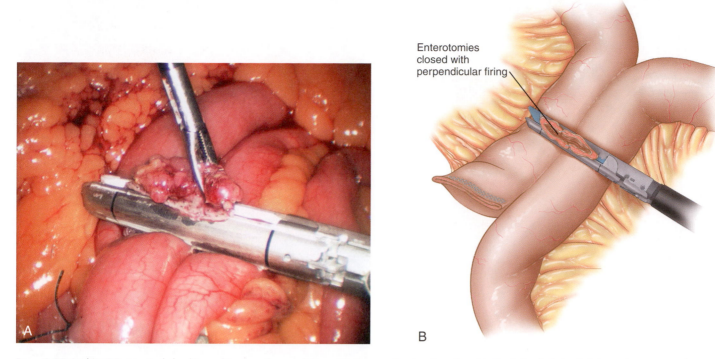

FIGURE 6-29 A white 2.5-mm staple load is used to close the remaining enterotomy and restore bowel continuity. **A,** Surgical site. **B,** Schematic representation.

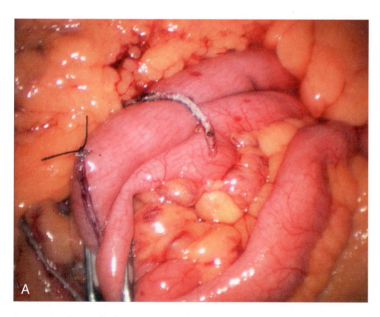 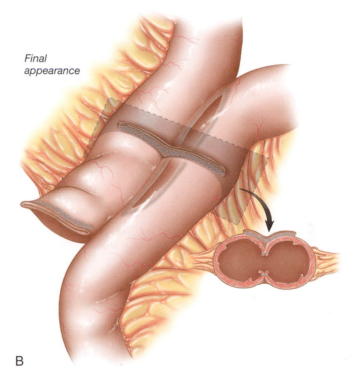

FIGURE 6-30 Perpendicular orientation of staple lines, and completed jejunojejunostomy utilizing the Frantzides-Madan triple-stapling technique. **A,** Surgical site. **B,** Schematic representation.

stapler is advanced into the jejunum (Fig. 6-32) until the head of the stapler is proximal to the divided mesentery. The post is then advanced through the antimesenteric side of the jejunum. The stapler head is joined to the anvil (Fig. 6-33), the two pieces of bowel are opposed, and the stapler is fired. It is important to make sure that there is no omentum trapped between the gastric pouch and jejunum, and that the pouch is not misaligned prior to firing. The stapler subsequently is removed and inspected for two complete "donut" rings. The plastic camera drape then is everted to cover the end of the EEA stapler prior to its removal from the abdomen (Fig. 6-34). The open-ended jejunum is closed using a white 60-mm × 2.5-mm staple load from trocar 6. The amputated

piece of jejunum then can be placed into an Endocatch device for removal. Having restored bowel continuity, multiple interrupted sutures of 3-0 absorbable or nonabsorbable suture are placed laterally, posterolaterally, and anteriorly in order to circumferentially reinforce the anastomosis.

Evaluation of the Anastomosis

A reliable method for evaluating the gastrojejunal anastomosis is to instill air and methylene blue (Fig. 6-35). An 18-F orogastric tube is positioned into the pouch. The Roux limb is occluded with an atraumatic grasper, and 40 to 60 mL of saline is instilled through the orogastric tube. The anastomosis is irrigated in this

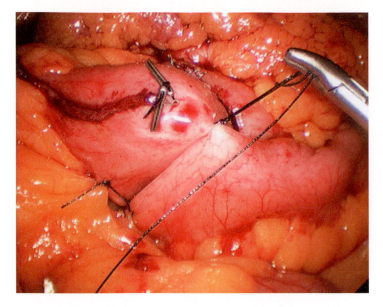

FIGURE 6-31 Closure of mesenteric defect. Two clips are placed for radiologic identification of the jejunojejunostomy.

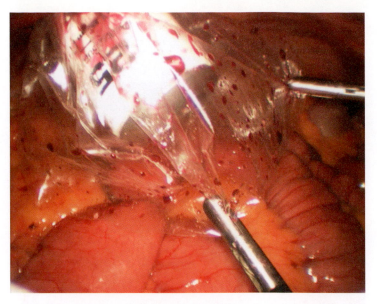

FIGURE 6-34 Everted camera drape, used to protect the anterior abdominal wall from contamination during removal of the EEA stapler.

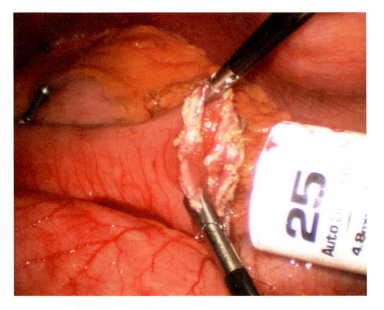

FIGURE 6-32 Introduction of 25-mm Autosuture EEA stapler into open end of jejunum.

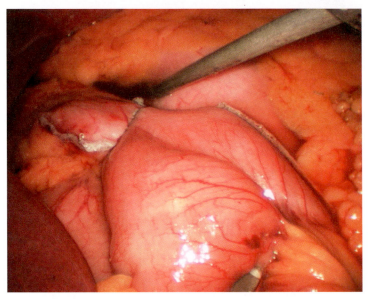

FIGURE 6-35 Completed gastrojejunal anastomosis.

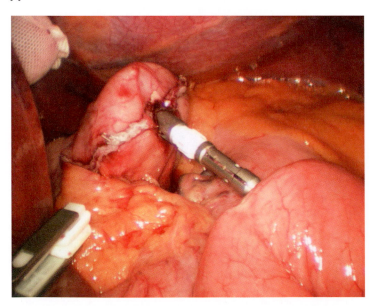

FIGURE 6-33 The post of the anvil is connected to the EEA stapler.

way until all clots are evacuated and the effluent is clear. The upper abdomen is flooded with irrigation to submerge the pouch. Air (40 mL) is insufflated into the pouch via the orogastric tube. If bubbling is noted, then interrupted reinforcement sutures should be placed to stop the air leak. Finally, 1 mL of methylene blue is added to 100 mL of saline, and 40 mL of this mixture is instilled into the pouch. There should be no evidence of dye extravasation. The stapled end of the Roux limb also should be evaluated during these maneuvers. The anastomosis also may be evaluated by endoscopy. The gastroscope is passed transorally into the pouch, where both the lateral gastric and the gastrojejunal staple line can be evaluated for hemostasis, patency, and leak. The anastomosis can be insufflated while the pouch is submerged under irrigation.

Prior to evacuation of the pneumoperitoneum, a laparoscopic fascial closure device is used to close the trocar sites with transfascial sutures of heavyweight absorbable braided suture. The pneumoperitoneum then may be evacuated and the skin incisions closed using an absorbable suture for a running subcuticular closure. Routine drainage of the abdomen is not necessary.

POSTOPERATIVE CARE

Routine telemetry monitoring and intensive care typically are not necessary. Early ambulation and mobilization are important for VTE prophylaxis. Disposition to a surgical floor is appropriate after meeting appropriate postanesthesia care unit (PACU) discharge criteria. If the patient has a diagnosis of obstructive sleep apnea (OSA) and utilizes a continuous positive airway pressure/bilevel positive airway pressure (CPAP/BiPAP) machine, a "step-down" unit (or surgical floor capable of monitoring cardiac telemetry and continuous pulse oximetry) should be utilized.

The patient should be instructed to ambulate with assistance on the evening of surgery. Incentive spirometry and routine respiratory aerosols also are beneficial. VTE prophylaxis should be continued after surgery (unless contraindicated). In addition to utilization of size-appropriate lower extremity intermittent pneumatic compression garments, subcutaneous unfractionated or low-molecular-weight heparin is recommended. Intraoperative or postoperative hemorrhage is a relative contraindication to anticoagulation therapy (refer to Chapter 10 for more discussion of VTE).

On the morning of postoperative day 1, a Gastrografin UGI swallow (Bracco Diagnostics, Princeton, NJ) may be performed in order to evaluate the esophagus, gastrojejunal anastomosis, Roux limb, and jejunojejunostomy. Gastrografin is administered (20 to 30 mL at a time) with the patient standing. There should be prompt emptying of the esophagus into the gastric pouch, and then into the Roux limb of the jejunum. Because the Gastrografin dilutes as it progresses distally, it may be difficult to identify extravasation of the contrast material at the jejunojejunostomy; however, contrast material passing distal to the marking clips should be apparent.

After the UGI swallow the morning after surgery, the Foley catheter may be removed and a gastric bypass clear liquid diet initiated. The latter diet includes fat-free and sugar-free chicken broth, gelatin, popsicles, and juices. Pain control is obtained with oral Darvocet or oral Vicodin, as well as scheduled IV ketorolac. It is recommended that the patient ambulate at least three times per day and continue incentive spirometry on an hourly basis. On the afternoon of postoperative day 2, the patient may be discharged home if hemodynamic parameters are normal, pain is well controlled, and there has been no dysphagia, nausea, or vomiting. Resolution of postoperative ileus is not necessary prior to discharge. The gastric bypass clear diet is continued until the first postoperative visit. At that time the diet is advanced to a diet of pureed and soft foods.

Patients are expected to follow-up in the office at 1 week and at 1, 3, 6, and 12 months after surgery, and thereafter every year. Nutritional counseling and screening laboratory work are important. Recommended postoperative vitamin supplementation includes a multivitamin fortified with iron (twice daily), calcium (1000 mg daily), vitamin D (800 IU daily), and vitamin B_{12} (1500 µg once per week, *sublingual* form). Protein supplementation (65–75 g/day) also is necessary. Immediately after surgery, extra protein will need to come in the form of "shake" supplements, but as the diet is advanced, more protein can come from meat and cheese.

Patients generally are hospitalized for a longer period of time after open surgery and, as such, many postoperative complications are identified during the hospitalization. As a result of the short length of stay after LRYGB, a variety of postoperative complications may occur after hospital discharge. It is important to educate the patient and the family regarding the signs and symptoms of postoperative complications including tachycardia, fevers, increasing abdominal pain, and persistent nausea or vomiting. Written instructions should be provided to the patient and the family instructing them to alert the surgeon or office staff should the patient's condition change or deteriorate.

PROCEDURE-SPECIFIC COMPLICATIONS

The most devastating postoperative complication is an anastomotic leak. Fever, sustained tachycardia, and low urine output are hallmarks of a leak at the anastomosis. These signs should be promptly evaluated with either a water-soluble UGI contrast study or a computed tomography (CT) scan. If symptoms persist despite a negative work-up, then a diagnostic laparoscopy or exploratory laparotomy may be considered. Leaks most frequently are identified 5 to 7 days after surgery. As the average length of stay following LRYGB diminishes, many different members of the bariatric team are asked to triage patients over the telephone. The office staff and allied health personnel that communicate with these patients should be educated regarding the signs and symptoms of the common postoperative complications.

The pouch, once created, should be handled gently with atraumatic graspers. The gastrotomy created for the anvil post should be as small as possible in order to prevent gaps after the EEA stapler is fired. The integrity of the donut rings should be evaluated, and if incomplete rings are identified, the anastomosis should be reinforced as described. Undue tension on the anastomosis can also lead to leaks. The mesentery of the small bowel should be divided sufficiently so as to prevent unnecessary tension when the Roux limb is brought cephalad to the gastric pouch. Care must also be taken to prevent rotation of the mesentery or the bowel of either the BPL or Roux limb.

Pulmonary embolism is one of the most common causes of death within 30 days (0.9%). In addition to routine VTE prophylaxis, temporary retrievable inferior vena cava (IVC) filters should be considered for high-risk patients with a personal or strong family history of pulmonary embolism. Patient positioning is very important in reducing lower extremity DVT. Historically this procedure has been performed in a modified lithotomy position with the knees flexed. This position may contribute to DVT formation in the popliteal fossa and lower extremities. The described technique, with the patient supine, may be less prone to lower extremity venous stasis, which may be a precursor to DVT formation.

Postoperative bleeding may occur in 4% to 6% of patients. Supportive care is important if there is evidence of anastomotic bleeding (rectal bleeding or vomiting blood after surgery). VTE prophylaxis and ketorolac should be discontinued. Blood transfusions will likely be necessary until the bleeding stops. Infrequently, upper endoscopy or reoperative surgical intervention will be necessary in order to stop the hemorrhage.

The gastrojejunostomy may be created with either a 21-mm or a 25-mm EEA stapler. An anastomosis created using the 21-mm EEA stapler has been associated with a higher rate of stricture; therefore, we prefer the 25-mm EEA stapler. If the transoral anvil technique is favored by the surgeon, then the Autosuture 25-mm EEA stapler allows the surgeon to deflect the platform of the anvil. This may be less traumatic to the esophagus during transoral anvil placement and result in fewer oral/esophageal complications.

Frequent vomiting at 4 to 6 weeks postoperatively should be evaluated with an UGI contrast study or UGI endoscopy, because an anastomotic stricture may occur 3% to 5% of the time. Balloon dilation can be performed safely as an outpatient procedure; two to three dilations typically are necessary to treat the stricture. After endoscopic dilation, the patient should take a sucralfate (Carafate) slurry every 8 hours and a proton pump inhibitor twice daily. This should be continued during the period of endoscopic dilations and for 6 weeks following the last treatment. The use of permanent sutures to reinforce the anastomosis, the use of a 21-mm EEA stapler, and untreated *Helicobacter pylori* infections have all been shown to increase stricture rates. Preoperative endoscopy with testing for *H. pylori* should be considered, because infection increases the stricture rate by nearly 30%.

Trocar site hernia has been described for 12-mm trocars, so it is advisable to close all such fascial defects at the conclusion of the procedure. There are many commercially available products to facilitate placement of transfascial sutures using a heavyweight braided absorbable suture. Should a Richter's hernia develop at a previous trocar site, the outcome may be devastating and difficult to diagnose in a patient with morbid obesity.

Both internal herniation and small bowel obstruction have been documented after gastric bypass. During the creation of a retrocolic Roux limb, it is possible for the small bowel to herniate through the defect of the transverse mesocolon. It is advisable to secure the jejunum to the mesocolon in order to prevent this complication. Similarly, hernias may develop at the mesenteric defect created after the jejunojejunostomy. Closing this defect may prevent postoperative internal hernia formation. Weight loss and reduction of intra-abdominal adipose tissue may cause this defect to enlarge over time and increase the likelihood of a small bowel obstruction. The third common site of internal obstruction is small bowel herniation posterior to the Roux limb. Patients often present years after surgery with waxing and waning abdominal pain and symptoms of intermittent small bowel obstruction. A CT scan may identify a classic "swirling" pattern of the small bowel and mesentery posterior to the Roux limb. If symptoms persist despite a negative CT, then diagnostic laparoscopy (or open laparotomy) may be required for diagnosis.

Wound-related complications of ORYGB occur as frequently as 50% of the time. Many open wounds require frequent packing and debridement and have a direct correlation with the development of incisional hernia. Wound-related issues after LRYGB are less common and have a lower morbidity rate. We believe that eversion of the camera drape over the contaminated stapler head has decreased postoperative wound infections at the third trocar position.

RESULTS AND OUTCOME

Mortality rate after LRYGB is in the range of 1%. This risk is increased for patients over age 65 and for patients with super-morbid obesity (greater than 50 kg/m^2). Complications and deaths occur less frequently at high-volume centers (more than 100 cases per year). The leak rate after LRYGB at high-volume centers is less than 0.15% (national published range is 1–3%). Other complications that have been documented after LRYGB include bowel obstruction (1.73%), gastrointestinal tract or anastomotic hemorrhage (1.93%), pulmonary embolus (0.41%), incisional hernia (0.47%), and anastomotic stricture (4.73%). These are all reasonable risks to assume, considering the lifetime risk of morbid obesity.

Laparoscopic gastric bypass can allow patients to lose 60% to 80% of their excess body weight. Numerous reports have documented the safety of the procedure, as well as the excellent resolution of medical comorbid conditions. A recent meta-analysis showed 86% of gastric bypass patients also had significant improvement or complete resolution of type II diabetes mellitus. Many patients with type II diabetes mellitus have demonstrated little or no need for antihyperglycemic medication after gastric bypass surgery.

There also has been dramatic resolution of hypertension after gastric bypass. A meta-analysis showed that hypertension is resolved or improved in 78.5% of patients. Another study of 500 patients who had successful gastric bypass concluded that there was a 92% resolution of hypertension. Similarly, 85.7% of those suffering from OSA had resolution of the disease and were able to discontinue CPAP therapy after successful gastric bypass surgery. Hyperlipidemia and hypercholesterolemia were improved in more than 93% of patients. Complete resolution of gastroesophageal reflux disease also has been documented in 98% of patients in one series.

Laparoscopic gastric bypass is a technically demanding procedure that requires appropriate training and instrumentation. While the field of bariatric surgery may be demanding on many fronts, it can be very satisfying to treat morbid obesity and its related comorbidities.

Suggested Reading

Abdel-Galil E, Sabry AA: Laparoscopic Roux-en-Y gastric bypass—Evaluation of three different techniques. Obes Surg 2002;12(5):639–642.

Brolin RE, LaMarca LB, Kenler HA, Cody RP: Malabsorptive gastric bypass in patients with superobesity. J Gastrointest Surg 2002;6(2):195–203.

Cho M, Carrodeguas L, Pinto D, et al: Diagnosis and management of partial small bowel obstruction after laparoscopic antecolic antegastric Roux-en-Y gastric bypass for morbid obesity. J Am Coll Surg 2006;202(2):262–268.

Fernandez AZ, Jr, DeMaria EJ, Tichansky DS, et al: Experience with over 3,000 open and laparoscopic bariatric procedures: Multivariate analysis of factors related to leak and resultant mortality. Surg Endosc 2004;18(2):193–197.

Frantzides CT, Carlson MA, Moore RE, et al: Effect of body mass index on nonalcoholic fatty liver disease in patients undergoing minimally invasive bariatric surgery. J Soc Laparoendosc Surg 2004;8(7):849–855.

Frantzides CT, Zeni TM, Madan AK, et al: Laparoscopic Roux-en-Y gastric bypass utilizing the triple stapling technique. J Soc Laparoendosc Surg 2006;10(2):176–179.

Higa KD, Boone KB, Ho T, Davies OG: Laparoscopic Roux-en-Y gastric bypass for morbid obesity: Technique and preliminary results of our first 400 patients. Arch Surg 2000;135(9):1029–1033.

Madan AK, Frantzides CT: Triple-stapling technique for jejunojejunostomy in laparoscopic gastric bypass. Arch Surg 2003;138(9):1029–1032.

National Institutes of Health Conference: Gastrointestinal surgery for severe obesity. Consensus Development Conference Panel. Ann Intern Med 1991;115:956–961.

Nguyen NT, Goldman C, Rosenquist CJ, et al: Laparoscopic versus open gastric bypass: A randomized study of outcomes, quality of life, and costs. Ann Surg 2001;234(3):279–289.

Podnos YD, Jimenez JC, Wilson SE, et al: Complications after laparoscopic gastric bypass: A review of 3464 cases. Arch Surg 2003;138(9):957–961.

Pories WJ, Swanson MS, MacDonald KG, et al: Who would have thought it? An operation proves to be the most effective therapy for adult-onset diabetes mellitus. Ann Surg 1995;222(3):339–350.

Schauer PR, Ikramuddin S, Gourash W, et al: Outcomes after laparoscopic Roux-en-Y gastric bypass for morbid obesity. Ann Surg 2000;232(4):515–529.

Scopinaro N, Adami GF, Marinari GM, et al: Biliopancreatic diversion. World J Surg 1998;22(9):936–946.

Sjostrom L, Lindroos A, Peltonen M, et al: Lifestyle, diabetes, and cardiovascular risk factors 10 years after bariatric surgery: N Engl J Med 2004;351:26.

Wittgrove AC, Clark GW: Laparoscopic gastric bypass, Roux-en-Y 500 patients: Technique and results, with 3–60 months follow-up. Obes Surg 2000;10(3):233–239.

Zeni TM, Frantzides CT, Mahr C, et al: Value of preoperative upper endoscopy in patients undergoing laparoscopic gastric bypass. Obes Surg 2006;16(2):142–146.

ATUL K. MADAN, JOHN G. ZOGRAFAKIS, AND
CONSTANTINE T. FRANTZIDES

Laparoscopic Adjustable Gastric Banding

Obesity has been increasing at a remarkable rate and has become a world-wide epidemic. The effects of obesity on the both the individual and the health care system are severe and dramatic. While medical treatment has had limited success, minimally invasive bariatric surgery has been demonstrated to be a successful long-term treatment for weight loss in the morbidly obese. Specifically, adjustable gastric banding has developed into a safe and reliable restrictive weight-loss procedure. Approval by the Food and Drug Administration (FDA) was obtained for the Lap-Band (Inamed Health, Santa Barbara, CA) in June 2001. Human trials have been performed in the United States since 1998. Early results were unsatisfactory secondary to band erosion and slippage. Since the transition from the perigastric technique to the pars flaccida approach for band placement, however, complication rates have decreased substantially (see "Suggested Reading"). The Lap-Band (or laparoscopic adjustable gastric band [LAGB]) is a 13-mm wide band (silicon elastomer) that is placed approximately 3 cm caudal to the gastroesophageal junction. An alternative system used in Europe is the Swedish adjustable gastric band (SAGB), which also is composed of a silicon elastomer. The SAGB allows for greater adjustability in the internal circumference. Approval of the SAGB by the FDA currently is pending.

OPERATIVE INDICATIONS

The National Institutes of Health (NIH) guidelines for bariatric surgery are used for placement of the LAGB. To meet operative criteria, patients should have a body mass index (BMI) greater than 40kg/m^2, or a BMI of 35 to 39.9kg/m^2 with an obesity-related comorbid condition (e.g., hypertension, diabetes, or obstructive sleep apnea). Some surgeons feel that the lower threshold for BMI should be decreased even further, possibly as low as 30kg/m^2. This would allow patients to intervene early and prevent weight-related comorbid conditions before they develop. Furthermore, because of the safety, ease of insertion, and potential reversibility, LAGB is being considered as a safe alternative for the adolescent population. Reports of its use in teenagers afflicted with morbid obesity are increasing. Currently, however, LAGB is not FDA approved for placement in patients younger than 18 years.

LAGB is a restrictive procedure that is efficacious in the appropriately selected patient. There are other options for bariatric surgery, including combined restrictive/malabsorptive procedures such as Roux-en-Y gastric bypass and biliopancreatic diversion

with or without duodenal switch. Both of these procedures can be performed laparoscopically (LRYGB and LBPD), but there is debate regarding the operative indications. To date, no randomized prospective trial has been performed comparing LRYGB or LBPD versus LAGB. Data from uncontrolled studies suggest that LRYGB and LBPD have higher perioperative morbidity and mortality rates than LAGB and that LAGB results in less short-term weight loss that LRYGB and LBPD. While long-term data are pending, it seems that LAGB is associated with less long-term weight loss than LRYGB, but the difference may be as little as 10% excess body weight. Many would agree that it is the patient and not the procedure that will ultimately determine long-term weight loss. A multidisciplinary team approach to weight loss is necessary for long-term success. Lifelong dietary and behavioral modifications, a structured exercise program, and nutritional and psychological counseling are essential to the outcome of a patient considering weight-loss surgery.

Some surgeons reserve LAGB for patients with multiple previous abdominal surgeries, advanced or young age, multiple medical comorbid conditions, strong preference, or inflammatory bowel disease. The LAGB, however, is not currently FDA-approved in patients with inflammatory bowel disease. Other surgeons recommend the LAGB as first-line surgical therapy for morbid obesity. Ideally, a prospective randomized trial comparing LAGB and LRYGB should be performed to address some of these issues.

PREOPERATIVE EVALUATION, TESTING, AND PREPARATION

Preoperative evaluation should include documentation of nonsurgical weight-loss attempts, along with evidence of psychological evaluation and dietary counseling. A variety of nonsurgical weight-loss options exist, but none have been shown to be successful over the long-term. The backbone of any medical weight loss program should include caloric restriction, protein supplementation, a structured exercise program, education and support from a dietitian, and psychological counseling. Counseling does not need to be provided by a psychologist or psychiatrist; however, it is important to identify and treat patients suffering from binge eating, overeating, or an undiagnosed major depressive disorder. Many insurance companies have utilized the NIH criteria of documented weight-loss attempts to delay or deny approval for potential bariatric surgery patients. Unfortunately, this practice sets standards for weight loss that are not based on scientific data and, in fact, may have detrimental effects on patients. These insurance restrictions often are the most difficult aspect of preoperative patient preparation.

Many surgeons disseminate a LAGB preoperative education book and written LAGB dietary guidelines. Some surgeons prefer to teach preoperative patient education classes themselves, and others prefer to have a bariatric dietitian complete the instruction. Education should continue during clinic follow-up and during adjustments. The patients should understand that bariatric surgery is not a "magic pill" and that they have to change not just what they eat but how they eat. The patient should continue to be informed of the importance of adjustments which provide restriction in food consumption along with the feeling of satiety.

Preoperative testing will depend on the patient's overall health condition and surgeon preference. Because morbid obesity commonly causes many cardiac and pulmonary ailments, preoperative testing may include a cardiac stress test, echocardiogram, pulmonary function tests, and arterial blood gas analysis. Sleep apnea also is common in morbid obesity, so all patients should be screened either via history or via a formal sleep study. Performance of routine esophageal manometry is controversial. Some type of evaluation of the upper gastrointestinal tract is helpful, however, in order to diagnose mucosal abnormalities of the esophagus and stomach and hiatal hernia. Failure to recognize and repair a hiatal hernia at the time of surgery may cause an enlarged pouch and postoperative gastroesophageal reflux. Evaluation of the esophagus and stomach should be undertaken either by upper gastrointestinal endoscopy or by a barium contrast study; each has its advantages.

After the patient has completed medical risk stratification and obtained appropriate insurance preauthorization, preoperative dietary preparation may begin. A high protein liquid diet for 2 weeks prior to surgery has been shown to decrease intra-abdominal adipose tissue and shrink the left lobe of the liver. These short-term weight loss benefits will facilitate laparoscopic exposure of the stomach and safe band placement. Venous thromboembolism (VTE) prophylaxis and a first-generation cephalosporin are given to the patient. A single dose of intravenous antibiotics administered prior to surgery is sufficient.

PATIENT POSITIONING

The LAGB procedure can be performed with the patient supine or in split-leg lithotomy. Regardless of the position, sequential compression devices should be utilized because morbid obesity is an independent risk factor for VTE (see discussion in Chapter 10). In the split-leg lithotomy position, the surgeon stands between the patient's legs. The operating table must have an adequate weight capacity and dimensions. If the lithotomy position is utilized, then properly sized stirrups or split-leg extensions are needed. Placing the patient in the reverse Trendelenberg position will help expose the gastroesophageal junction; therefore, the patient should be well secured to the operating table. Options include bean bags and extremity straps. Depending on the table and the size of the patient, the surgeon and the assistants may need to use standing stools.

INSTRUMENTATION

Commonly employed instruments for this procedure include bariatric-length Debakey forceps (both locking and nonlocking),

a padded atraumatic grasper (Atraugrip, Specialty Surgical Instrumentation, Nashville, TN), hook electrocautery, a Lap-Band tightener, and a fine curved dissector. Occasionally, 5-mm Babcock forceps and ultrasonic shears are necessary. Most surgeons prefer to place a 10-cm Lap-Band; occasionally, however, a larger VG band may be needed for patients with severe central obesity or thicker gastric walls. Prior to initiating the procedure, the integrity of the tubing and the balloon are checked, the tubing and band are primed with saline, and any air in the system should be purged.

TROCAR PLACEMENT

Five trocars are utilized (Fig. 7-1). Prior to placing the trocars, each site is infiltrated with local anesthetic. Access to the abdominal cavity is gained using a 12-mm trocar with an optical obturator placed in the left upper quadrant below the costal margin at the lateral edge of the rectus sheath. This technique allows the surgeon to view the layers of the abdominal wall during initial trocar placement. This trocar site (1) will also serve as the band insertion and port placement site. The current gastric band does not fit through a 12-mm trocar, however, so the trocar will need to be removed prior to inserting the band into the abdomen (using a Ponce Lap-Band Introducer or a long Kelly clamp). The right upper quadrant trocar (2) is either a 5-mm or a 10-mm trocar; the remaining trocars are 5 mm. Trocar 3 is placed lateral and caudad to Trocar 1. Trocar 4 is placed in the subxiphoid position; this trocar can be upsized in case a larger liver retractor is required. The final trocar (5) is placed between the umbilicus and the xiphoid process. The laparoscope is placed through trocar 5. The first assistant utilizes trocar 3 to retract the stomach and trocar 4 to retract the left lobe of the liver. The surgeon stands between the patient's legs, and operates through trocars 1 and 2 (right and left hand, respectively).

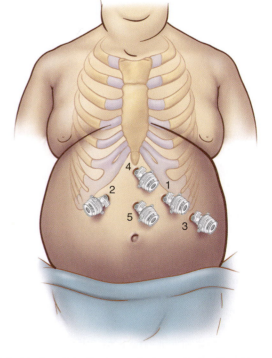

FIGURE 7-1 Positioning of the five trocars for laparoscopic adjustable gastric band (LAGB) placement.

OPERATIVE TECHNIQUE

The minimally invasive approach for the LAGB is straightforward, but this procedure can be quite treacherous for the novice laparoscopic surgeon. The presence of a large pre-esophageal "fat pad" and an enlarged left lobe of the liver can make the operation quite challenging. Two techniques have been utilized for placement of the band: (1) the perigastric dissection and (2) the pars flaccida technique. The perigastric method led to many technical failures (slippage and erosions), so it rarely is performed today. For this reason, only the pars flaccida technique will be described here.

Exposure

With a relatively small liver, retraction of the left lobe can be done with a palpation probe. At times an atraumatic balloon retractor, fan retractor, or a Nathanson liver retractor may be needed. After retracting the left lobe of the liver trough trocar 4, the omentum is grasped and retracted caudally, exposing the angle of His. The first assistant can retract the stomach or gastrosplenic ligament caudad through trocar 3 to help with this exposure. The left hand of the surgeon should retract the stomach posterior and caudad, without grasping the stomach itself, using an atraumatic grasper placed through trocar 2. The phrenoesophageal ligament and angle of His should be opened and dissected with a blunt esophageal retractor through trocar 1. At this point, it is important to determine the presence of a hiatal hernia, which, if present, should be repaired.

If the patient has a large pre-esophageal fat pad or large gastrohepatic ligaments, then removal of the fat pad may be necessary. This is needed in fewer than 10% of patients, especially when a 10-cm band is utilized. Some surgeons, however, routinely remove the anterior fat pad in order to facilitate placement of the fixation sutures. Removal of the fat pad may require electrocautery or ultrasonic shears. Care should be taken to avoid damaging the serosa of the stomach, as this may lead to subsequent erosion. The entire fat pad need not be removed, rather just enough to ensure the band is not too tight and that the fixation sutures maybe placed on the stomach.

Retrogastric Dissection

The lesser sac is entered by dividing the pars flaccida, the avascular plane of the gastrohepatic ligament noted superficial to the caudate lobe (Fig. 7-2). This may be divided utilizing the hook electrocautery through trocar 1. Even in the massively obese, this area often is thin and free of blood vessels. After opening the pars flaccida, three important structures can be seen: the caudate lobe, the vena cava, and the right bundle of the right crus of the diaphragm. The liver retractor can retract the caudate lobe so that the vena cava can be exposed. The right bundle of the right crus will be to the left of the vena cava. Identification of the esophagus or stomach is not needed at this point. The right bundle of the right crus should be followed to its base where a fat pad passes transversely. An esophageal retractor then is placed through trocar 2 (left hand), and an atraumatic grasper is placed through trocar 1 (right hand). The atraumatic grasper provides upward retraction on the side of the stomach. The esophageal retractor is placed just anterior to the right bundle of the right crus (Fig. 7-3) and gently is inserted toward the angle of His. During this time, any resistance should alert the surgeon that the retractor is not in the correct plane. The instrument should not be twisted or turned during this part of the dissection. Ideally, this instrument should "fall" into the retrogastric space. After the tip of the esopha-

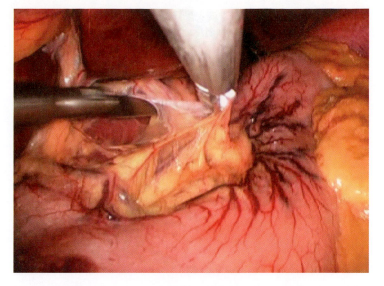

FIGURE 7-2 The lesser sac is entered by bluntly dividing the avascular plane of the gastrohepatic ligament (pars flaccida).

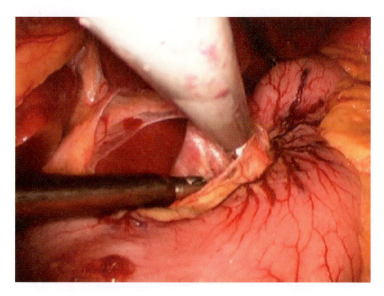

FIGURE 7-3 The esophageal retractor is used to divide the peritoneum along the right crus of the diaphragm, posterior to the gastroesophageal junction.

geal retractor has been positioned at the angle of His, the fat overlying the tip of the instrument can be cleaned off by the assistant with a blunt grasper. Occasionally the fundus may roll over the tip of the esophageal retractor. If this happens, then the retractor should be straightened and adjusted to avoid the fundus. When the tip of the esophageal retractor is plainly visible at the angle of His, the retrogastric dissection is complete.

Band Placement

The band can be inserted into the abdomen either through a 15-mm trocar or directly through the abdominal wall after removing trocar 1. There is a commercially available device for introduction of the band (Ponce Lap-Band Introducer); however, a Kelly clamp may be utilized as well. Care should be taken not to grasp the balloon directly, as this may injure the band. Once the band is placed into the abdomen, the tip of the tubing is placed on a locking Debakey grasper, at an acute angle to the jaws of the grasper. This acute angle facilitates placement of the tip of the tubing into the opening at the end of the esophageal retractor (Fig. 7-4). Once the tubing is positioned, the assistant grasps

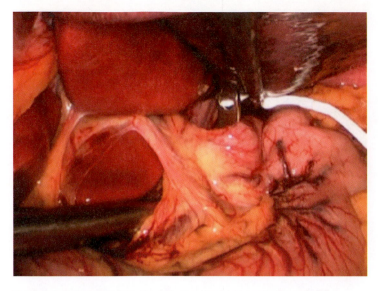

FIGURE 7-4 Placement of the tip of the Lap-Band tubing into the end of the esophageal retractor.

the tubing and pulls several centimeters of the tubing through the esophageal retractor. Aggressive maneuvers at this point can damage the tubing. The surgeon straightens out the esophageal retractor and withdraws it from behind the stomach, pulling the tubing from left to right.

As the esophageal retractor (with the tip of the band) is pulled from the retrogastric space, the tip of the tubing is grasped and removed from the esophageal retractor. At this point, only non-locking instruments are utilized to grasp the tubing of the band, as locking instruments may place undue force on the tubing, which in turn may cause injury to the band. Using a continuous hand-over-hand motion, the tubing is pulled through behind the stomach until the band follows. The buckle of the band may get caught on the tissue along the right bundle of the right crus. Gentle retraction of the band and tubing toward the spleen will expose this tissue and allow easier passage.

Once the band has been pulled from left to right behind the stomach and is freely mobile behind the stomach, the end of the tubing is inserted through the buckle of the band (Fig. 7-5). Before fastening the band, the Gastric Balloon Calibration Tube (BioEnterics, Carpinteria, CA) can be inserted transorally. This

device is a flexible gastric tube designed for gastric and bariatric surgical procedures, and facilitates pouch identification and sizing. The tube should be placed by an anesthesiologist and positioned into the stomach at 45 cm. Once the sizing balloon is positioned, 20 mL of air can be inflated into the balloon port, inflating the balloon in the stomach, distal to the band. The calibration tube then is withdrawn, pulling the balloon cephalad toward the gastroesophageal junction. Once inflated, the balloon may be seen in the stomach. The band should be positioned along the equator of the balloon. The balloon then is deflated, and the calibration tube is removed before the band is tightened. Utilization of the calibration tube allows for correct placement of the band; however, appropriate dissection also can ensure that the band is in correct position. Many surgeons have abandoned the use of the calibration tube, as there is little benefit of this device after the learning curve is complete; in addition, there is a small but real risk of perforation.

In order to securely fasten the band, a Lap-Band Closure Tool may be used. The Lap-Band Closure Tool has a hook that is placed into the hole of the buckle. The tip of the closure tool fits at the end of the thickened area of the tubing, just distal to the band. By pulling on the tubing, the band is locked in place with minimal effort (Fig. 7-6). Alternatively, two atraumatic graspers can be used to accomplish the same effect, also with minimal effort. It is imperative that the band is not placed too tightly around the stomach. The band should be loose enough so that another instrument can be passed between the secured band and the stomach. If the band is too tight, removing the anterior fat pad with electrocautery may loosen the fit. This can be done with the band in place. If the band still is too tight after removing the anterior fat pad, then the adipose tissue along the lesser curvature and gastrohepatic ligament may be divided. Care must be taken not to damage either the vascular supply to the lesser curvature of the stomach or the nerve of Latarjet. For some large men or in those patients with significant perigastric adipose tissue, a VG Band may be considered. This band has a larger inner diameter, allowing for more flexibility in the patient with thicker gastric walls and excessive fat near the gastroesophageal junction.

Gastric fixation sutures (gastrogastric sutures) then are placed to secure the stomach over the band. Interrupted heavyweight nonabsorbable sutures incorporate the stomach caudal (first) and cephalad to the band; the first suture is placed anterolateral

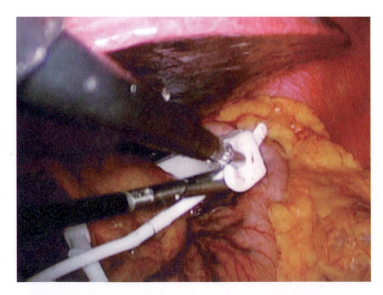

FIGURE 7-5 The end of the tubing is placed through the buckle, in order to fasten the Lap-Band.

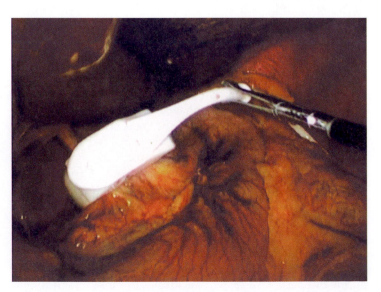

FIGURE 7-6 Completed closure of the Lap-Band.

to the buckle. The sutures should be placed so that the stomach "wrap" around the band is not too tight. The first bite of the suture is taken on the stomach caudad to the band. The second bite of the suture is taken after the fat pad is grasped and pulled up cephalad so that a good bite of the stomach can be taken. The suture is tied, creating a wrap around the band. It is important to be sure that the sutures are placed far enough from the band so that, when secured, the wrap is not too tight. A loose wrap is helpful in preventing erosions. Once the first stitch is placed and secured, it is utilized to rotate the stomach to the patient's right, which will reveal the area of the band that is not covered. Further sutures (1 to 3) are placed to prevent the band from slipping at the angle of His (Fig. 7-7). The last suture should be placed high on the angle of His in order to prevent gastric prolapse or an anterior "slip" of the band. As long as a suture is placed high on the fundus near the angle of His, the risk of gastric prolapse is low. Furthermore, gastrogastric sutures should not be placed over the buckle of the band, as this has been shown to lead to band erosion. After the wrap is performed, the band still should rotate along its circumference without any difficulty, and allow for passage of an instrument between the band and the stomach. If the wrap is too tight, then it should be taken down and redone. The new wrap should be made looser by incorporating the stomach more caudal to the band.

Port Placement

After the band is placed, the tubing is grasped and pulled out through trocar 1. The pneumoperitoneum is evacuated and the trocars are removed. It is not necessary to close the fascial defects if nonbladed trocars have been utilized. After infiltration of local anesthetic into the subcutaneous tissues, the incision from trocar 1 is extended and a subcutaneous pocket is created to allow for the access port. It is important to identify the anterior rectus sheath fascia; this can be quite challenging in a patient with a large amount of subcutaneous fat. Once the anterior fascia is found, four sutures are placed to correspond with the four quadrants of the access port.

The tip of the tubing is cut so that the tubing of the band may be attached to the tubing of the access port. The two components are joined with the stainless steel tubing connector, which

is attached to the access port. Constant steady pressure is needed to connect the two. If too much pressure is applied and the tubing suddenly kinks, it can cause a tear in the tubing. If this occurs, the tubing may be cut from the metal connector and reconnected. Gauze may be utilized for traction on the tubing. The stainless steel tubing connector also can be dipped in saline to serve as lubrication. The components should be joined together so that the stainless steel tubing connector is no longer visible.

The access port then is sutured onto the fascia utilizing the four suture holes in the port base. Heavyweight nonabsorbable monofilament suture may be used. Each suture is tied with the assistant holding the port on the anterior fascia. At this point it is important to ensure that the tubing is fed back into the abdomen, and that there is no kink in the tubing as it passes back through the fascia. Once satisfactory placement of the access port and tubing is confirmed, the wound should be irrigated and closed in at least two layers.

POSTOPERATIVE CARE

The patients can be extubated immediately after surgery. If the patient has obstructive sleep apnea, then it is important to have a continuous positive airway pressure machine available. Most patients should be able to transition from the postanesthesia care unit to a surgical ward. The patient is assisted with ambulation the day of surgery; early mobilization after surgery is imperative in order to reduce the risk of postoperative VTE events. Typically the intensive care unit is not needed, unless there are specific indications for such monitoring. The patient is kept NPO during the first night. Pain management consists of intermittent intravenous morphine augmented by scheduled intravenous ketorolac. The morning after surgery, an upper gastrointestinal (UGI) radiograph with water-soluble contrast material is performed to assure that there has been no injury to the stomach or leakage of contrast agent. It also is important to document the position of the band and esophageal emptying distal to the band. If the study is satisfactory, then the patient may be started on a bariatric liquid diet (sugar-free, no carbonated beverages). The patient may be discharged home later that day if the patient can tolerate oral intake and has adequate oral pain control. Some surgeons discharge patients to home on the day of the procedure, and this has been shown to be safe. The authors prefer overnight observation, however, with a contrast study performed the morning after surgery. While an UGI radiograph can be done the day of surgery, most patients tolerate it better the next morning.

The patient is required to stay on a bariatric liquid diet for 2 weeks after surgery to help prevent any retching or vomiting. All patients are seen 1 week after surgery to ensure there is no dysphagia or vomiting. The wounds, especially at the site of the access port, should be inspected for any signs of infection. The first balloon adjustment is performed 6 weeks after surgery. Earlier adjustments may lead to a dysphagia from a tight band, slippage, or erosions. After the first adjustment, the patients are seen monthly and evaluated for further adjustments. Goals for weight loss are 1 to 2 pounds per week. If this weight-loss goal is not met and hunger persists after eating 4 ounces of food, the band should be adjusted. It is important to integrate daily exercise, dietary restrictions, and behavioral modification into the routine of the postoperative patient. This combination of an aggressive band adjustment strategy and patient cooperation will allow for maximum health benefit and weight loss. Adjustments can be performed under

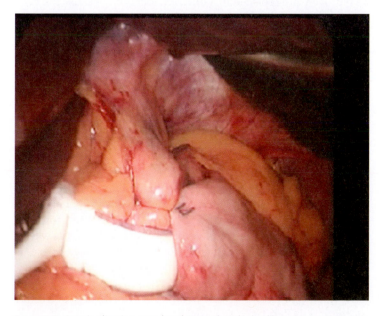

FIGURE 7-7 Gastric plication completed. Note that the buckle is not incorporated into the plication.

fluoroscopy or in the office. Routine use of fluoroscopy allows for prompt access of the subcutaneous port and allows for verification of band position, which minimizes the risk of overtightening of the band. The presence of pouch or esophageal dilation also may be determined with fluoroscopy. Early diagnosis of pouch dilation with subsequent reduction of the band volume will decrease the risk of gastric prolapse or band slippage.

PROCEDURE-SPECIFIC COMPLICATIONS

Infection

Superficial infections of the wound overlying the access port should be monitored carefully. Hospital admission and intravenous antibiotics may be necessary to prevent port or band infections. Port site infection, if unable to be managed conservatively, may require surgical therapy. If the infection is isolated to the port (without evidence of intra-abdominal infection), an attempt to salvage the band should be considered. The tubing can be divided laparoscopically, and left loose in the abdomen. The port site then can be opened so that the port can be removed. After the infection has resolved and the wound is healed, the patient can have a new port inserted. The tubing can be identified laparoscopically and brought out to the new port. If there is evidence of an intra-abdominal infection, then both the band and port should be removed to allow for resolution of the process.

Gastroesophageal Reflux

Most patients who have gastroesophageal reflux prior to surgery find relief of their symptoms after LAGB. Unfortunately, however, some patients may experience an increase in their reflux after surgery. This reflux frequently is related to overfilling of the band. The symptoms may be ameliorated by removing fluid from the band. Occasionally, the reflux is due to failure to recognize and repair a hiatal hernia during the initial operation. A laparoscopic reoperation can be performed for the hiatal hernia repair; however, the band will have to be repositioned at this time. Therefore, the surgeon should be vigilant in the diagnosis and repair of any hiatal hernias prior to the LAGB procedure.

Enlarged Pouch or Slippage

An enlarged pouch may occur if a band is too tight and the patient continues to overeat. If this occurs, then the band should be loosened. An enlarged pouch eventually will lead to slippage. As the pouch increases in size, it can push the band distally, inducing slippage. Thus, radiographic evidence of an enlarging pouch should prompt the surgeon to loosen the band, which will minimize the risk of band slippage. A slip can be caused by a variety of reasons. Technical errors, rapid weight loss, as well as overeating all have been suggested to contribute to a slipped band. When the perigastric technique for band placement was utilized, posterior slippage was common. With the transition to the pars flaccida approach for band placement, anterior slips have been identified most frequently. There is little chance of developing a posterior slip with the pars flaccida technique because minimal dissection is required in the retrogastric space. An anterior slip may occur at the angle of His secondary to placement of band fixation sutures too caudal along the greater curvature. It is imperative that the fixation sutures be placed high on the fundus of the stomach, which should minimize the risk of an anterior slip. In addition, forceful vomiting or retching can cause the sutures to tear, which also can cause a slip.

A slippage can be diagnosed on plain abdominal x-rays. Instead of the normal diagonal orientation of the band (2 o'clock to 8 o'clock position), the band is seen in a horizontal position (left to right) on x-ray. Surgical intervention is required to fix a slippage. This can be done laparoscopically. With an anterior slip, the fundus of the stomach will be cephalad to the band (gastric prolapse). Once the left lobe of the liver is dissected free of the band and pouch, the fixation sutures are identified and divided to separate the wrap. It may be possible to reduce the stomach through the band at this point. If this is not possible, then the band should be unfastened and the stomach reduced. The band then can be positioned and new gastrogastric fixation sutures placed. Attention should be directed to the fundus near the angle of His in order to prevent further slips.

Erosion

The rate of erosion is approximately 1%; there is little data, however, as to the etiology of a band erosion. Any foreign body can have the tendency to erode, so it is imperative to be vigilant in all steps of the LAGB procedure. Serosal tears should be avoided, but repaired if identified. The band should not be fastened too tight around the stomach. In addition, the fixation sutures should not be placed too tight. All sutures should be tied to approximate the tissue rather than constrict. Lastly, the first adjustment should not be performed until 6 weeks after operation. This will give the edema from the procedure a chance to subside. A late port site infection often is the presenting sign of an erosion. This should be treated with band removal, which can be done with endoscopic assistance or laparoscopically. After removal of the band and closure of the perforation, another type of bariatric procedure may be performed, or another band may be placed at a later date.

Port-Related Concerns

Port-related issues are not uncommon after LAGB. It is imperative that the port be sutured to the fascia using all four available holes. This will help prevent migration and slippage; despite this anchorage, however, port displacement still can occur. If the port is not accessible via fluoroscopy, then reoperation may be needed. This usually can be done under local anesthesia. The port should be removed and replaced in a different location, because the capsule may make it difficult to place appropriate fascial fixation sutures. The tubing of the band also can be kinked at the fascial entry site. If the tubing is kinked, then it will not be possible to adjust the band. Reoperation will be necessary to move the port and readjust the tubing so that there is a more direct route into the fascia and peritoneal cavity.

RESULTS AND OUTCOME

The results of LAGB in the United States initially were poor. Some factors implicated in these poor results include the procedural learning curve, technical issues, and postoperative management of the gastric band. Recent data have demonstrated, however, that gastric banding can result in impressive weight loss as well as resolution of obesity-related comorbidities. Percentage of excess body weight lost has been reported to be over 50% at 3 years. This is less than what has been reported for the gastric bypass; however, the adjustable gastric banding is associated with a lower mortality rate (<0.1%) compared to gastric bypass. In addition, resolution or improvement in type II diabetes, hypertension, and obstructive sleep apnea has been demonstrated. Long-term data in randomized groups of patients are not yet available to compare LAGB with LRYGB, so a debate continues regarding the relative merits of these two bariatric procedures. Nevertheless, it has been well established that LAGB can produce excellent results in the motivated patient who is closely followed in a structured bariatric program.

Suggested Reading

Ahroni JH, Montgomery KF, Watkins BM: Laparoscopic adjustable gastric banding: Weight loss, co-morbidities, medication usage and quality of life at one year. Obes Surg 2005;15(5):641–647.

Fielding GA, Duncombe JE: Laparoscopic adjustable gastric banding in severely obese adolescents. Surg Obes Relat Dis 2005;1(4):399–405.

Fielding GA, Ren CJ: Laparoscopic adjustable gastric band. Surg Clin North Am 2005;85(1):129–140.

O'Brien PE, Dixon JB, Laurie C, Anderson M: A prospective randomized trial of placement of the laparoscopic adjustable gastric band: Comparison of the perigastric and pars flaccida pathways. Obes Surg 2005;15(6):820–826.

Parikh MS, Fielding GA, Ren CJ: U.S. experience with 749 laparoscopic adjustable gastric bands: Intermediate outcomes. Surg Endosc 2005;19(12):1631–1635.

Ponce J, Haynes B, Fromm R, et al: Effect of Lap-Band-induced weight loss on type 2 diabetes mellitus and hypertension. Obes Surg 2004;14(10):1335–1342.

Provost DA: Laparoscopic adjustable gastric banding: An attractive option. Surg Clin North Am 2005;85(4):789–805.

Ren CJ, Fielding GA: Laparoscopic adjustable gastric banding: Surgical technique. J Laparoendosc Adv Surg Tech A 2003;13(4):257–263.

Ren CJ, Weiner M, Allen JW: Favorable early results of gastric banding for morbid obesity: The American experience. Surg Endosc 2004;18(3):543–546.

Tolonen P, Victorzon M, Makela J: Impact of laparoscopic adjustable gastric banding for morbid obesity on disease-specific and health-related quality of life. Obes Surg 2004;14(6):788–795.

Watkins BM, Montgomery KF, Ahroni JH, et al: Adjustable gastric banding in an ambulatory surgery center. Obes Surg 2005;15(7):1045–1049.

Weiner R, Blanco-Engert R, Weiner S, et al: Outcome after laparoscopic adjustable gastric banding—8 years experience. Obes Surg 2003;13(3):427–434.

TALLAL M. ZENI

Minimally Invasive Sleeve Gastrectomy

Both the National Institutes of Health and the World Health Organization have acknowledged that bariatric surgery is beneficial in the treatment of morbid obesity. The recent expansion in laparoscopic bariatric surgery mostly has involved two surgical procedures, the laparoscopic Roux-en-Y gastric bypass (LRYGB) and the laparoscopic adjustable gastric band (LAGB). These procedures accounted for more than 150,000 cases in 2005 in the United States. Although LRYGB can effect long-term weight loss, it may have side effects that include iron deficiency anemia, osteoporosis and osteomalacia secondary to calcium malabsorption, marginal ulceration, and internal herniation. The potential for malabsorption with the biliopancreatic diversion/duodenal switch procedure is even greater and has limited its widespread adoption. The LAGB procedure required insertion of a foreign body, which may erode into the gastric lumen or may slip and require revision. The need for frequent adjustments of the adjustable gastric band and typically less weight loss (compared to LRYGB) also hinder the overall efficacy of the LAGB procedure.

An alternative bariatric procedure is the laparoscopic sleeve gastrectomy. The mechanism of weight loss with this operation mainly is caloric restriction secondary to decreased capacity of the stomach. Sleeve gastrectomy generally is a less efficacious weight-loss operation compared to the gastric bypass, but the former does not produce the side effects of the latter. Normal gastrointestinal continuity is maintained, thus eliminating the risk of malabsorption. In addition, the ghrelin hormone and hunger both have been shown to be decreased after a sleeve gastrectomy, which may contribute to the weight-loss effect of this procedure. This putative hormonal effect may be an important differentiating factor between the sleeve gastrectomy and the vertical banded gastroplasty or Magenstrasse and Mill operation. Although long-term data are not complete, it appears that laparoscopic sleeve gastrectomy may produce weight loss that is at least comparable to the LAGB, if not greater. Some surgeons who perform sleeve gastrectomy might consider it a first-stage procedure to be used in select patients (e.g., super-morbidly obese); however, there now is some evidence which has documented the efficacy of sleeve gastrectomy by itself as a definitive bariatric operation.

OPERATIVE INDICATIONS

Sleeve gastrectomy initially was introduced as a component of the BPD operation. The realization that patients with a body mass index (BMI) greater than $60 kg/m^2$ are at increased mortality risk

compared to those with a BMI less than $60 kg/m^2$ led to staging of these two procedures, with the sleeve being done first, then followed by the BPD at a later date, after the patient's BMI had decreased. It became apparent, however, that impressive weight loss was possible with the sleeve gastrectomy alone. The current indications for sleeve gastrectomy include a BMI above $60 kg/m^2$, severe comorbidity (such as poor cardiorespiratory status or cirrhosis), arthritis with a dependence on nonsteroidal anti-inflammatory drugs (in order to avoid marginal ulceration from a LRYGB), and conversion of a failed LAGB procedure. Some patients elect to have a sleeve gastrectomy done in order to avoid the long-term complications associated with the LRYGB procedure. In addition, the surgeon may elect to perform this procedure if faced with the probability of a "frozen" or "hostile" abdomen secondary to dense adhesions.

PREOPERATIVE EVALUATION, TESTING, AND PREPARATION

The preoperative evaluation for a laparoscopic sleeve gastrectomy is similar to that for a LRYGB. Patients with cardiac risk factors or a BMI above $60 kg/m^2$ should undergo a cardiac stress test; a pulmonary evaluation also may be necessary. Endoscopy is performed routinely in order to rule out Barrett's esophagus, ulceration, or a tumor that may alter the medical or surgical management of these patients. Patients with severe gastroesophageal reflux disease should not undergo sleeve gastrectomy, as it may exacerbate their reflux symptoms. Abdominal ultrasonography also is performed; if cholelithiasis is diagnosed, then a concomitant cholecystectomy is performed. A low-calorie diet is initiated several weeks preoperatively in order to reduce the size of the liver. A bowel preparation consisting of one half-gallon of polyethylene glycol 3350 (NuLytely) and oral antibiotics (neomycin and erythromycin base) is given the day before surgery, along with a clear liquid diet. Alternatively, a Fleet Phospho-soda laxative also can be utilized. The patient should be hydrated in the preoperative area, in order to minimize the occurrence of intraoperative hypotension.

PATIENT POSITIONING AND PLACEMENT OF TROCARS

The patient is placed in the French position with the surgeon standing between the patient's legs, as described in Chapter 6 for LRYGB. The camera operator stands on the right side of the

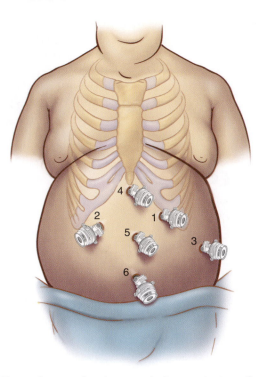

FIGURE 8-1 Trocar placement for a laparoscopic sleeve gastrectomy. Trocar 2 and trocar 6 are 15 mm; the rest are 12 mm.

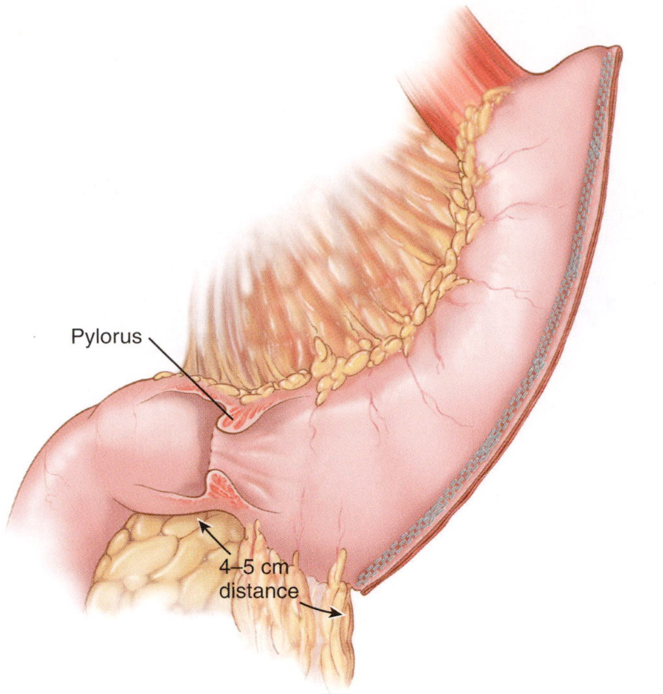

FIGURE 8-2 Diagramatic representation of a laparoscopic sleeve gastrectomy.

patient, while the assistant stands on the left. Four to six trocars may be utilized; however, placement of six trocars will facilitate the dissection and creation of the sleeve. Two 15-mm trocars and four 12-mm trocars are used, as shown in Figure 8-1. Entry into the peritoneal cavity is obtained using a 12-mm optical blade-less trocar at the left subcostal midclavicular line. The other trocars are placed under direct visualization at the sites depicted in Figure 8-1.

OPERATIVE TECHNIQUE

The liver is retracted using an inflatable balloon, and the phreno-esophageal ligament overlying the gastroesophageal junction is divided with the hook electrocautery. Delineation of the left crus of the diaphragm at the angle of His is crucial. The short gastric vessels are divided using an ultrasonic (harmonic) scalpel, beginning at the midpoint of the greater curvature and close to the gastric wall. This dissection proceeds cephalad toward the angle of His. As with any procedure involving mobilization of the gastric fundus, the surgeon should exercise caution near the upper pole of the spleen to avoid injury to this organ. If bleeding from a short gastric vessel occurs, then this may be compressed with the balloon retractor (Soft-Wand, Gyrus-ACMI, Southborough, MA) while a clip applier or other hemostatic device is prepared. Once the fundus and the upper corpus of the stomach have been mobilized, the dissection proceeds caudad along the greater curvature up to but not reaching the pylorus. Some surgeons advocate stopping the greater curve mobilization/beginning the gastric transection 2 cm from the pylorus, while other surgeons utilize an 8-cm distance. The author prefers to end the mobilization of the greater curvature 4 to 5 cm from the pylorus, so as to preserve some antral emptying capacity.

Since the distal antrum can be quite thick, it is reasonable to use 45-mm cartridges with 4.8-mm staples for the gastric transection. The linear stapler-cutter first is placed via the right-sided port in order to transect the distal antrum to a point approximately 1 cm away from the lesser curvature. If the stapler fails because of the thickness of the antrum, then the surgeon should be prepared to place sutures to repair the staple line. A 48-F esophageal bougie (preferred size by the author) then is placed transorally into the distal antrum. The next two 45-mm/4.8-mm stapler cartridges are fired to maneuver around the incisura angularis. ePTFE staple line reinforcement material (Gore Seamguard, W. L. Gore & Associates, Flagstaff, AZ) may be used to reduce the incidence of staple line bleeding, but supportive data for this are limited.

After these first three stapler loads have been fired, the surgeon then can utilize 60-mm/4.8-mm cartridges (or 3.5-mm staples without the ePTFE reinforcement material) along the length of the bougie. Three such cartridges are needed to complete the sleeve gastrectomy, for a total (typically) of six stapler loads. In the region of the fundus, it is helpful to exert posterior traction before firing the stapler to help prevent redundant stomach in this region. Any bleeding along the staple line should be controlled with clips or sutures rather than cautery. The staple line may be oversewn (with the bougie still in place) if the surgeon prefers. A completed sleeve gastrectomy is shown in Figure 8-2. The gastric specimen is placed into a 15-mm specimen retrieval bag and is removed through the umbilical port, which may need a minimal amount of extension to get the specimen out. Methylene blue (~100 mL) then is instilled into the stomach via an orogastric tube (with distal luminal compression) in order to test the gastric staple line; this solution is aspirated out after the test. A closed suction drain may be placed along the length of the staple line, and all ports are closed with size 0 polyglactin suture.

POSTOPERATIVE CARE

Patients are maintained NPO except for ice chips during the first night. They undergo an upper gastrointestinal series with water-soluble contrast material on postoperative day 1 (Fig. 8-3). If the contrast study is without leak, then the patient is advanced to a clear liquid diet. The patient is typically discharged on postopera-

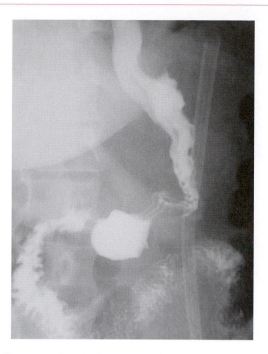

FIGURE 8-3 Upper gastrointestinal contrast study after a laparoscopic sleeve gastrectomy.

tive day 2. The Jackson-Pratt drain is removed prior to discharge. We maintain all patients on liquids for the first 2 weeks; thereafter, soft foods are initiated. Emphasis is placed on limiting intake to 2 to 3 oz at a time. Each patient also should take a daily multivitamin and calcium supplement and also a weekly sublingual vitamin B_{12} supplement. In addition, each patient is followed at routine intervals similar to those for other postoperative bariatric patients.

PROCEDURE-SPECIFIC COMPLICATIONS

Dissection posterior to the stomach should be kept to a minimum. Posterior adhesions should be divided only if they are felt to interfere with the line of transection. Preservation of those adhesions will maintain the gastric tube in place and minimize the risk of twisting or volvulus. In addition, aggressive dissection of the posterior stomach may result in a left gastric artery injury, which can devascularize the sleeve, thus making a total gastrectomy necessary. If the gastric transection is begun too close to the pylorus (generally more than 2 cm away), then abnormal antral emptying may result with resultant gastroesophageal reflux disease. For this reason the author prefers to begin the transection 4 to 5 cm proximal to the pylorus. During the first stapler firing, the surgeon should remain about 1 cm away from the incisura angularis in order to prevent stenosis at the incisura. Once the incisura is traversed, the posterior wall should be retracted in a cephalad and lateral fashion in order to avoid leaving behind a redundant gastric tube posteriorly. Another recognized complication of this

surgery is esophageal injury; the surgeon should avoid catching the esophagus in the staple line, as this will increase the risk of a staple-line leak. The published leak rate from the gastric staple line is 1%. Utilization of the ePTFE staple-line reinforcement in the presence of thick tissue (as in the antrum, during the first stapler firing) may compromise the integrity of the staple line, as the ePTFE adds about 0.5 mm of material to be compressed within each staple.

RESULTS AND OUTCOME

Overall, there are a limited number of studies that address the concept of sleeve gastrectomy as a sole and definitive procedure for induction of weight loss. The available data indicate that laparoscopic sleeve gastrectomy can produce a 33% to 45% excess weight loss at 1 year in patients with a BMI over 60 kg/m². The percentage of excess weight loss in short-term follow-up after sleeve gastrectomy may be even higher in patients with a BMI in the range of 40. Additional weight loss may be possible if the patient has a staged LRYBG 1 year after the sleeve gastrectomy (i.e., the sequence of operative events originally intentioned for the sleeve procedure). There also is a small amount of controlled data which suggest that laparoscopic sleeve gastrectomy produces more short-term weight loss than the LAGB procedure. Although limited, the available data support the notion that laparoscopic sleeve gastrectomy has short- and mid-term effectiveness as a sole bariatric procedure. Nevertheless, it still may be prudent not to advocate sleeve gastrectomy as the definitive bariatric procedure in the patient with a BMI greater than 50, as the resultant weight loss may not be adequate; the final answer is not yet known on this issue. Whether the loss of excess weight after a sleeve procedure will endure beyond short-term follow-up also needs to be determined. The patient- and surgeon-related advantages of sleeve gastrectomy, however, will ensure that this procedure will continue to be used in the future.

Suggested Reading

Baltasar A, Serra C, Perez N, et al: Laparoscopic sleeve gastrectomy: A multipurpose bariatric operation. Obes Surg 2005;15:1124–1128.

Cottam D, Qureshi FG, Mattar SG, et al: Laparoscopic sleeve gastrectomy as an initial weight-loss procedure for high risk patients with morbid obesity. Surg Endosc 2006;20:859–863.

Himpens J, Dapri G, Cadiere GB: A prospective randomized study between laparoscopic gastric banding and laparoscopic isolated sleeve gastrectomy: Results after 1 and 3 years. Obes Surg 2006;16:1450–1456.

Langer FB, Reza Hoda MA, Bohdjalian A, et al: Sleeve gastrectomy and gastric banding: Effects on plasma ghrelin levels. Obes Surg 2005;15:1024–1029.

Mognol P, Chosidow D, Marmuse JP: Laparoscopic sleeve gastrectomy as an initial bariatric operation for high-risk patients: Initial results in 10 patients. Obes Surg 2005;15:1030–1033.

Regan JP, Inabnet WB, Gagner M, Pomp A: Early experience with two-stage laparoscopic Roux-en-Y gastric bypass as an alternative in the super-super obese patient. Obes Surg 2003;13:861–864.

MANISH PARIKH, MICHEL GAGNER, AND
ALFONS POMP

Minimally Invasive Biliopancreatic Diversion with Duodenal Switch

Laparoscopic biliopancreatic diversion with duodenal switch (BPD-DS) is one of the most effective weight-loss procedures currently available. Both short-term and long-term weight loss exceed that of any other bariatric operation. This procedure evolved from the classic biliopancreatic diversion for morbid obesity, first introduced in 1979 by Nicolas Scopinaro. The Scopinaro BPD was a combination of gastric restriction and intestinal malabsorption: a horizontal gastrectomy (resulting in a 200- to 300-mL pouch) and a long Roux-en-Y configuration, consisting of a 200-cm alimentary limb, a 50-cm common absorptive channel, and a gastroileal anastomosis (Fig. 9-1).

Although satisfactory weight loss was achievable with the BPD procedure, long-term complications such as vitamin and protein deficiencies, bone demineralization, and marginal ulcers were problematic. The majority of these complications were thought to be secondary to the elimination of the pylorus and proximal duodenum from the digestive tract, and the relatively short length of the common absorptive channel. In an effort to reduce the side effects of the BPD without compromising weight loss, Hess and Marceau both independently modified the BPD by adding a duodenal switch as well as lengthening the common absorptive channel. DeMeester's group first described the "duodenal switch" as a suprapapillary Roux-en-Y duodenojejunostomy to treat bile reflux gastritis without creating an ulcerogenic state or prolonging gastric emptying. They observed that the incidence of jejunal ulceration was decreased by preserving the proximal duodenum.

As it is known today, the BPD-DS involves a 150- to 200-mL sleeve or vertical gastrectomy, a duodenoileal anastomosis, and a long Roux-en-Y with a 150-cm alimentary limb and a 100-cm common channel (Fig. 9-2). The key features of this operation are that the lesser curvature, antrum, pylorus, first portion of the duodenum, and vagal innervation are all spared, while parietal cell mass is reduced. This configuration improves digestive behavior while decreasing the likelihood of the dumping syndrome and marginal ulceration. Furthermore, by placing the ileoileal anastomosis 100 cm proximal to the ileocecal junction (instead of 50 cm as in the classic BPD), metabolic disturbances and the number of surgical revisions for malnutrition or diarrhea are less common. The laparoscopic BPD-DS combines the effective weight-loss results of the open BPD-DS with the reduced morbidity of a laparoscopic approach in the morbidly obese population. Although most data on the laparoscopic BPD-DS are preliminary, it is reasonable to assume that the same benefits derived from other laparoscopic bariatric procedures, such as shorter hospitalization, decreased analgesic requirements, decreased wound complications, and shorter recovery period, will apply to laparoscopic BPD-DS.

OPERATIVE INDICATIONS AND CONTRAINDICATIONS

Numerous studies have shown that bariatric surgery is the only modality that can induce and maintain long-term weight loss, thus prolonging patient survival. The criteria from the National Institutes of Health Consensus Development Conference state that patients who are either morbidly obese with body mass index (BMI) greater than $40\,kg/m^2$ or those who have BMI greater than $35\,kg/m^2$ with severe obesity-related comorbidities are eligible for bariatric surgery. We consider morbidly obese patients with BMI less than $40\,kg/m^2$ poor candidates to undergo the BPD-DS, however, as they may become malnourished with this operation. At our institution, a patient must have a BMI above $40\,kg/m^2$ to be considered for laparoscopic BPD-DS. More particularly, the super-obese (BMI greater than $50\,kg/m^2$) and super-super-obese patient (BMI greater than $60\,kg/m^2$) are excellent candidates for this procedure. It has been shown that the BPD-DS procedure provides superior weight-loss outcomes in these patients compared to the Roux-en-Y gastric bypass (RYGB). Patients who do not wish to undergo the significant dietary or volume restrictions imposed by the RYGB may prefer a BPD-DS because the latter leaves the patient with a substantially larger stomach pouch. Other potential candidates for BPD-DS are patients considering gastric bypass but who require chronic high-dose anti-inflammatory medications (e.g., for severe arthritis). Such gastric irritants would be contraindicated in both RYGB and BPD because of the fragile mucosa at the gastroenterostomy. Such a patient would benefit from the less ulcerogenic BPD-DS. The patient who requires periodic surveillance of the stomach (e.g., secondary to *Helicobacter pylori* infection, gastritis, ulcers, neoplasm, or intestinal metaplasia) also is an appropriate candidate, because the entire stomach remains accessible via upper endoscopy. Finally, a patient who has failed vertical-banded gastroplasty, gastric banding, or gastric bypass may be considered for conversion to BPD-DS.

BPD-DS should be avoided in patients who are bedridden, who are strict vegans (because of the need to ingest at least 80 to 100 g protein daily), who have had a prior gastrectomy, or who have inflammatory bowel disease. In addition, patients who have

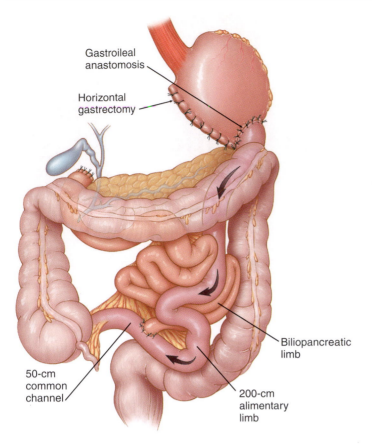

FIGURE 9-1 Classic Scopinaro biliopancreatic diversion: horizontal gastrectomy, gastroileal anastomosis, a long Roux-en-Y with a 200-cm alimentary limb and a 50-cm common channel.

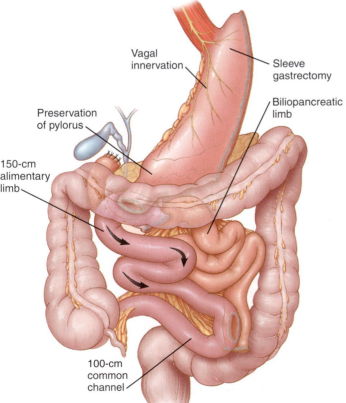

FIGURE 9-2 Laparoscopic biliopancreatic diversion with duodenal switch: sleeve gastrectomy, duodenoileostomy and a long Roux-en-Y, with a 150-cm alimentary limb and 100-cm common channel.

undergone colon resection may not be good candidates because they may be more prone to develop diarrhea. The patient with severe gastroesophageal reflux and morbid obesity may be better served with a RYGB rather than a BPD-DS, because the former is an excellent antireflux operation, and also because it is impossible to perform an antireflux procedure after sleeve gastrectomy. The patient with Barrett's esophagus is not a good candidate for the BPD-DS, because the greater curvature should be preserved in case these patients require an esophagectomy. In the latter two groups, however, a possible alternative is laparoscopic adjustable gastric banding with duodenal switch, which eliminates the need for a vertical sleeve gastrectomy.

PREOPERATIVE EVALUATION, TESTING, AND PREPARATION

In addition to undergoing medical clearance, each patient should undergo a psychiatric evaluation and instruction by a registered dietician/nutritionist. Patient compliance can help minimize the risk of metabolic complications after bariatric surgery, especially with BPD-DS; thus, preoperative screening and education are vital. We routinely perform esophagogastroduodenoscopy to exclude gastric or duodenal disease, including *H. pylori* infection. If *H. pylori* is present, then the patient is treated prior to surgery. All patients above age 50 undergo screening colonoscopy. Sleep studies are used liberally to evaluate for obstructive sleep apnea. The patient usually is placed on a clear liquid diet the day prior to surgery; a bowel preparation is unnecessary.

PATIENT POSITIONING AND TROCAR PLACEMENT

The patient is placed in the "French" position (legs split and abducted, but not flexed), and then properly secured to the operating table (Fig. 9-3). The surgeon stands between the patient's

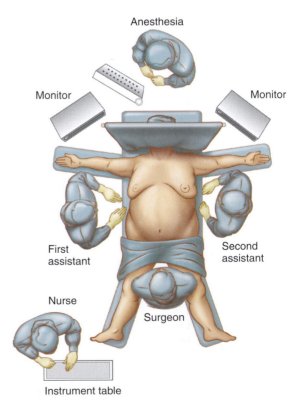

FIGURE 9-3 The patient is in the split-leg position with the surgeon between the patient's legs; the first assistant (camera operator/liver retractor) is on the patient's right and the second assistant is on the patient's left.

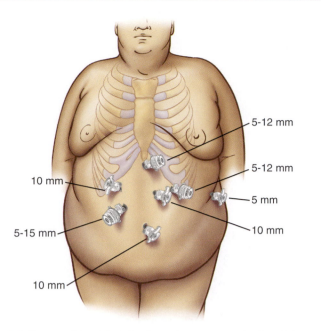

FIGURE 9-4 Trocar positions. The left subcostal port may need to be a 5-15 mm Versaport, depending on the type of stapler used for the sleeve gastrectomy.

legs, the first assistant (liver retractor and camera holder) stands on the patient's right, and the second assistant stands on the patient's left. We prefer the Alphastar table (Maquet, Rastatt, Germany) with footplate attachments.

Seven trocars are used (Fig. 9-4). We prefer an open technique at the umbilicus to enter the peritoneal cavity. Once pneumoperitoneum has been established with carbon dioxide to 15 mm Hg, the 10-mm 30-degree laparoscope is introduced, and a diagnostic laparoscopy is performed. Two 10-mm trocars are placed, one in the epigastric left paramedian position and one in the right subcostal position in the midclavicular line (for liver retraction). Two 5-12–mm ports (Versaport, U.S. Surgical, Norwalk, CT) are placed, one in the subxiphoid position and one in the left midclavicular line, approximately 4 fingerbreadths inferior to the costal margin. The left subcostal port may need to be a 5-15–mm port, depending on the type of stapler used for the sleeve gastrectomy. A 5-mm port is placed in the left anterior axillary line, lateral to the 5-12–mm port. A 5-15–mm port is placed in the right midclavicular line, just superior to the umbilicus. A second insufflator is attached to facilitate maintenance of the pneumoperitoneum in case an aspirator needs to be used.

OPERATIVE TECHNIQUE

Sleeve Gastrectomy

We prefer to start with the sleeve (vertical) gastrectomy rather than the distal ileoileostomy, because occasionally patients cannot tolerate pneumoperitoneum and may require a shorter procedure. In these cases, a sleeve gastrectomy alone provides an effective procedure without compromising the patient. Several months later (after significant weight loss has taken place), the patient may return for a completion duodenal switch.

The patient is placed in steep reverse Trendelenburg position, and the table is tilted right side down in order to optimize visualization of the gastroesophageal junction. The laparoscope is placed through the 10-mm left epigastric paramedian trocar. If the stomach is distended, then the anesthesiologist should decompress the stomach with an orogastric tube; this tube should

be removed as soon as the stomach is decompressed. A 10-mm fan-type liver retractor is placed through the right subcostal port to retract the liver anteriorly, and the entire stomach and gastroesophageal junction is exposed. The surgeon's working ports are the subxiphoid and the left subcostal 5-12–mm ports. The second assistant retracts the omentum laterally with a bowel grasper through the 5-mm left lateral port.

The dissection begins along the distal greater curvature by dividing the branches of the gastroepiploic artery near the gastric wall with an ultrasonic scalpel. It is important to avoid injury to the gastroepiploic vessels which can produce hemorrhage into the omentum that obscures the dissection planes. The greater curvature is devascularized to the level of the left crus. The second assistant's grasper is frequently repositioned superiorly to maximize retraction. As the dissection proceeds toward the spleen and left crus, the exposure may become difficult, especially in males with thick abdominal walls and abundant mesenteric fat. The short gastric vessels may be exposed by placing the second assistant's grasper on the lateral folds of omentum (consistently in the middle of the gastrosplenic ligament) and retracting this toward the spleen. Other helpful maneuvers include temporarily increasing the pneumoperitoneum to 20 mm Hg, placing the patient in maximal reverse Trendelenburg position, tilting the patient more toward the right side, and ensuring an appropriate level of paralysis.

All posterior attachments of the stomach to the pancreas should be lysed, taking care not to injure the splenic artery. Placing the second assistant's graspers on the posterior fundus and retracting this toward the patient's right shoulder will expose these attachments. If these posterior attachments are not divided prior to stapling, then tearing with bleeding may occur during the stapler applications. The surgeon should be cautious near the lesser curvature, however, because the gastric sleeve is supplied solely by the lesser curve vasculature.

The left crus can be visualized by lifting the stomach anteriorly. The ligaments attaching the stomach and diaphragm should be divided. The anterior perigastric fat just to the left of the gastroesophageal junction should be cleared in order to minimize the amount of tissue in the stapler jaws during the subsequent steps. The surgeon should avoid dissection to the right of the gastroesophageal junction, however, because of risk of injury to the vagus nerve. If the patient has a hiatal hernia, then this should be reduced and repaired; failure to recognize a herniated fundus may lead to weight-loss failure after sleeve gastrectomy.

The greater curvature then is liberated distally to a point 2 cm beyond the pylorus. The second assistant retracts the greater curvature anteriorly and toward the patient's right shoulder. The surgeon's left hand grasps the fat of the gastrocolic ligament (via the right midclavicular port) and retracts it inferiorly. The surgeon's right hand manipulates the ultrasonic scalpel. The remainder of the gastrocolic ligament between the antrum and gastroepiploic arcade is divided with the ultrasonic scalpel. The surgeon should avoid any antral injury or burns, especially while dissecting its posterior aspect, because the antrum will be vital for gastric emptying.

Palpation with an instrument is used to confirm the position of the pylorus. Approximately 6 to 8 cm proximal to the pylorus (at the level of the last branch of the vessel from the lesser curve, just distal to the incisura angularis), the sleeve gastrectomy is begun along the greater curvature (Fig. 9-5). Initiating the sleeve less than 6 cm proximal to the pylorus will compromise the antrum, and likely will lead to gastric emptying problems. The surgeon's left hand holds the linear stapler (4.8-mm staples, 60-mm length) through the right midclavicular 5-12–mm port, while the second

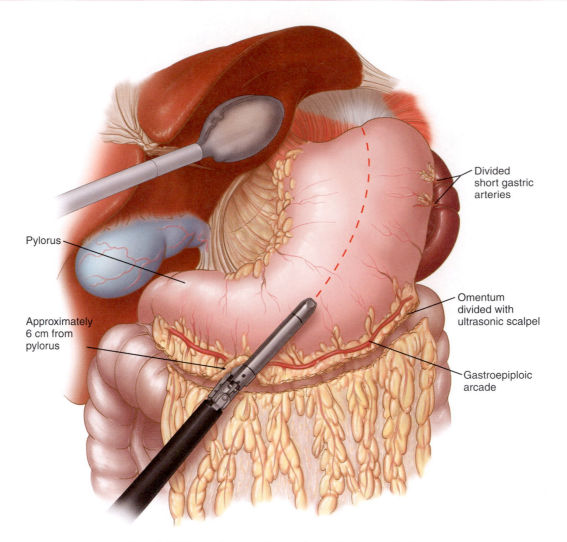

Pylorus

Approximately
6 cm from
pylorus

Divided
short gastric
arteries

Omentum
divided with
ultrasonic scalpel

Gastroepiploic
arcade

FIGURE 9-5 Initial application of the stapler for the sleeve gastrectomy.

assistant retracts the body of the stomach toward the patient's left. Although we have used the 3.5-mm staples in the past, we believe that it is safest to use the 4.8-mm staples for the entire sleeve gastrectomy because of the relative thickness of the stomach in morbidly obese patients. The stapler should be positioned so that at least 2 cm of anterior stomach serosa are visible between the stapler and lesser curvature. The first two firings of the stapler are performed, aiming approximately 2 cm away from the lesser curvature. These firings should be done slowly, because the stomach is the thickest in this area. Additional sutures may be required if the tissue is too thick for the stapler. We routinely use a buttress material (Bioabsorbable Seamguard, W. L. Gore & Associates, Flagstaff, AZ) similar to the Maxon suture (U.S. Surgical), which is sandwiched between, over, and below the anterior and posterior gastric wall. This bioabsorbable material reduces staple-line hemorrhage and possibly the leakage rate. We have abandoned the use of bovine pericardial strips as buttressing material after some patients were noted to vomit these strips after apparent intraluminal migration.

After these initial stapler applications, the anesthetist inserts a 60-F orogastric bougie which, under laparoscopic vision, is directed medially along the lesser curvature into the duodenum. Two bowel graspers can be used to position the bougie posteriorly into the lesser curve of the sleeve toward the pylorus. Inserting the bougie after the first two stapler firings helps align the bougie along the lesser curvature (Fig. 9-6). For all BPD-DS cases, we currently use a 60-F bougie to ensure gastric volume for adequate protein intake; for a primary sleeve gastrectomy, we use a 32- to

40-F bougie. The remainder of the sleeve gastrectomy is completed with sequential firings of the linear stapler (4.8-mm staples) along the bougie toward the angle of His (Fig. 9-7). The surgeon's right hand holds the stapler via the left midclavicular 5-12–mm port and aims toward the left crus; the surgeon's left hand (via the subxiphoid port) grasps the anterior wall of the stomach and retracts this toward the patient's right side. The second assistant holds the posterior stomach wall and retracts this toward the patient's left side. At the gastroesophageal junction, the transection line deviates slightly from the bougie to avoid a stenosis. About 5 to 6 stapler applications typically are required to complete the sleeve. The anesthetist should monitor the bougie so that it does not retract during stapling and have its tip imbricated in the staple line.

Upon completion of the sleeve stapling, the anesthetist removed the bougie, and the surgeon places figure-of-eight 3-0 Maxon sutures at a number of high-risk points: the apex of the sleeve gastrectomy; the intersections of the staple lines; and the distal end of the staple line. The second assistant can retract the stomach toward the patient's right side to help expose the apex of the sleeve. If there is any doubt regarding the integrity of the staple line, then a methylene blue test should be performed prior to proceeding to the next stage. While the surgeon clamps near the pylorus, the anesthetist instills approximately 120 mL of methylene blue mixed with saline through an 18-F orogastric tube. Another option for checking the sleeve is to insert a gastroscope and inspect for a leak (and intraluminal bleeding) via air insufflation; this latter option may be suboptimal because of

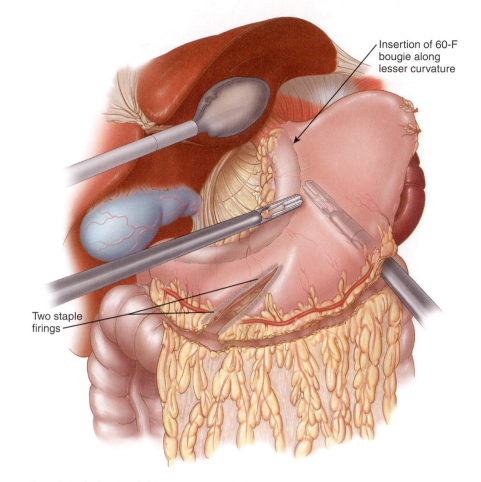

FIGURE 9-6 The bougie is held in apposition to the lesser curve with anterior and posterior pressure.

Insertion of 60-F
bougie along
lesser curvature

Two staple
firings

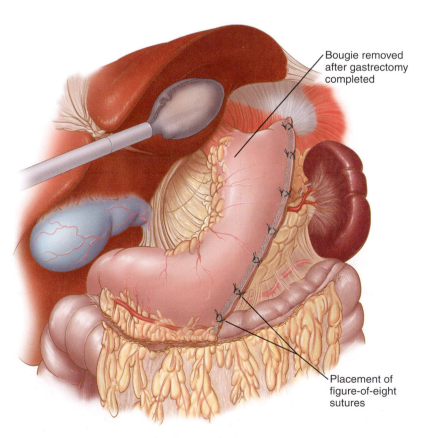

Bougie removed
after gastrectomy
completed

Placement of
figure-of-eight
sutures

FIGURE 9-7 The laparoscopic sleeve gastrectomy is created by sequential firings of the 4.8-mm stapler along a 60-F bougie. At the gastroesophageal junction, the staple line deviates slightly from the bougie to avoid stenosis.

the tendency of the air to pass through the pylorus and distend the small bowel. After these maneuvers, the right midclavicular trocar site is enlarged, the abdominal wall is dilated with an atraumatic clamp (the circular stapler will be introduced through this site later), a large impermeable bag is introduced, and the specimen is extracted. Grasping the end of the sleeve on a staple line and applying progressive traction may make extraction easier, and require less abdominal wall dilation.

Duodenal Transection and Preparation for Duodenoileostomy

The pylorus and first portion of duodenum are palpated with a laparoscopic probe. Any remaining branches from the gastroepiploic arcade to the antrum and pylorus are divided with the ultrasonic scalpel. Typically, this vessel ligation extends just beyond the vascular complex inferior to the pylorus. It is important to avoid hemostatic clips in this area (especially on the duodenal side) so that the clips will not get caught in the staple line. It usually is not necessary to perform a Kocher maneuver. Any adhesions to the duodenum from a prior cholecystectomy must be divided at this time.

The retroduodenal and supraduodenal attachments are divided with the ultrasonic scalpel. The second assistant retracts the stomach laterally and anteriorly so that the surgeon can see both the greater curvature and posterior stomach for the retroduodenal dissection. The gastroduodenal artery, which lies posteriorly between the first and second portion of duodenum, marks the distal aspect of the dissection. Using a 10-mm right-angle dissector, the surgeon creates a 1-cm window (enough to accommodate the linear stapler) posterior and superior to the first portion of the duodenum, medial to the common bile duct (Fig. 9-8). Ideally, the supraduodenal window is between the serosa of the duodenum and the pyloric branches of the right gastric artery, thus maximizing blood supply to the subsequent anastomosis.

The duodenum then is transected with a linear stapler (3.5-mm staples, 60-mm length, buttressed), leaving a 2- to 5-cm duodenal cuff; typically this stapler is inserted through the left midclavicular 5-12–mm port (Fig. 9-9). The second assistant retracts the antrum toward the patient's left side in order to facilitate this step. The

buttressing material should obviate the need to oversew the duodenal stump. If the surgeon is unable to complete the supraduodenal window, then an alternate method is to transect the inferior two thirds of the duodenum with the linear stapler, complete the supraduodenal window, and then transect the remaining duodenum with an additional stapler application.

We prefer to use a 21-mm circular stapler for the duodenoileostomy, specifically the CEEA 21 (U.S. Surgical); a 25-mm stapler is too large for the ileum, and frequently will tear the bowel during insertion. The anvil of the 21-mm stapler is delivered transabdominally through the right midclavicular trocar site. Note that it is somewhat difficult to deliver this anvil transorally with a modified nasogastric tube-anvil apparatus (as is done with conventional gastric bypass), because the anvil of the 21-mm stapler cannot flex as it traverses the pylorus. After the anvil is introduced into the abdomen, the ultrasonic scalpel is used to remove 1 to 2 cm of the proximal duodenal staple line, the base of the anvil is placed into the duodenal lumen, and the anvil is secured with a 3-0 Prolene purse-string suture (Fig. 9-10).

The surgeon then should assess the ability of the ileum to be brought up to the duodenum in an antecolic fashion, without tension. If the patient has a bulky omentum, then the surgeon should divide the omentum along its right lateral third to facilitate the passage of the ileum toward the duodenum. This division should be performed on the right side of the omentum (and not on the left side, as commonly is done in gastric bypass), because an oblique line runs from the ileocecal valve toward the pylorus.

Small Bowel Measurement

The surgeon and first assistant move to the patient's left side, and the patient is placed in the Trendelenburg position with the left side down for exposure of the ileocecal region. With the laparoscope in the left epigastric paramedian trocar and the surgeon's working hands in the subxiphoid and umbilical ports, a point on the ileum 100 cm proximal to the ileocecal valve is marked with clips on the mesentery (the site of the future common channel anastomosis). This distance is measured with a 50-cm length of umbilical tape applied to the antimesenteric border of the bowel; we prefer umbilical tape for measuring small intestine, because

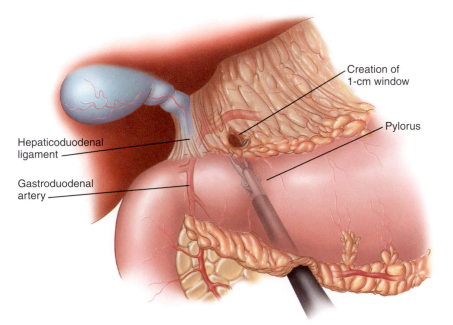

Labels: Creation of 1-cm window; Pylorus; Hepaticoduodenal ligament; Gastroduodenal artery

FIGURE 9-8 Creation of a window posterior to the first portion of the duodenum, medial to the hepatoduodenal ligament and gastroduodenal artery.

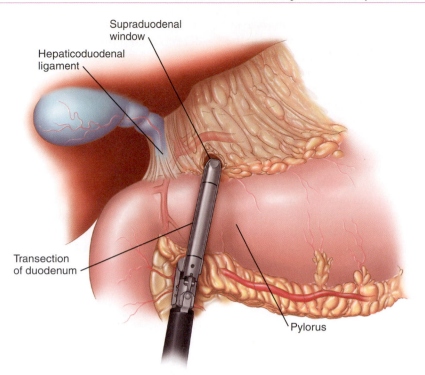

FIGURE 9-9 Duodenal transection with linear stapler.

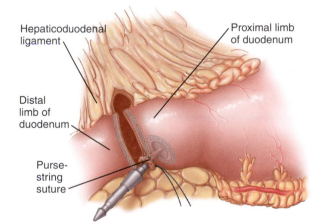

FIGURE 9-10 The anvil has been inserted into the proximal duodenum and secured with a purse-string suture.

the tape is more reliable compared to estimating distances with a bowel grasper. Any adhesions that prevent proper measurement of the small intestine (e.g., prior lower abdominal or pelvic surgery) must be divided. The small bowel is marked again at 250 cm proximal to the ileocecal valve (future alimentary limb). At this second mark, a window is made in the ileal mesentery with a 10-mm right-angle clamp, about 1 cm away from the bowel wall.

The ileum then is transected with the linear stapler (2.5-mm staples, 45-mm cartridge, buttressed) via the left midclavicular 5-12–mm port. The ultrasonic scalpel is used to divide another 1 to 2 cm of mesentery at the two ends of the divided bowel. Dividing more than 1 to 2 cm of mesentery is unnecessary and places the subsequent anastomosis at risk for ischemia. The grasper remains on the distal bowel (with the umbilical tape) to maintain proper orientation. The staple line and buttress material on the distal ileum are excised to permit entry of the 21-mm circular stapler. The umbilical tape then is removed. The surgeon should ensure that there is no mesenteric twisting or bowel limb misidentification by running the bowel again from the ileocecal valve to the transected ileum.

Duodenoileal Anastomosis

A suture is attached to the spike of the 21-mm circular stapler for easy retrieval. The stapler is secured to a plastic camera drape (for wound protection) with an adhesive strip, and the stapler then is introduced through the right midclavicular trocar site. Three graspers are used to triangulate the opened end of ileum. The stapler is maneuvered into the distal ileum and advanced cephalad by rotating in a clockwise manner toward the duodenal cuff, which contains the anvil (Fig. 9-11). Two graspers are removed, but the third continues to maintain traction on the ileum from the 6 o'clock position so that the stapler does not slip out of the

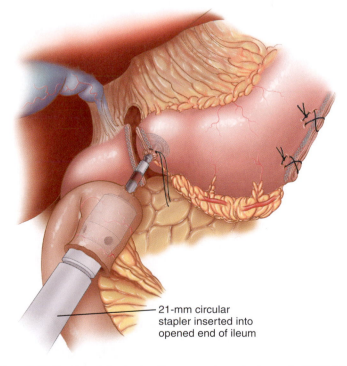

FIGURE 9-11 Creation of the duodenoileostomy using a circular stapler (CEEA 21).

85

bowel. It is critical that the ileum is brought up to the duodenum (and not vice versa) under minimal or no tension. Division of the omentum, as described earlier, will facilitate this maneuver.

With the stapler in position, the first assistant moves between the patient's legs, and the surgeon remains on the patient's left (the second assistant remains on the right in order to retract the liver). The plastic perforator of the 21-mm circular stapler is advanced through the antimesenteric wall of ileum at a point 6 to 7 cm distal to the opened end. The spike then is removed by grasping the attached suture. The anvil in the duodenum subsequently is mated to the stapler. The surgeon should check that there is no tissue between the ileum and duodenum nor pinching of the bowel wall (which can create an obstruction). The stapler then can be fired to create an end-to-side anastomosis. The 21-mm circular stapler is not a flipped-top, so two to three rotations of the stapler are required along with countertraction on the antrum in order to pull the stapler back through the anastomosis. Next the adhesive strip holding the wound protector is removed, and the stapler is extracted from the trocar site while advancing the wound protector over the tip of the stapler, in order to prevent it from contacting the wound.

The surgeon returns to the position between the patient's legs, and the first assistant returns to the patient's right side. The right midclavicular 5-12–mm port is reinserted. The open ileal limb is inspected for bleeding; any oozing from the enterotomy may indicate bleeding from the duodenoileostomy and should be evaluated. If there is no bleeding from the open limb, then a 2.5-mm linear stapler (buttressed) inserted via the subxiphoid or the left midclavicular 5-12–mm port is used to close the blind limb of ileum. The tips of the stapler must be in the ileal mesentery to ensure that the ileum has been completely closed. The resulting specimen then is extracted from the right midclavicular trocar site.

The duodenoileostomy staple line (including the upper and lower corners) is reinforced with a running 3-0 Maxon suture. We prefer monofilament absorbable suture for this because permanent suture (e.g., silk) has been associated with marginal ulcer and stricture. One helpful maneuver to provide adequate exposure of the superior corner (where leaks are prone to occur) is to place the second assistant's graspers on the antrum and retract this to the patient's left, which pulls the anastomosis toward the midline. In order to expose the posterior aspect of the staple line, the second assistant should grasp the posterior antrum and gently retract this toward the patient's right shoulder.

After the duodenoileostomy is complete, the anesthetist inserts an 18-F orogastric tube just proximal to the anastomosis and instills approximately 120 mL of methylene blue mixed with saline while the surgeon clamps the ileum distal to the anastomosis. The area around the anastomosis is irrigated with saline to help identify any methylene blue. Once the test has been completed and no leak has been identified, the gastric sleeve is completely aspirated and the orogastric tube is removed.

Distal Ileoileostomy

The surgeon and first assistant return to the patient's left side, and the laparoscope is placed through the left epigastric paramedian trocar. The table is tilted left side down, and the patient is placed in slight Trendelenburg position. The surgeon runs the alimentary limb from the duodenoileostomy distally to the level of the previously placed clips on the ileal mesentery (at 100 cm proximal to the ileocecal valve). For the ileoileostomy, we prefer the M triple-staple technique, which provides a widely patent,

completely stapled anastomosis that avoids lumenal narrowing during enterotomy closure (Fig. 9-12). The clips on the ileal mesentery are removed first, and then an enterotomy is made with the ultrasonic scalpel on the antimesenteric side of the marked (distal) ileum. Another enterotomy is made approximately 1 to 2 cm from the stapled end of the proximal ileum. The stapled proximal ileum (biliopancreatic limb) should be on the patient's left side, and the distal ileum (alimentary limb) should be on the patient's right. After ensuring that there is no mesenteric twisting, the surgeon advances a linear stapler (2.5-mm staples, 60-mm length) through the subxiphoid 5-12–mm port and, aiming toward the pelvis, inserts the larger jaw of the stapler into the proximal ileum and the smaller jaw into the distal ileum. The stapler then is fired along the antimesenteric border of each limb, creating a standard side-to-side anastomosis between the biliopancreatic and alimentary limbs which leads into the 100-cm common channel. Through the same enterotomy, the linear stapler (2.5-mm staples, 60-mm length) is fired again between the alimentary limb and the common channel. A third firing of the linear stapler (via the left midclavicular 5-12–mm port) closes the enterotomy transversely. The specimen then is removed without contaminating the wound. An alternate option for enterotomy closure is suturing with running 2-0 silk, either in one or two layers.

Closure of Mesenteric Defects

We recommend complete closure of all mesenteric defects to avoid internal hernias and their associated complications. With the same position (surgeon and first assistant on the patient's left side), the ileoileostomy mesenteric defect is closed with a running 2-0 silk suture. We prefer to incorporate the serosa of the ileum into the last stitch of this closure. The surgeon then returns to stand between the patient's legs in order to close Petersen's defect (Fig. 9-13). The patient is placed in slight reverse Trendelenburg position; sometimes it is necessary to insert an additional 5-mm trocar in the left lower quadrant to optimize suturing angles. The omentum is retracted superiorly, and the first assistant grasps an epiploic appendage of the transverse colon and retracts it cephalad. The space between the transverse colon mesentery and the ileal mesentery then is closed with a running 2-0 silk suture. We prefer to close this from the patient's left side, because exposure is better from this side, and seeing the ligament of Treitz from this angle helps the surgeon avoid incorporating the proximal jejunum into the closure. The final stitch should approximate the transverse colon serosa to the ileum serosa, because closure of mesenteric fat alone may result in a defect after a large amount of weight loss. It is important to meticulously close these defects, especially at the root of the mesentery, because a small defect may be more susceptible to incarceration than a large one.

Inspection and Closure

The sleeve gastrectomy staple line, duodenoileostomy, and ileoileostomy are all inspected for any evidence of bleeding or leakage. The final anatomic configuration is shown in Figure 9-2. The biliopancreatic limb must be coming from the patient's left, and the alimentary limb and common channel must be on the patient's right side. We do not routinely place any drains or a nasogastric tube. All fascial defects larger than 5 mm are closed with a suture-passing device with size 0 Vicryl sutures. The umbilical wound usually is closed under direct vision with a 1 Prolene suture. Skin incisions are closed with subcuticular absorbable monofilament sutures.

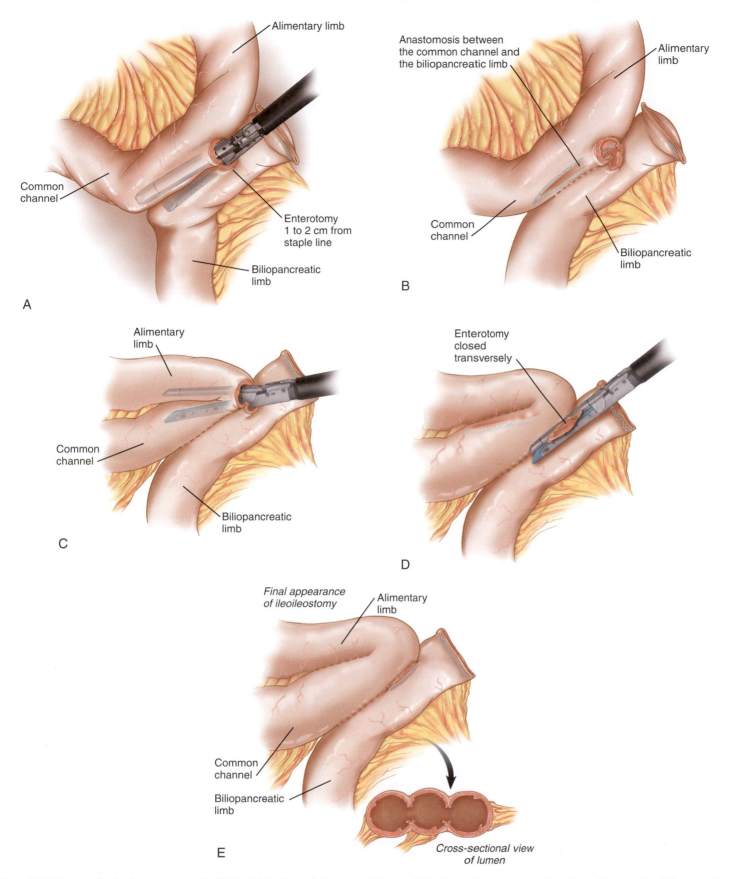

FIGURE 9-12 Creating the ileoileostomy using the "triple-M" stapling technique. **A** and **B**, A standard side-to-side anastomosis is performed between the biliopancreatic limb and the last 100 cm of distal ileum (i.e., the common channel). **C**, Through the same enterotomy, the linear stapler is fired between the alimentary limb and the common channel. **D**, A third firing of the linear stapler closes the enterotomy. **E**, Final appearance of the ileoileostomy, including a cross section of the widely patent M anastomosis.

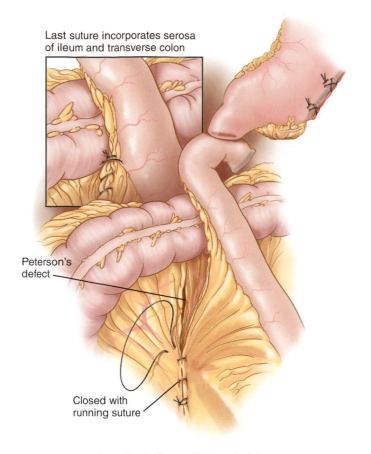

Last suture incorporates serosa of ileum and transverse colon

Peterson's defect

Closed with running suture

FIGURE 9-13 Closure of Petersen's defect.

POSTOPERATIVE CARE

Patients have their vital signs checks at an increased frequency for at least 6 hours. They are placed on continuous positive airway pressure (CPAP) if sleep apnea is present or suspected. Maintenance intravenous fluids are continued to ensure urine output of at least 0.5 to 1 mL/kg/hour. Early ambulation is critical; the majority of our patients ambulate the same evening after surgery.

We use postoperative upper gastrointestinal contrast studies selectively, for example, in cases of any intraoperative technical difficulties (e.g., positive methylene blue test requiring additional sutures) or for patients who manifest signs and symptoms of a leak (fever higher than 38.5°C, with tachycardia, tachypnea, somnolence, or failure to thrive). Patients usually require an intravenous patient-controlled analgesic pump for the first 2 days. They receive a clear liquid diet on the first postoperative day. If they do well, their Foley catheters are removed and they are weaned off the intravenous fluids. Patients are advanced to a pureed diet the next day. Our nutritionist sees all patients postoperatively, and their dietary recommendations are reviewed. They usually are discharged home by the third postoperative day on a pureed diet and oral analgesics.

Patients are seen 4 weeks after discharge, and they receive follow-up nutritional counseling for a protein-enriched diet. They are given twice-daily multivitamins, oral calcium supplements, iron, and fat-soluble vitamins. Patients with intact gallbladders are prescribed ursodiol 300 mg twice daily for 6 months for gallstone prophylaxis. At 3 months postoperatively, a thorough nutritional evaluation is performed including serum levels of iron, ferritin, vitamin B_{12}, folate, albumin, parathyroid hormone, calcium, phosphorus, alkaline phosphatase, zinc, selenium, lipids, vitamins A and D, total protein, and hematology panels.

PROCEDURE-SPECIFIC COMPLICATIONS

The overall mortality rate following open BPD-DS ranges from 0.5% to 1.6% in most large series. As surgeons become more experienced with the laparoscopic technique, we expect the published mortality rates after laparoscopic BPD-DS to be even lower. The most dreaded complication after BPD-DS is leakage from the gastric staple line, the duodenoileostomy, or the ileoileostomy. As with all bariatric procedures, the surgeon should have a low threshold to re-explore if the patient manifests any signs of an anastomotic leak (e.g., tachycardia, fever, severe abdominal pain, mental status changes). We previously have shown that the use of a staple-line buttressing material (e.g., Seamguard) is effective at reducing staple-line hemorrhage and leakage along the sleeve gastrectomy staple line. We now use this material routinely in our practice. Routine intraoperative testing of the duodenoileostomy (with methylene blue) also is important to detect leakage that can be repaired at the time of operation. The most critical factor that results in a leak at the duodenoileostomy is excess tension at the anastomosis. Maneuvers to reduce this tension include dividing the omentum along its right lateral aspect on the transverse colon and dividing some of the blood vessels superior to the pylorus. The surgeon must be cautious when performing the latter maneuver, because this may compromise the blood supply to the anastomosis. We have not found it necessary to perform a retrocolic duodenoileostomy; we generally avoid retrocolic constructions due to their association with an increased incidence of internal hernias.

The surgeon should consider the two-stage approach in the high-risk patient, such as the super-obese. In our early series of laparoscopic BPD-DS we found that after stratifying by BMI, the complication rate was 38% in patients with BMI above 65 kg/m², and 8% in patients with BMI below 65 kg/m². Therefore, separating the restrictive and malabsorptive aspects of the procedure into two operative stages (laparoscopic sleeve gastrectomy and laparoscopic duodenoileostomy and ileoileostomy 6 to 12 months later) may reduce the complication and mortality rate compared to the traditional one-stage approach. Other criteria for considering the two-stage approach include intolerance of pneumoperitoneum, extensive intra-abdominal adhesions prolonging the operative time, or lack of adequate working space despite higher pneumoperitoneum pressures. We prefer to keep the total operative time to less than 4 hours in order to avoid the attendant risks (pulmonary embolism, thromboembolism, and rhabdomyolysis) of prolonged general anesthesia, especially in the high-risk bariatric population.

Although nutritional side effects exist with the BPD-DS, they are significantly less compared to the classic BPD. The vast majority of nutritional markers—iron, corrected calcium, alkaline phosphatase, albumin, total protein, aspartate aminotransferase, alanine aminotransferase, and bilirubin—will remain within the normal range. Only the mean hemoglobin and parathyroid hormone have been shown to depart from the normal range, but they both can normalize with appropriate supplementation. It is imperative that the common channel of the BPD-DS be at least 100 cm, because nutritional side effects (comparable to the classic BPD) can occur with a 50-cm common channel.

Internal hernias carry an incidence of 2% to 3% after laparoscopic BPD-DS. We recommend complete closure of all mesenteric defects to avoid internal hernias and their associated complications. Furthermore, we prefer to incorporate a superficial bite in the bowel serosa during the final closure stitch, because mesenteric closure alone may eventually (with loss of mesenteric fat) enlarge and lead to an internal hernia. It is imperative to completely close these mesenteric defects, especially at the root of the mesentery, because a small defect may be even more susceptible to incarceration than a large patent defect.

RESULTS AND OUTCOMES

The BPD-DS, if properly performed, has the best long-term weight loss of any bariatric operation. Most current data involve the open BPD-DS. In one series of over 1400 cases of open BPD-DS, excess weight loss (EWL) was 75% at 10 years (92% follow-up), and 94% of the patients achieved more than 50% EWL. All diabetics were off medications by 6 months. Complication statistics included a 0.7% leak rate, a 0.6% mortality rate, and a 3.7% revision rate. The majority of revisions were for excess weight loss and protein deficiency (requiring lengthening of the common channel). Another report in 701 patients undergoing open BPD-DS with an average BMI of 53kg/m^2 had morbidity and mortality rates of 2.9% and 1.4%, respectively, and EWL at 1, 2, and 3 years was 69%, 73%, and 66%, respectively. Mean number of bowel movements was less than three daily. At 3 years, levels remained normal for serum albumin in 98% of patients, hemoglobin in 52%, and calcium in 71%. No patients reported dumping, and no marginal ulcers were seen. Overall, patient satisfaction is high with the BPD-DS—up to 86% in some series.

In our published series of completely laparoscopic BPD-DS patients ($n = 40$, median BMI 60kg/m^2), we reported a 58% EWL at 9 months, 2.5% mortality rate ($n = 1$), 15% morbidity rate, and a 4-day median length of stay. The majority of the perioperative complications were bleeding-related issues at the gastrectomy staple line. This problem has been reduced by the routine use of buttressing material at the sleeve gastrectomy staple line, and by reevaluating our prophylactic heparin use. More recently, we have reviewed our experience with 248 laparoscopic BPD-DS patients, with a mean BMI of 54kg/m^2. Two intraoperative leaks were identified and corrected with sutures. One conversion was required from severe adhesions secondary to a prior open cholecystectomy. Major morbidity was encountered in 15% of patients, with sepsis and bowel obstruction being the most frequent; the 30-day mortality rate was 0.8% ($n = 2$; both from respiratory failure in male patients with BMI greater than 60kg/m^2). The majority of patients were discharged home by the third postoperative day. These data suggest that the laparoscopic approach is feasible with an acceptable morbidity rate.

There are very few large series directly comparing the BPD-DS to the RYGB. In an extensive meta-analysis of all bariatric procedures, BPD (with and without DS) was compared to RYGB, with the following (respective) numbers: EWL, 70% versus 62%; 30-day mortality rate, 1.1% versus 0.5%; resolution of diabetes, 99% versus 84%; hyperlipidemia, 99% versus 97%; hypertension, 83% versus 68%; and obstructive sleep apnea, 92% versus 80%. Statistically, the BPD $\pm$ DS appeared to have an edge over the RYGB. In the super-obese patient, the BPD-DS has been shown to produce greater EWL and greater decrease in BMI compared to RYGB.

The BPD-DS is one of the most effective bariatric procedures currently available. The long-term efficacy is well established, and the operation has been adopted by a number of surgical practices. Patients must understand the malabsorptive component of the surgery and must be compliant with supplement use and postoperative visits. The BPD-DS may be the procedure of choice for some bariatric patients, particularly those who are super-obese.

Suggested Reading

Anthone G, Lord R, DeMeester T, et al: The duodenal switch operation for the treatment of morbid obesity. Ann Surg 2003;238:618–628.

Buchwald H, Avidor Y, Braunwald E, et al: Bariatric surgery. A systematic review and meta-analysis. JAMA 2004;292:1724–1737.

Comeau E, Gagner M, Inabnet W, et al: Symptomatic internal hernias after laparoscopic bariatric surgery. Surg Endosc 2005;19:34–39.

DeMeester T, Fuchs K, Ball C, et al: Experimental and clinical results with proximal end-to-end duodenojejunostomy for pathologic duodenogastric reflux. Ann Surg 1987;206:414–424.

Dolan K, Hatzifotis M, Newbury L, et al: A clinical and nutritional comparison of biliopancreatic diversion with and without duodenal switch. Ann Surg 2004;240:51–56.

Gagner M: Laparoscopic biliopancreatic diversion with duodenal switch. In Inabnet W, DeMaria E, Ikramuddin S (eds): Laparoscopic Bariatric Surgery. Philadelphia, Lippincott Williams & Wilkins, 2005, pp 133–142.

Gagner M, Inabnet W, Pomp A: Laparoscopic sleeve gastrectomy with second stage biliopancreatic diversion and duodenal switch in the superobese. In Inabnet W, DeMaria E, Ikramuddin S (eds): Laparoscopic Bariatric Surgery. Philadelphia, Lippincott Williams & Wilkins, 2005, pp 143–150.

Marceau P, Hould F, Simard S, et al: Biliopancreatic diversion with duodenal switch. World J Surg 1998;22:947–954.

Prachand V, Davee R, Alverdy J: Duodenal switch provides superior weight loss in the super-obese (BMI >50 kg/m^2) compared with gastric bypass. Ann Surg 2006;255:611–619.

Ren C, Patterson E, Gagner M: Early results of laparoscopic biliopancreatic diversion with duodenal switch: a case series of 40 consecutive patients. Obes Surg 2000;10:514–523.

Scopinaro N, Adami G, Marinari G, et al: Biliopancreatic diversion. World J Surg 1998;22;936–946.

JOSEPH A. CAPRINI

Risk Assessment as a Guide to Thrombosis Prophylaxis in Bariatric Surgical Patients

10

Surgery for morbid obesity has become a popular and successful approach to the escalating problems of obesity and its complications. It has been well documented that the morbidly obese patient undergoing a bariatric surgical procedure is at an elevated risk for developing venous thromboembolism (VTE) compared to the average surgical patient, and that this risk is proportional to the patient's body mass index (BMI). The incidence of fatal pulmonary emboli following bariatric surgery has been estimated to be 1%. In 2002, about 900,00 cases of VTE were documented in U.S. hospitals, and pulmonary embolism was the cause of death in nearly 300,000 patients. About 34% of these latter individuals presented as sudden death, thereby denying the clinician any opportunity for treatment. Nearly one third of these cases occurred in the community following hospital discharge. Chronic pulmonary hypertension occurred in at least 4% of patients who survived a pulmonary embolus and has especial importance in the bariatric group, because they often have underlying pulmonary abnormalities. In light of these notable morbidity and mortality statistics, and the fact that the bariatric patient is at a high risk for this complication, this chapter will be devoted to the prophylaxis of VTE.

THE PROBLEM OF VENOUS THROMBOEMBOLISM

A recent analysis determined that only 85% of surgical patients with four or more VTE risk factors received any sort of postoperative thrombosis prophylaxis. This fact is concerning when one considers that the American College of Chest Physicians (ACCP) chest guidelines have estimated that patients with more than four risk factors for thrombosis have a postoperative mortality rate as high as 5%. These guidelines, which have been published every other year for over a decade, are based on the data from about 900 scientific articles. It is conceivable that the lack of compliance with VTE prophylaxis is secondary to the clinician's fear of postoperative bleeding when anticoagulant prophylaxis is used. The available data do not support this concern, though; a controlled trial in 2005 which employed 23,000 surgical patients and compared postoperative LMWH (low-molecular-weight heparin) versus unfractionated heparin did not document any deaths from bleeding; furthermore, anticoagulant prophylaxis using either drug reduced the incidence of death. In retrospect it is not clear why some clinicians do not use VTE prophylaxis more uniformly. Sudden death from VTE is not treatable, while

bleeding complications from anticoagulant use are almost always treatable, and the risk of death is exceedingly low.

There are a number of other reasons to employ thrombosis prophylaxis in addition to mortality prevention. The post-thrombotic syndrome is a serious condition that affects 25% of individuals following a deep vein thrombosis (DVT). A permanent disability occurs in 7% of these patients, and it is estimated that 2 million workdays are lost annually secondary to this complication. Moreover, about two thirds of patients with a history of DVT will suffer another DVT if they undergo a subsequent operative procedure. Another DVT complication is paradoxic stroke, which may occur if the patient has a patent foramen ovale (present in 25% of the population). If a clot forms in the legs or pelvis and embolizes to the right ventricle, then the right atrium may become dilated. This event can open the foramen so that the clot is able to migrate into the left atrium and then to the brain, causing a nonhemorrhagic stroke. At least one autopsy study implicated the presence of a patent foramen ovale in 50% of patients suffering this type of stroke who were younger than 60 years of age.

Morbidly obese surgical patients are at increased risk of VTE; this risk is increased further by the presence of venous stasis syndrome, a comorbid condition common to this patient group. Venous stasis syndrome, as defined by pitting leg edema, venous stasis ulcers, or pretibial bronze edema, has been associated with a 4% incidence of fatal pulmonary emboli (PE). The fatal PE rate in patients without this syndrome has been shown to be 0.2%. Patients with venous stasis syndrome have a markedly elevated mortality risk secondary to VTE, and their overall perioperative mortality rate is double that seen in patients without the syndrome. In addition, the incidence of postoperative leak, peritonitis, major wound infection, and incisional hernia has been shown to be significantly higher in patients with venous stasis syndrome.

Interestingly, the presence of morbid obesity may exacerbate the manifestations of venous stasis syndrome. For example, a venous stasis ulcer in a morbidly obese patient which fails to heal with compression therapy or skin grafting commonly will heal after major weight loss is achieved. It has been postulated that the increased pressure of the abdominal pannus reduces venous return to the heart, thereby increasing venous pressure in the extremities. In support of this idea is the observation of increased urinary bladder pressure in morbidly obese patients that typically returns to normal 1 year after a bariatric procedure. The interplay of morbid obesity with venous stasis syndrome, and the associated risk for VTE, emphasizes the need to inform patients about the consequences of the venous stasis syndrome, as well as the clinician's need to minimize the thromboembolic complications of this syndrome.

The incidence of VTE in hospitalized patients has attracted the attention of national groups such as The National Quality Forum, which introduced a policy (Safe Practice 17) stating that "each patient should be evaluated upon admission, and periodically thereafter, for the risk of developing deep vein thrombosis and/or pulmonary embolism. Furthermore clinicians should utilize clinically appropriate methods to prevent DVT and PE." Currently, the Joint Commission on Accreditation of Healthcare Organizations is piloting measures to document compliance with Safe Practice 17, and mandatory measures soon may be introduced. The goal of the Surgical Care Improvement Project is to reduce rates of preventable surgical morbidity and mortality by 25% by the year 2010. This organization has endorsed voluntary hospital reporting on (1) the proportion of patients who receive recommended VTE prophylaxis, and on (2) the proportion of patients who receive recommended VTE prophylaxis within 24 hours before or after surgery. Currently only voluntary reporting is required, but mandatory reporting soon may be necessary. In addition, the next step likely will be a pay-for-performance clause; so if compliance with VTE prophylaxis is not achieved, then reduced payments for services will occur for both the hospital and physician.

TECHNIQUES OF VTE PROPHYLAXIS

Current prophylactic measures to prevent VTE in bariatric patients include intermittent pneumatic compression, anticoagulation, and the vena cava filter. The primary intention of the first two treatments is to prevent thrombotic events, while the intention of filter placement is to prevent pulmonary embolism.

Intermittent Pneumatic Compression

Intermittent pneumatic compression (IPC) is an essential prophylactic modality in the morbidly obese patient undergoing a bariatric procedure. The value of IPC has been demonstrated in clinical trials both when used alone and when combined with anticoagulants. When combination therapy is used, very low thrombosis rates have been achieved in the general surgical patient. There are specialized IPC sleeves designed for the bariatric surgical patient; these devices should be fitted before the start of anesthesia and should be continued until the patient is discharged from the hospital. The IPC sleeves may be removed for ambulation only; at all other times the patient should wear them.

Anticoagulation

Studies in general surgery cancer patients demonstrated that the administration of a LMWH for the first 30 days postoperatively produces a reduction in total VTE compared to 7 days of LMWH. At least 12 trials in orthopedic patients demonstrated that using a variety of anticoagulants for 30 days produced a lowered incidence of deep venous thrombosis. The use of small doses of unfractionated heparin for thrombosis prophylaxis in general surgery has been employed since the 1970s. The advantages of this drug include a short half-life, the ability to measure the drug's effect, the ability to reverse the drug's effect, and the familiarity

of the drug among clinicians. The disadvantages of unfractionated heparin include poorly predictable bioavailability, resistance in some patients, need for frequent administration, and the development of the relatively rare but potentially disastrous complication known as heparin-induced thrombocytopenia (HIT). In this syndrome the heparin actually causes the platelets to clump, resulting in widespread thrombosis (and occasionally even death). The incidence of HIT in a recent meta-analysis was 2.6% for unfractionated heparin and 0.2% for LMWH. LMWH agents have increased the utilization of thrombosis prophylaxis. Compared to unfractionated heparin, these heparin derivatives have improved bioavailability when injected subcutaneously and show stable dose-response curves; these qualities improve the clinical utility of these drugs compared with unfractionated heparin. Although the proper dosing scheme has yet to be worked out, it is likely that the usual dose for prophylaxis in the typical general surgical patient will not be adequate for the typical bariatric surgical patient (see the section, Recommendations).

Vena Cava Filter

The indications for preoperative vena cava filter insertion in the bariatric surgical patient has included those with a past history of VTE or pulmonary hypertension. The concept of routine filter utilization in the super-morbidly obese bariatric patient (variably defined as BMI over $50 \, kg/m^2$), however, has represented a change in clinical practice; but this additional indication has been supported by data that indicate a 10% incidence of fatal pulmonary emboli in the subgroup of patients with a BMI greater than $55 \, kg/m^2$. If vena cava filter placement is routine in this patient group, then the incidence of fatal pulmonary emboli drops to zero. Filter placement is not a benign procedure, however, and some protection from PE is offset by the morbidity associated with the placement. The size of the patient (including a massive abdominal pannus), the difficulty in obtaining good-quality fluoroscopic images, and the need to selectively catheterize the renal veins are some of the issues that complicate filter placement in these patients. Further study is needed to help resolve these issues.

RECOMMENDATIONS

In order to tailor prophylaxis to the individual patient, including the modality and length of prophylaxis, individual risk assessment for VTE is important. We use a form that summarizes a comprehensive history and physical examination, outlining the factors that could predispose the patient to thrombosis. Each factor is weighted according to the relative incidence of thrombosis seen with that factor in controlled trials. A prospective validation of this treatment schema is underway at our institution. Variants of this form for the preoperative assessment of VTE risk have been in use by the author since 1988; in addition, this form is easily modified for the bariatric surgical patient (Fig. 10-1).

All patients should be fitted preoperatively with appropriate antiembolism stockings and intermittent pneumatic compression devices. These devices should be worn at all times before, during, and after surgery, unless the patient is fully ambulatory. All patients should receive LMWH (40 mg once every 12 hours), beginning 12 hours after completion of the procedure and lasting for at least 10 days. We recommend the 40-mg dose of LMWH in all bariatric surgical patients unless a contraindication exists. Those individuals with additional risk factors but no venous stasis or past history of VTE (high-risk group) should receive this LMWH therapy for at least 30 days. A bilateral leg duplex scan should be done on postoperative day 30 as a survey for asymptomatic clots. Finally, the highest risk patients (i.e., those with a past history of VTE, a family history of VTE with positive markers, multiple risk factors, BMI greater than 50 kg/m² , or venous stasis syndrome) should undergo preoperative insertion of a permanent vena cava filter, in addition to 30 days of LMWH. We do not yet recommend removable filters, because long-term results are not available in the bariatric surgical group.

VENOUS THROMBOEMBOLISM RISK FACTOR ASSESSMENT

Patient's Name:_____ Age: ___ Sex: ___ Wgt:___ pounds

Choose all that apply

Each risk factor represents 1 point

- ☐ Age 41–60 years
- ☐ Minor surgery planned
- ☐ History of prior major surgery
- ☐ Varicose veins
- ☐ History of inflammatory bowel disease
- ☐ Swollen legs (current)
- ☐ Obesity (BMI > 30 kg/m²)
- ☐ Acute myocardial infarction (<1 month)
- ☐ Congestive heart failure (<1 month)
- ☐ Sepsis (<1 month)
- ☐ Serious lung disease incl. pneumonia (<1 month)
- ☐ Abnormal pulmonary function (COPD)
- ☐ Medical patient currently at bed rest
- ☐ Leg plaster cast or brace
- ☐ Other risk factors _____

Each risk factor represents 3 points

- ☐ Age over 75 years
- ☐ Major surgery lasting 2–3 hours
- ☐ BMI >50 (venous stasis syndrome)
- ☐ History of SVT, DVT/PE
- ☐ **Family history of DVT/PE**
- ☐ Present cancer or chemotherapy
- ☐ Positive factor V Leiden
- ☐ Positive prothrombin 20210A
- ☐ Elevated serum homocysteine
- ☐ Positive lupus anticoagulant
- ☐ Elevated anticardiolipin antibodies
- ☐ Heparin-induced thrombocytopenia (HIT)
- ☐ Other thrombophilia Type _____

Each risk factor represents 2 points

- ☐ Age 60–74 years
- ☐ Major surgery (>60 min)
- ☐ Arthroscopic surgery (>60 min)
- ☐ Laparoscopic surgery (>60 min)
- ☐ Previous malignancy
- ☐ Central venous access
- ☐ Morbid obesity (BMI > 40 kg/m²)

Each risk factor represents 5 points

- ☐ Elective major lower extremity arthroplasty
- ☐ Hip, pelvis or leg fracture (<1 month)
- ☐ Stroke (<1 month)
- ☐ Multiple trauma (<1 month)
- ☐ Acute spinal cord injury (paralysis) (<1 month)
- ☐ Major surgery lasting over 3 hours

For women only (each represents 1 point)

- ☐ Oral contraceptives or hormone replacement therapy
- ☐ Pregnancy or postpartum (<1 month)
- ☐ History of unexplained stillborn infant, recurrent spontaneous abortion (≥3), premature birth with toxemia or growth-restricted infant

Total risk factor score ☐

Please see following page for prophylaxis safety considerations

VTE risk and suggested prophylaxis for surgical patients

Total risk factor score	Incidence of DVT	Risk level	Prophylaxis regimen	Legend
0–1	<10%	Low risk	No specific measures; early ambulation	ES–Elastic stockings IPC–Intermittent pneumatic compression LDUH–Low-dose unfractionated heparin LMWH–Low-molecular-weight heparin FXa I–Factor X inhibitor
2	10–20%	Moderate risk	ES, IPC, LDUH (5000U BID), LMWH (<3400 U)	
3–4	20–40%	High risk	IPC, LDUH (5000U TID), or LMWH (>3400U)	
5 or more	40–80% 1–5% mortality	Highest risk	Pharmacological: LDUH, LMWH (>3400 U),* Warfarin,* or FXa I* alone or in combination with ES or IPC	

* Use for major orthopedic surgery

FIGURE 10-1 Form for the preoperative risk assessment and prophylaxis of venous thromboembolism (VTE). DVT, deep vein thrombosis; PE, pulmonary embolism; SVT, superficial vein thrombosis.

Continued

Prophylaxis safety considerations: Check box if answer is 'YES'

Anticoagulants: Factors associated with increased bleeding
☐ Is patient experiencing any active bleeding?
☐ Does patient have (or has had history of) heparin-induced thrombocytopenia?
☐ Is patient's platelet count <100,000/mm^3?
☐ Is patient taking oral anticoagulants, platelet inhibitors (e.g., NSAIDs, clopidogrel, salicylates)?
☐ Is patient's creatinine clearance abnormal? If yes, please indicate value _____
If any of the above boxes are checked, the patient may not be a candidate for anticoagulant therapy and you should consider alternative prophylactic measures: elastic stockings and/or IPC
Intermittent pneumatic compression (IPC)
☐ Does patient have severe peripheral arterial disease?
☐ Does patient have congestive heart failure?
☐ Does patient have an acute superficial/deep vein thrombosis?
If any of the above boxes are checked, then patient may not be a candidate for intermittent compression therapy and you should consider alternative prophylactic measures.

Based on Geerts WH et al: Prevention of venous thromboembolism. Chest 2004;126(suppl 3):338S-400S; Nicolaides AN et al: 2001 International Consensus Statement: Prevention of Venous Thromboembolism, Guidelines According to Scientific Evidence; Arcelus JI, Caprini JA, Traverso CI: International perspective on venous thromboembolism prophylaxis in surgery. Semin Thromb Hemost 1991;17(4):322-5; Borow M, Goldson HJ: Postoperative venous thrombosis. Evaluation of five methods of treatment. Am J Surg 1981;141(2):245-51; Caprini JA, Arcelus I, Traverso CI et al: Clinical assessment of venous thromboembolic risk in surgical patients. Semin Thromb Hemost 1991;17(suppl 3):304-12; Caprini JA, Arcelus JI et al: State-of-the-art venous thromboembolism prophylaxis. Scope 2001;8:228-240; Caprini JA; Arcelus JI, Reyna JJ: Effective risk stratification of surgical and nonsurgical patients for venous thromboembolic disease. Semin Hematol 2001;38(2)Suppl 5:12-19; Caprini JA: Thrombosis risk assessment as a guide to quality patient care. Dis Mon 2005; 51:70-78; Oger E: Incidence of venous thromboembolism: A community-based study in Western France. Thromb Haemost 2000; 657-660; Turpie AG, Bauer KA, Eriksson BI et al: Fondaparinux vs. Enoxaparin for the prevention of venous thromboembolism in major orthopedic surgery: A meta-analysis of 4 randomized double-blind studies. Arch Intern Med 2002;162(16):1833-40; Ringley et al: Evaluation of intermittent pneumatic compression boots in congestive heart failure. Am Surg 2002;68(3):286-9; Morris et al: Effects of supine intermittent compression on arterial inflow to the lower limb. Arch Surg 2002;137(11):1269-73; Sugerman HJ et al: Ann Surg 2001;234(1):41-46.
REVISED NOVEMBER 4, 2006.
THIS DOCUMENT IS FOR EDUCATIONAL PURPOSES ONLY AND THE OPINIONS EXPRESSED ARE SOLELY THOSE OF THE AUTHOR.

Examiner _____ Date _____

FIGURE 10-1 CONT'D.

Suggested Reading

Bergqvist D, Agnelli G, Cohen AT: Duration of prophylaxis against venous thromboembolism with enoxaparin after surgery for cancer. N Engl J Med 2002;346(13):975–980.

Caprini JA (guest editor): Venous thromboembolism. Disease-a-Month Monograph 2005;51(2–3):68–69.

Carmody BJ, Sugerman HJ, Kellum JM, et al: Pulmonary embolism complicating bariatric surgery: Detailed analysis of a single institution's 24-year experience. J Am Coll Surg 2006;203(6):831–837.

Gargiulo NJ, Veith FJ, Lipsitz EC, et al: Experience with inferior vena cava filter placement in patients undergoing open gastric bypass procedures. J Vasc Surg 2006;44(6):1301–1305.

Geerts WH, Pineo GF, Heit JA, et al: The seventh ACCP conference on antithrombotic and thrombolytic therapy. Chest 2004;126(Suppl 3):338S–400S.

Hamad GG, Choban PS: Low molecular weight heparin prophylaxis (PROBE study). Obesity Surg 2002;15:1368–1374.

Martel N, Lee J, Wells P: Risk for heparin-induced thrombocytopenia with unfractionated and low molecular weight heparin thromboprophylaxis: A meta-analysis. Blood 2005;106(8):2710–2715.

Scholten DJ, Hoedema RM, Scholten SE: A comparison of two different prophylactic dose regimens of low molecular weight heparin in bariatric surgery. Obes Surg 2002;12:19–24.

Sugerman HJ, Sugerman EL, Wolfe L, et al: Risks and benefits of gastric bypass in morbidly obese patients with severe venous stasis disease. Ann Surg 2001;234(1):41–46.

Small Bowel

TALLAL M. ZENI, WILLEM A. BEMELMAN, AND
CONSTANTINE T. FRANTZIDES

Minimally Invasive Procedures on the Small Intestine

11

Minimally invasive small bowel and colorectal operations have gained widespread acceptance as large case series, randomized trials, and systematic reviews have indicated that the laparoscopic approach is feasible, safe, and beneficial. In experienced hands, these procedures can have low conversion rate, acceptable operative times, shorter hospital stays, and faster postoperative recoveries. A higher conversion rate may be seen in patients with prior laparotomy, obesity, enterocutaneous fistula, adhesions, large inflammatory masses, and an emergency operative indication. In general, the transition to a laparoscopic approach to intestinal surgery has not been as complete as it has been with, say, laparoscopic cholecystectomy; this probably is secondary to the increased complexity and technical difficulty of the intestinal procedures. It seems apparent, however, that the transition is ongoing, and the proportion of intestinal operations performed with minimally invasive technique likely will increase in the future.

OPERATIVE INDICATIONS

Laparoscopic operations upon the small intestine include enterectomy, adhesiolysis, Meckel's diverticulectomy, and stricturoplasty. For any of these procedures, the surgeon should be prepared to perform a minimally invasive small bowel resection if indicated. Laparoscopic adhesiolysis for acute bowel obstruction has been described by numerous authors; this procedure remains somewhat controversial, though. If the degree of abdominal distention does not prohibit the laparoscopic approach, then, in general, laparoscopic adhesiolysis can be performed. Other less common indications for laparoscopic small bowel surgery include intussusseption (Fig. 11-1), gallstone ileus (Fig. 11-2), and foreign body removal (Fig. 11-3). A more controversial indication for minimally invasive small bowel surgery is laparoscopy for chronic abdominal pain. A randomized trial has demonstrated that only 27% of the patients undergoing laparoscopy for this indication had subsequent improvement.

Nearly 70% of patients with Crohn's disease will ultimately require surgery; a decision to operate should be considered with long-term medical management. Indications for surgery in patients with Crohn's disease typically include obstruction, fistula, perforation, or simply symptom intractability with inadequate response to medical management. Most often the distal ileum is involved, which would require ileocolic resection of the grossly involved segment only. Intraoperatively, the surgeon may encounter a thickened mesentery, phlegmon, abscess or fistula; any of these can make the procedure more difficult. Nonetheless, these complicating factors are only relative contraindications for laparoscopic resection. Crohn's disease also may be associated with long and short intestinal strictures. Short strictures are best treated with stricturoplasty, and long strictures typically require segmental resection. Nearly 50% of patients will need reoperation within 10 to 15 years and therefore limited resection to only those margins grossly involved is warranted.

Meckel's diverticulum is a congenital abnormality which occurs if the connection between the yolk sac and the midgut (the omphalomesenteric duct) fails to obliterate during gestation. The estimated incidence is 2%; a diverticulum is usually found on the antimesenteric wall of the distal ileum, approximately 10 to 150 cm from the ileocecal valve. Its length and thickness may vary, and there may or may not be a separate mesentery supplied by an abnormal remnant of the distal right vitelline duct artery. The Meckel's diverticulum may contain ectopic tissue such as gastric mucosa, pancreatic tissue, and colonic tissue. A frequent complication of a Meckel's diverticulum is obstruction secondary to intussusception, volvulus, or incarceration within a femoral or inguinal hernia. Another common symptom is bleeding, secondary to acid secretion of ectopic gastric tissue. Diverticulitis also can occur in a Meckel's diverticulum. If any of these complications occur, the diverticulum should be resected. If an asymptomatic Meckel's diverticulum is found incidentally, then the indication to resect is more relative.

Malignant tumors of the small bowel account for less than 1% of gastrointestinal malignancies. Nearly half of these tumors are not diagnosed preoperatively. Carcinoid tumors typically are located in the ileum and, less commonly, in the duodenum. Only 10% of carcinoids are symptomatic, thus making preoperative diagnosis difficult. Lymphomas and sarcomas most commonly are located in the jejunoileum. On the other hand, adenocarcinomas usually are located in the duodenum, and may require pancreaticoduodenectomy. Jejunoileal adenocarcinomas, lymphomas, and carcinoid tumors require wide mesenteric resection and lymphadenectomy, but sarcomas do not because they generally do not metastasize to the lymph nodes. Benign tumors, including leiomyomas, adenomas, lipomas, and Peutz-Jeghers polyps, are less common indications for small bowel resection.

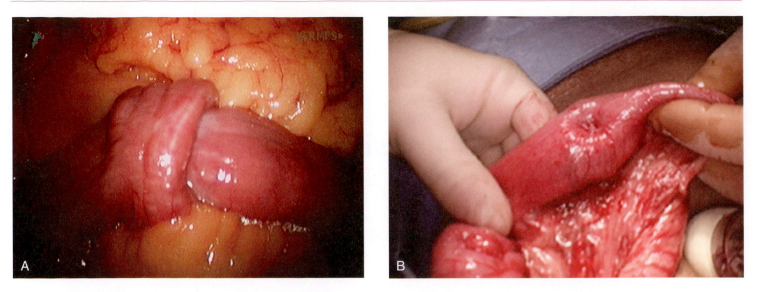

FIGURE 11-1 **A,** Small bowel intussusception. **B,** Small intestinal leiomyoma, which was the lead of the intussusceptum in part A.

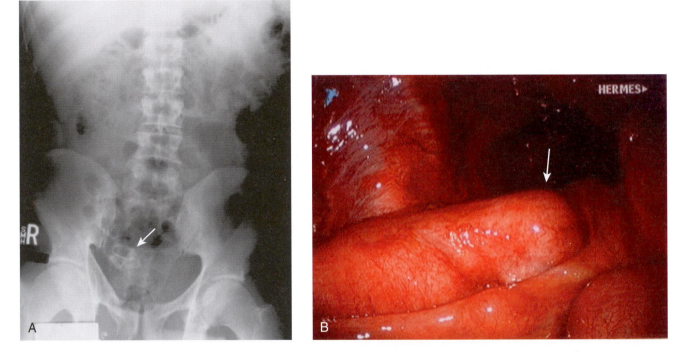

FIGURE 11-2 **A,** Abdominal plain film showing gallstone ileus; note the air-fluid levels and the radiopaque stone in the right lower quadrant *(arrow)*. **B,** Laparoscopic view of the terminal ileum with large intraluminal gallstones *(arrow)*.

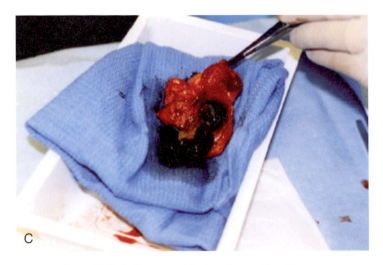

FIGURE 11-2 **C,** The resected ileal specimen with gallstones.

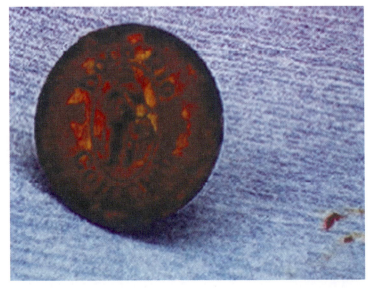

FIGURE 11-3 Foreign body (golf ball marker) extracted laparoscopically from the small intestine.

PREOPERATIVE PREPARATION

Preoperative evaluation of the small bowel in the setting of chronic partial bowel obstruction may be done using small bowel fluoroscopic or computed tomographic (CT) enteroclysis. This is particularly important in Crohn's disease to assess the number and extent of diseased sites. Gastric mucosa in a Meckel's diverticulum may be identified with a ^{99m}Tc-pertechnetate scan, although this investigation has been known to produce false negative results. Small bowel tumors may be diagnosed preoperatively with a CT scan, but these tumors often are an incidental finding at operation. Patients may be prepared for surgery with a Condon-Nichols bowel preparation. Crohn's patients who are on chronic steroids may be given stress doses, if indicated.

PATIENT POSITIONING AND TROCAR PLACEMENT

The patient is placed supine with the legs separated (French position), which enables the surgeon to stand between the patient's legs. The patient's arms should be tucked to allow mobility around the operating table. An infraumbilical cutdown (Hasson technique) is performed for the first trocar. Extension of this incision can be done later for removal of the specimen, if necessary. If an ileocecal or ileal resection will be performed, then two or three additional trocars may be placed in the left upper, left lower, and right upper quadrants. The table is put into a slight Trendelenburg position in order to displace the transverse colon and omentum cephalad. Use of atraumatic instrumentation in handling the small bowel (especially if it is distended) is important to avoid enterotomies. We prefer to use 10-mm atraumatic graspers (Atraugrip, Teleflex Medical, Horsham, PA) for handling the bowel. Certain medications, such as steroids and colchicine, may cause the small bowel to be more friable, so the surgeon should exercise caution.

OPERATIVE TECHNIQUE

Ileocecal Mobilization

A 30-degree scope is inserted via the umbilical port. The omentum is retracted above the transverse colon using atraumatic graspers and with the help of Trendelenburg position. The entire small bowel is run from the ligament of Treitz to the terminal ileum in order to identify the pathologic area. If it is difficult to expose the ligament of Treitz, then the examination may begin at the ileocecal valve. Lateral tilt (rotation) to the right or to the left can be helpful when running the small bowel. The ileocecal area may be mobilized by incising the white line of Toldt from the ileocecal peritoneum up to the hepatic flexure. This may be done with electrocautery (Fig. 11-4) or the harmonic scalpel. After this incision, mobilization of the right colon may be performed bluntly with a sweeping motion of an inflatable balloon retractor (Soft-Wand, Gyrus-ACMI, Southborough, MA) (Fig. 11-5). This maneuver will allow subsequent exteriorization of the small bowel specimen through an extension of the umbilical incision. Adhesions may be lysed with laparoscopic scissors. Aggressive use of the harmonic scalpel or electrocautery for adhesiolysis may result in advertent enterotomy or delayed leak from the site of injury.

Laparoscopic Enterectomy

Segmental small bowel resection can be done totally laparoscopically or in a laparoscopically assisted fashion. Although a totally

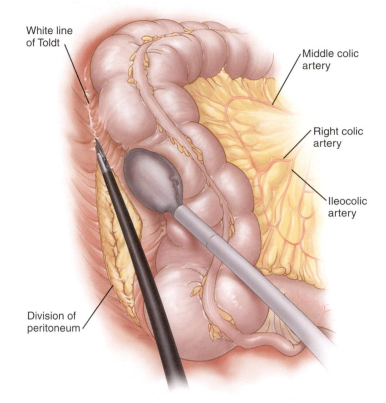

FIGURE 11-4 Incision of the line of Toldt for mobilization of the cecum for an ileocecal resection.

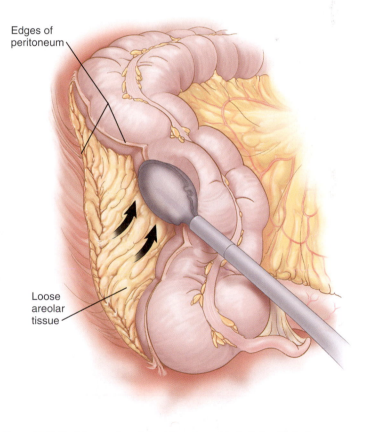

FIGURE 11-5 Medial sweeping of the right colon with the inflatable balloon retractor.

laparoscopic approach may require more time and instrumentation, this technique also may result in a shorter incision; in addition, the surgeon may be able to perform a resection near the ligament of Treitz with a totally laparoscopic approach. For patients with diffuse Crohn's disease, however, evaluation of the small intestine is best done extracorporeally in order to assess strictures. A Baker tube passed into the small bowel can be used to diagnose strictures in areas that may appear grossly normal. Unfortunately, thickening and shortening of the mesentery with Crohn's disease may make exteriorization of the bowel quite difficult, which would necessitate a totally laparoscopic approach. A fistula between small bowel segments may be addressed extracorporeally; a fistula involving the bladder or sigmoid colon, however, may be better handled with intracorporeal stapler division of the involved intestine, with subsequent intracorporeal suture repair as necessary. The ultimate approach depends on the type and extent of the disease, the available instruments, and the comfort level and experience of the surgeon.

Totally Laparoscopic Resection

Use of 12-mm trocars facilitates passage of laparoscopic stapler-cutters; typically, four trocars are required for this approach in order to place the intestine on proximal and distal traction for stapler placement. The bowel may be transected using a 45-mm cartridge with 2.5-mm staples in most circumstances. If the bowel is thickened, then 3.5-mm staples may be more appropriate. Intracorporeal ligation of the small bowel mesentery is done using bipolar or ultrasonic shears (Fig. 11-6). Alternatively, the laparoscopic stapler-cutter may be used to transect the mesentery with vascular cartridges, with or without staple line reinforcement (Seamguard, W. L. Gore & Associates, Flagstaff, AZ). A side-to-side anastomosis can be created with 60-mm, 2.5-mm cartridges of the laparoscopic stapler-cutter. After firing of the stapler, the enterotomy from the stapler can be closed either with another stapler cartridge or by intracorporeal suturing. The specimen is placed in a plastic specimen retrieval bag and is brought out through the umbilical incision.

Laparoscopically Assisted Resection

The assisted approach can help minimize the difficult angles often required for total laparoscopic performance. After full inspection of the small bowel, an atraumatic grasper grasps the affected part of the bowel. The periumbilical incision is extended just large enough (typically 5 cm, but possibly longer in some cases of Crohn's disease) to enable exteriorization of the affected bowel with its mesentery. Once exteriorized, vascular ligation, transection, and the anastomosis can be done in a conventional manner. The abdominal wall should remain completely relaxed until the fresh anastomosis is placed back into the abdomen. Muscle contraction around the incision can narrow the minilaparotomy, resulting in venous congestion of the mesentery with subsequent bleeding.

Laparoscopically Assisted Stricturoplasty

The affected part of the small bowel is exteriorized via an extended infraumbilical incision. The stricture is incised longitudinally and closed transversally using a running suture, as described in conventional operative atlases. A Baker tube should be advanced through this repair and then run through the small bowel both proximally and distally to detect any further strictures.

Laparoscopic Meckel's Diverticulectomy

If the base of the diverticulum is not too broad, then the diverticulum may be transected with a laparoscopic stapler-cutter. The trocar in the left lower quadrant should be a 12-mm port in order to accommodate this instrument. Using an atraumatic grasper inserted in the right lower quadrant, the diverticulum is elevated in order to expose its base. If the diverticulum has a separate mesentery, then this should be transected with a suitable device. A 60-mm, 2.5-mm stapler cartridge is positioned axially in order to create a longitudinal staple line (Fig. 11-7). This stapler orientation makes it easier to perform a complete resection of the diverticulum. The staple line is checked for integrity and bleeding; if necessary, the staple line can be oversewn laparoscopically (with caution, so as to not narrow the lumen). The specimen is

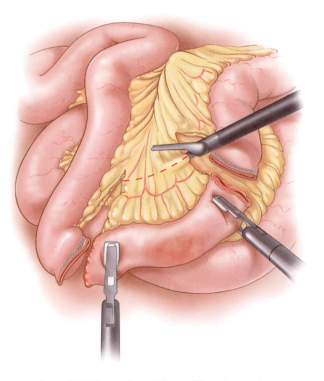

FIGURE 11-6 Transection of the small bowel mesentery.

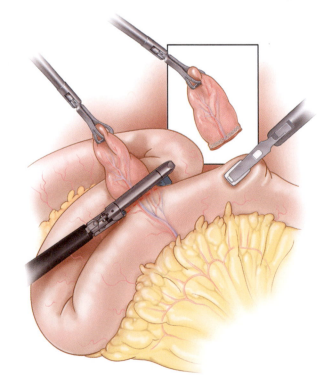

FIGURE 11-7 Application of the laparoscopic stapler-cutter to resect a Meckel's diverticulum.

removed and checked for ectopic tissue on the suture line; some authors advocate a frozen section for this purpose. If the patient with a Meckel's diverticulum has (1) severe bleeding, (2) ectopic tissue, (3) a broad-based diverticulum, or (4) a discrepancy in the bowel diameter, then the diverticulum probably should be treated with a segmental resection, as described earlier.

POSTOPERATIVE CARE

At the end of surgery, both the orogastric tube and indwelling urinary catheter are removed. Patients are started on a liquid diet and encouraged to walk on the day of surgery. Patients without a major resection typically are advanced to a regular diet on postoperative day 1 and discharged as tolerated. For patients who have undergone a resection a liquid diet may be started on postoperative day 1, and then they may be advanced to a regular diet once flatus/bowel movement has occurred. This protocol may need to be adjusted for complicated Crohn's disease patients. The surgeon should always have a high level of suspicion for a missed enterotomy after an extensive adhesiolysis. A low threshold for diagnostic laparoscopy should be maintained, particularly in those patients who have excessive postoperative pain or who fail to resolve their ileus.

PROCEDURE-SPECIFIC COMPLICATIONS

Enterotomy may occur during any laparoscopic procedure on the small bowel. Use of atraumatic graspers is imperative while manipulating the small bowel. Often manipulation of the mesentery in running the bowel is preferable, particularly when the bowel is friable. If an enterotomy is encountered, then the surgeon should be prepared to do intracorporeal repair. Furthermore, repair of serosal injuries should be considered in order to reduce the possibility of a delayed leak. Adhesions should be divided primarily with scissors; electrocautery and the ultrasonic scalpel should be used sparingly to avoid thermal injury to the bowel wall, which can manifest as a delayed leak. Finally, if the surgeon is not satisfied with an intracorporeal anastomosis, then the anastomosis should be exteriorized for inspection and correction.

RESULTS AND OUTCOME

Crohn's disease is the most common indication for small bowel resection. The available data from experienced centers in these patients indicate that pulmonary dysfunction, complication rates, and length of stay in patients undergoing laparoscopically assisted resection are decreased compared to patients undergoing an open resection; operative times tend to be slightly longer in the laparoscopic patients. There does not appear to be much difference in quality of life between the laparoscopic and open surgery patients at later follow-up though. In the hands of experts, laparoscopically assisted resection also has been feasible with a low conversion in the setting of fistulous Crohn's disease, even in the presence of abscess or phlegmon disease. Laparoscopic adhesiolysis for acute small bowel obstruction has a relatively high conversion rate, but patients who have their operation completed laparoscopically typically have a shorter length of stay compared to patients undergoing laparotomy. Of course, patients who can be completed laparoscopically tend to have less extensive adhesions.

Suggested Reading

Bemelman WA, Hugenholtz E, Heij HA, et al: Meckel's diverticulum in Amsterdam: Experience in 136 patients. World J Surg 1995;19(5):734–736.

Canin-Endres J, Salky B, Gattorno F, Edye M: Laparoscopically assisted intestinal resection in 88 patients with Crohn's disease. Surg Endosc 1999;13:595–599.

Khaikin M, Schneidereit N, Cera S, et al: Laparoscopic vs. open surgery for acute adhesive small-bowel obstruction: Patients' outcome and cost-effectiveness. Surg Endosc 2007;21:742–746.

Maartense S, Dunker MS, Slors FM, et al: Laparoscopic-assisted versus open ileocolic resection for Crohn's disease. Ann Surg 2006;243:143–149.

Milsom JW, Hammerhofer KA, Böhm B, et al: Prospective, randomized trial comparing laparoscopic vs. conventional surgery for refractory ileocolic Crohn's disease. Dis Colon Rectum 2001;44(1):1–8.

Regan JP, Salky BA: Laparoscopic treatment of enteric fistulas. Surg Endosc 2004;18(2):252–254.

Swank DJ, Swank-Bordewijk SCG, Hop WCJ, et al: Laparoscopic adhesiolysis in patients with chronic abdominal pain: A blinded randomized controlled multicenter trial. Lancet 2003;361:1247–1251.

Tilney HS, Constantinides VA, Heriot AG, et al: Comparison of laparoscopic and open ileocecal resection for Crohn's disease: A meta-analysis. Surg Endosc 2006;20(7):1036–1044.

Young-Fadok TM, HallLong K, McConnell EJ, et al: Advantages of laparoscopic resection for ileocolic Crohn's disease: Improved outcomes and reduced costs. Surg Endosc 2001;15(5):450–454.

CEDRIC S. F. LORENZO AND
KENRIC M. MURAYAMA

Laparoscopic Feeding Gastrostomy and Jejunostomy

CHAPTER 12

INTRODUCTION

The Importance of Nutrition in Surgical Patients

Operating on malnourished patients is associated with higher morbidity and mortality rates. Inadequate nutrition lasting 5 to 10 days in the surgical patient can manifest as alterations in physiologic function, increased susceptibility to infection, multiorgan system failure, poor wound healing, and death. This is of particular concern when considering 15% to 65% of patients entering a hospital have some degree of malnutrition. Twelve percent of these patients can be classified as severely malnourished. Ultimately, because of ongoing disease states or medically required fasts, 50% to 100% of hospitalized patients become malnourished during their hospitalization. Malnourished surgical patients have up to a 90% longer hospital stay, resulting in 35% to 75% higher hospital charges when compared to their well-nourished counterparts. In most healthy individuals, there are ample nutritional reserves to help avert the effects of malnutrition; however, in those with preexisting or expected prolonged malnutrition, efforts to optimize nutrition should be a priority.

Nutritional supplementation should be provided to patients whose illness is expected to last longer than 5 to 10 days (e.g., pancreatitis, extensive burns, major trauma, sepsis, and peritonitis) and to patients already presenting with a greater than 10% to 15% loss of their usual body weight over 3 months. Nutritional supplementation should also be provided to patients who are unable to eat or who are unable to meet their nutritional requirements.

It is widely accepted that nutritional supplementation utilizing the gastrointestinal tract is preferred over parenteral delivery of nutrients. Intraluminal nutrition promotes intestinal epithelial desquamation and turnover, gut motility, release of many trophic gut hormones, and the maintenance of intestinal villous height and crypt cell production. In turn, this helps maintain host defenses in the gut including the prevention of the translocation of toxic substances and microbes. For these reasons, the gastrointestinal tract should be provided with intraluminal nutrition. Conversely, parenteral nutrition is associated with increased cost, immune suppression, creation of more inflammatory mediators, and gut atrophy and carries the risk of catheter-associated infections. Enteric routes of nutrition are also easier to maintain than parenteral access

devices and allow patients or their caregivers to administer feeding at home and with minimal training. Finally, tube feeds are also cheaper and easier to store than parenteral formulations.

Enteral Access

Providing nutrition through surgically obtained portals into the gastrointestinal (GI) tract was pioneered in 1837 by Egeberg who conceptualized the idea of a surgical gastrostomy. In 1849, Sedillot performed the first successful gastrostomy. Currently, the Stamm method, which uses two concentric purse-string sutures to secure the catheter into the stomach, is the most commonly performed surgical gastrostomy. However, the open surgical gastrostomy largely has been supplanted by the percutaneous endoscopic gastrostomy (PEG) technique described by Gauderer and Ponsky in 1980. This approach utilizes an endoscope to visually guide and assist in the percutaneous placement of a gastrostomy tube over a wire. The PEG technique is a safe and quick procedure that avoids the use of a general anesthetic; furthermore, a PEG can be placed at the bedside with intravenous sedation and local anesthesia. Unfortunately, patients with facial trauma, an inaccessible oral cavity, tumors of the head and neck, an esophageal stricture or obstruction, a large hiatal hernia, or a gastric volvulus are frequently not candidates for a PEG and instead require a surgical gastrostomy.

Alternatively, in patients requiring enteral access for nutrition who are not candidates for a gastrostomy (e.g., gastroparesis, gastric outlet obstruction, severe gastroesophageal reflux, and increased aspiration risk), a surgical jejunostomy may be performed. Various techniques have been described using an open approach. The first jejunostomy was performed by Bush in 1858. In 1878, Surmay de Harve was the first to introduce a feeding catheter by way of an enterostomy. The more commonly used technique today is that described by Witzel in 1891.

In 1990, O'Regan and Scarrow described the first laparoscopic jejunostomy. In 1991, Edelman and Unger described the first laparoscopic gastrostomy. Since then, advances in laparoscopic technology and refinements in technique have resulted in a variety of methods for the laparoscopic placement of gastrostomy and jejunostomy tubes. The safety and efficacy of laparoscopic enteral access have also been validated and is an important adjunct to patient care.

OPERATIVE INDICATIONS

The laparoscopic approach has the potential advantages of smaller incisions, less postoperative pain, decreased wound complications, and better visualization of the peritoneal cavity. Cost analysis also show there is no significant difference between a laparoscopic or open approach to feeding tube placement. Although performing these procedures using conscious sedation and local anesthesia has been described, the laparoscopic approach typically requires general anesthesia with its associated risks. Other less invasive nonsurgical alternatives exist for accessing the gastrointestinal tract for feedings, and these alternatives may be considered prior to a jejunostomy.

Temporary methods for enteral feeding include the placement of a nasogastric (NG) or an orogastric (OG) tube. In a patient with adequate gastric emptying, tube feeds can be initiated on a temporary basis through NG or OG tubes until the patient is able to eat or until more permanent methods of enteral access are obtained. Postpyloric feedings can also be initiated with the nasal or oral placement of specially designed feeding catheters into the duodenum, should gastric emptying be impaired. When prolonged enteral feedings (>4 weeks) are required, a more permanent means of enteral access should be established to avoid the complications of prolonged placement of NG or OG tubes (e.g., pressure ulcers, sinus infections, oronasopharynx irritation, patient discomfort, and poor oral hygiene).

The preferred option for long-term enteral access in patients with a functional stomach and who are candidates for a gastrostomy tube should be a PEG. Feeding gastrostomy tubes should be avoided in patients with a high risk for aspiration, gastroparesis, or gastric outlet obstruction. A PEG can easily be placed at bedside without a general anesthetic. The PEG method has a 96% success rate and has been proved to be safe; this procedure may be difficult, however, in a morbidly obese patient. Furthermore, caution should be taken with patients in whom there may be loops of bowel or a large left liver lobe anterior to the stomach, which places the patient at risk for inadvertent organ injury. Aside from the problems with access secondary to a head/neck malignancy, there also is the risk that a PEG technique may result in seeding of tumor cells into the stomach or the anterior abdominal wall. In patients who are not candidates for a gastrostomy tube placement, a jejunostomy tube is preferred.

The general indications for a gastrostomy or jejunostomy are listed in Table 12-1. In situations in which gastric emptying is problematic and long-term gastric decompression is required, a gastrostomy tube may be placed in order to avoid the complications and drawbacks of long-term NG or OG tube placement.

If long-term gastric decompression is required in conjunction with long-term enteral access for feedings, then both a gastrostomy and jejunostomy tube should be placed.

Simple means of assessing gastric function include monitoring NG or OG tube output over several days. Generally, if NG or OG tube output exceeds 600 to 1000 mL per day, the stomach may not be a suitable conduit for enteral feeding. Most patients also undergo a brief period of enteral feedings through an NG or OG tube. During this period residual gastric contents should be checked every 4 hours. If 50% or more of the total volume of feed delivered remains in the stomach, then the stomach may not have adequate emptying ability. Scintigraphy studies to determine gastric emptying may also be employed for more quantitative data.

Specific indications for the laparoscopic placement of a gastrostomy or jejunostomy tube are summarized in Table 12-2. There are few absolute contraindications to the laparoscopic placement of a gastrostomy or jejunostomy tube, and these essentially are the same reasons a patient would not be a candidate for a feeding tube regardless of the placement method, including overwhelming ascites, carcinomatosis, and an inability to tolerate tube feedings. A contraindication unique to the laparoscopic approach is the inability to tolerate abdominal insufflation and extreme head-up or head-down positioning. Factors which could make the laparoscopic approach difficult include previous abdominal surgery and morbid obesity. An algorithm summarizing the indications for enteral access is shown in Figure 12-1.

PREOPERATIVE EVALUATION, TESTING, AND PREPARATION

Patients requiring placement of a gastrostomy or a jejunostomy tube should be evaluated for surgical risk as in any patient undergoing an operation. Patients or their surrogate decision makers are made aware of the potential risks of the procedure. These include the risks associated with general anesthesia, bleeding, infection, conversion to an open approach, leakage around the tube, and the risk of tube dislodgement. Patients are generally made NPO at least 6 hours before their procedure. In patients with poor gastric emptying, this period may be longer and may require decompression with the placement of an NG or OG tube. Preoperative antibiotics should be given to reduce the risk of wound infection. In particular, antibiotic coverage should

---

Table 12-1 General Indications for Gastrostomy and Jejunostomy Tubes

Gastrostomy Tube
To prevent or treat malnutrition
Long-term gastric decompression
   Inability to swallow due to neurologic deficits
   Head and neck neoplasms

Jejunostomy Tube
To treat malnutrition in patients who are not candidates for a gastrostomy tube
   Gastric outlet obstruction
   Gastroparesis
   Gastroesophageal reflux disease with aspiration
   Difficult or failed gastrostomy

Table 12-2 Specific Indications for Laparoscopic Feeding Tube Placement

Gastrostomy Feeding Tube
Difficult or contraindicated PEG placement
   Large hiatal hernia
   Large Zenker's diverticulum
   Morbid obesity
   Large left liver lobe or overlying bowel
   Failed PEG
   Esophageal obstruction or stricture
   Facial trauma with wired mandible
Early catheter dislodgement with a free gastric perforation
Concomitant laparoscopy or general anesthesia for another procedure

Jejunostomy Feeding Tube
All patients with indications for a jejunostomy (see Table 12-1)
Concomitant laparoscopy or general anesthesia for another procedure
Difficult laparoscopic gastrostomy

PEG, percutaneous endoscopic gastrostomy.

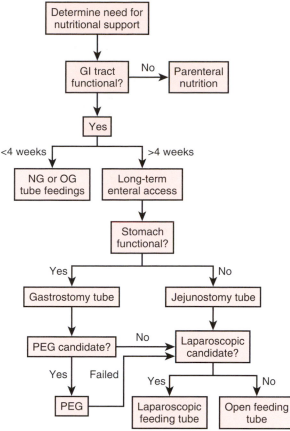

FIGURE 12-1 Algorithm for obtaining enteral access. GI, gastrointestinal; NG, nasogastric; OG, orogastric; PEG, percutaneous endoscopic gastrostomy.

include *Staphylococcus aureus* and beta-hemolytic streptococci (see Chapter 31). Deep venous thrombosis prophylaxis should be based on established guidelines. In general, lower extremity sequential compression devices should be placed on the patient prior to induction of anesthesia. In appropriate cases, heparin should be administered.

OPERATIVE TECHNIQUE

Many methods for the laparoscopic placement of gastrostomy and jejunostomy tubes have been described. We will describe a commonly performed technique that is simple, reproducible, and standardized and which utilizes a prepackaged kit incorporating T-fastener technology (Fig. 12-2). This method obviates the need for any special laparoscopic instrumentation, is relatively simple, and does not require laparoscopic suturing skills.

Gastrostomy Tube

Abdominal access is obtained using either a closed or open technique with abdominal insufflation of carbon dioxide to 10 to 12 mm Hg. A 10-mm, 30-degree laparoscope then is inserted at the umbilicus. The stomach is identified and a 5-mm port is placed directly over this organ in the left upper quadrant. This port site eventually will become the exit site for the gastrostomy tube. An atraumatic grasper then is used to select an appropriate site on the anterior wall of the stomach for insertion of the gastrostomy tube. The site selected should reach the anterior abdominal wall at the site of the 5-mm port without undue tension. A standard prepackaged percutaneous gastrostomy kit (Ross Laboratories, Columbus, OH) is used. Specially designed T-fasteners are passed through the abdominal wall and through

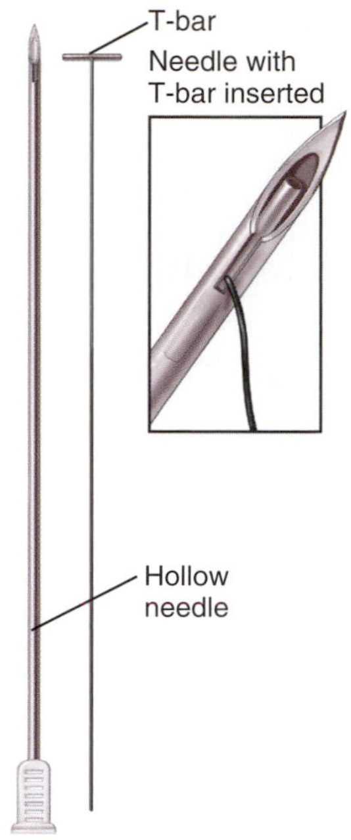

FIGURE 12-2 T-fastener and introducer needle.

the anterior wall of the stomach (Fig. 12-3). Insufflating the stomach using an NG or OG tube may help prevent placement of the T-fasteners through the posterior wall of the stomach. Four T-fasteners are placed around the 5-mm port site. This creates a "four corners" support of the stomach (Fig. 12-4) which then is used to elevate the anterior wall of the stomach to the abdominal wall. The 5-mm port then is removed, and an 18-gauge introducer needle is placed through the same hole and into the lumen of the stomach (Fig. 12-5). A guidewire then is passed through the needle, and the tract is serially dilated from 12 to 22 F. An 18-F laparoscopic gastrostomy tube is passed over the wire (Fig. 12-6). The gastrostomy tube's anchoring balloon then is inflated with 15 mL of normal saline. Once completed, special metal crimps included with each T-fastener are secured to ensure the anterior wall of the stomach remains in contact with the anterior abdominal wall. Cotton bolsters are situated between the skin and the metal

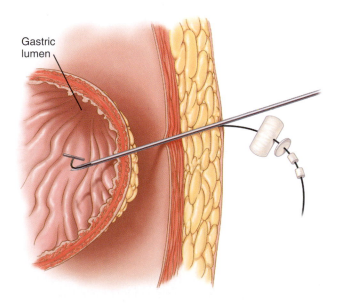

FIGURE 12-3 T-fastener being placed transabdominally and into the stomach.

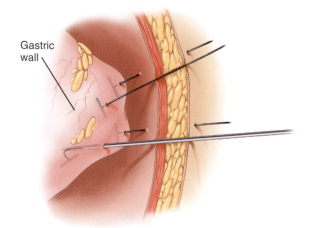

Gastric wall

FIGURE 12-4 Four T-fasteners elevating the anterior abdominal wall of the stomach.

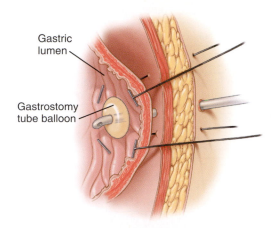

Gastric lumen

Gastrostomy tube balloon

FIGURE 12-6 Four T-fasteners with the gastrostomy tube placed in the elevated stomach.

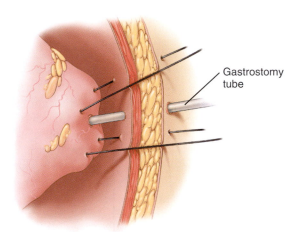

Gastrostomy tube

FIGURE 12-5 Four T-fasteners elevating the anterior wall of the stomach with the Seldinger needle penetrating the wall of the stomach.

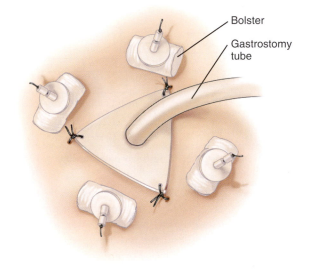

Bolster

Gastrostomy tube

FIGURE 12-7 External view of the completed gastrostomy tube with the four cotton bolsters in place and the metal crimps just external to the bolsters.

crimps to alleviate any undue pressure on the patient's skin. The external appearance of the completed laparoscopic gastrostomy is demonstrated in Figure 12-7. The laparoscope and the 10-mm port are then removed and the pneumoperitoneum released. The fascia at the umbilical incision is closed, followed by skin closure of all ports.

Jejunostomy Feeding Tube

With the patient in the supine position, abdominal access is obtained using an open or closed technique followed by abdominal insufflation with carbon dioxide to 10 to 12 mm Hg. A 10-mm laparoscope then is inserted at the umbilicus. If possible, the stomach should be decompressed using an NG or OG tube. A 5-mm port then is inserted in the lower midline followed by a second 5-mm port about two fingerbreadths below the left subcostal margin, at about the midrectus position. The patient is placed in the Trendelenburg position, which aids in the reflection of the omentum and transverse colon cephalad. The ligament of Treitz then is identified, and the small bowel is measured using a "hand-over-hand" technique. An appropriate site is identified about 30 to 40 cm distal to the ligament of Treitz. The small bowel should be brought to the anterior abdominal wall at the projected site of the jejunostomy tube without

any tension. A site to the left and slightly superior to the umbilicus is often adequate. A prepackaged laparoscopic jejunostomy kit (Ross Laboratories) provides a simple and reproducible enteral access method. The first T-fastener is placed approximately 2 cm proximal to the selected site on the bowel for jejunostomy placement (Fig. 12-8). Four T-fasteners are placed in a linear fashion along the antimesenteric wall of the small bowel. Two T-fasteners proximal and two distal should flank the projected site of the tube (Fig. 12-9). Although the T-fasteners can be placed in a diamond-shaped configuration around the tube site, we favor the linear pattern in order to minimize the risk of small bowel volvulus around the tube. Using the T-fasteners, the small bowel then is brought in contact with the abdominal wall, where it is cannulated using an 18-gauge introducer needle. A guidewire is passed through the needle into the jejunum, and the needle then is exchanged for an introducer with a peel-away sheath via the Seldinger technique. The feeding tube is passed through the introducer into the lumen of the bowel, and the peel-away sheath is removed. The feeding tube should be observed going distally without coiling or kinking. The feeding tube can be flushed to assess for patency or problems with the placement. An intraoperative fluoroscopic examination can be obtained if there is any doubt regarding the feeding tube location or position. Once

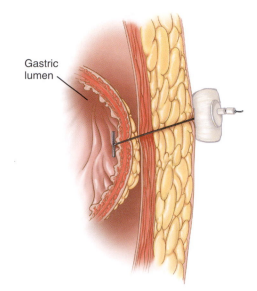

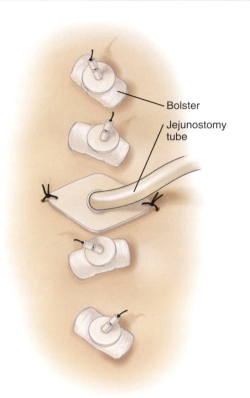

FIGURE 12-8   Cross section of T-fastener elevating the jejunum to the anterior abdominal wall.

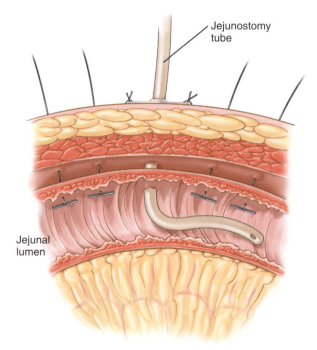

FIGURE 12-9   Jejunostomy tube in the jejunum with four T-fasteners in place.

FIGURE 12-10   External view of the completed jejunostomy tube with the four in-line cotton bolsters of the T-fasteners in place.

completed, special metal crimps included with each T-fastener are secured to ensure the small bowel remains in contact with the anterior abdominal wall. Cotton bolsters are situated between the skin and the metal crimps to alleviate any undue pressure on the patient's skin. The external view of the completed laparoscopic jejunostomy is demonstrated in Figure 12-10. The laparoscope and all ports are removed, and the pneumoperitoneum released. The laparoscope port fascia then is closed, followed by closure of the skin at all port sites.

POSTOPERATIVE CARE

Simple wound care should be implemented after surgery. The skin site frequently should be inspected for infection and leakage. Leakage around the catheter may indicate inadequate apposition of the viscera to the anterior abdominal wall. This may be resolved with tightening of the plastic bolster against the skin surface while gently pulling up on the catheter to appose the viscera and abdominal wall. At about 2 weeks after surgery, the cotton bolsters accompanying each T-fastener should be removed by cutting the nylon suture at the skin site and allowing the T-bar to either remain in the submucosa or pass into the lumen. If these cotton bolsters are left in place they tend to collect debris and cause localized wound infections.

Feedings can usually be initiated on the first postoperative day. The volume of tube feedings gradually should be increased to the patient's goal rate over a few days. Frequent assessments of the patient's ability to tolerate tube feeds should be made, and the rate of feedings adjusted accordingly. Routine water flushes should be done before and after tube feedings in order to prevent the clogging of the feeding tubes. For patients on continuous tube feedings, water flushes every 6 hours should be done. Medications ideally should be converted to a liquid formulation. When this is not possible, pills should be thoroughly crushed and administered as a slurry followed by a water flush in order to prevent clogging. Patients who can tolerate head elevation should have the head of the bed elevated at least 30 degrees at all times. This simple adjunct can help minimize the risk of aspiration. Furthermore, the use of promotility agents such as metoclopramide may be beneficial in appropriate patients in order to promote gastric emptying.

PROCEDURE-SPECIFIC COMPLICATIONS

The most common intraoperative complication encountered using T-fasteners is penetration of the gastric or jejunal backwall. All attempts should be made to identify this at the time of surgery, which then will allow for repair of the defect using a laparoscopic approach or, if necessary, with conversion to an open approach. Insufflation of the stomach prior to placement of the T-fasteners may help prevent this complication.

The most common complications after laparoscopic jejunostomy or gastrostomy tube placement include infection and leakage at the tube exit site. Most local wound infections can be managed conservatively without hospitalization. Death within the first 30 days attributed directly to the procedure is a rare complication, and most commonly is attributed to aspiration pneumonia. This complication may be avoided by keeping the patient's head slightly elevated, administering prokinetic agents when appropriate, and continuing to monitor tolerance to tube feedings.

Complication rates from laparoscopic gastrostomy tube placement range from 5% to 10%, which compares favorably with complication rates reported for open gastrostomy. Complication rates for laparoscopic jejunostomy range from 0% to 26%; this includes a reoperation rate of 1% to 2%, most commonly for jejunal volvulus or early tube dislodgement. Another cause for reoperation is unrecognized bowel injury. Complication rates for laparoscopic jejunostomy also compare favorably to open jejunostomy. Late tube dislodgements for both gastrostomy and jejunostomy tubes frequently can be resolved with simple replacement of the feeding tube through a mature tract, which sometimes requires radiographic guidance.

Results and Outcome

Preventing and treating malnutrition in the surgical patient should be a top priority. Efforts toward supplemental nutrition should be directed toward utilizing the patient's own digestive tract when possible, optimizing nutritional status while promoting gastrointestinal health and avoiding the complications of parenteral nutrition. When eating becomes impaired, the surgeon has the ability to obtain enteral access using several methods. When indicated, the laparoscopic placement of gastrostomy and jejunostomy tubes has been shown to be safe, economic, and effective. In addition, the benefits of laparoscopic surgery also are realized in these patients, including faster recovery time, decreased postoperative pain, and minimal wound complications. The method described is a simple, reproducible technique that all surgeons with basic laparoscopic skills and instrumentation can keep in their armamentarium.

Suggested Reading

Duh Q, Senokozlieff-Englehart AL, Choe YS, et al: Laparoscopic gastrostomy and jejunostomy. Arch Surg 1999;134:151–156.

Gauderer MWL, Ponsky JL, Izant RJ: Gastrostomy without laparotomy: Percutaneous endoscopic technique. J Pediatr Surg 1980;15:872–875.

Han-Geurts IJM, Lim A, Stijnen T, et al: Laparoscopic feeding jejunostomy. Surg Endosc 2005;19:951–957.

Ho HS, Ngo H: Gastrostomy for enteral access: A comparison among placement by laparotomy, laparoscopy, and endoscopy. Surg Endosc 1999;13:991–994.

Murayama KM, Johnson TJ, Thompson JS: Laparoscopic gastrostomy and jejunostomy are safe and effective for obtaining enteral access. Am J Surg 1996;172:591–595.

Murayama KM, Schneider PD, Thompson TJ: Laparoscopic gastrostomy: A safe method for obtaining enteral access. J Surg Res 1995;58:1–5.

Nagle AP, Murayama KM: Laparoscopic gastrostomy and jejunostomy. J Long Term Eff Med Implants 2003;14(1):1–11.

Rolandelli RH, Gupta D, Wilmore DW: Nutritional management of hospitalized patients. In: Souba WW, Wilmore DW, Fink MP, et al (eds): ACS Surgery: Principles and Practice 2007. New York, WebMD Professional Publishing, 2007. Accessed at www.acssurgery.com.

Colon and Rectum

CHAPTER

KIRK A. LUDWIG

Hand-Assisted Minimally Invasive Right Colectomy

13

A minimally invasive right colectomy has two basic approaches: (1) the standard lateral to medial approach, in which the ileocolic artery is taken near its origin as the initial maneuver; (2) the retroperitoneal approach, in which the peritoneum is incised at the base of the small bowel mesentery from the right lower quadrant up to the duodenum, and then the ileal and right colon mesentery are lifted off the retroperitoneum to the hepatic flexure, while the lateral attachments are left in place. It is valuable for the laparoscopic surgeon to be facile with each approach, because they each have their advantages. The approach to minimally invasive right colectomy for this chapter, however, will be the hand-assisted technique. This choice is based on the fact that this technique can be applied in everyday practice by the average surgeon. The hand-assisted approach helps overcome most of the common problems associated with laparoscopic colon surgery, as discussed below.

Laparoscopic colon surgery has a steep and long learning curve, requiring around 20 to 50 cases for proficiency. Given that the average general surgeon in the United States performs fewer than 20 colectomies a year of which 50% may not be candidates for laparoscopy, it might take 5 to 10 years to ascend the learning curve. Operative times for laparoscopic colectomy tend to be long, and there is a fairly high conversion rate. In both the COST and CLASSIC trials (see Suggested Reading), the average operative time for laparoscopic colectomy was almost an hour longer than for open colectomy; the conversion rates were greater than 20%. There has been no argument that minimally invasive colectomy is a technically demanding procedure.

Hand-assisted laparoscopic surgery has several characteristics that may make minimally invasive colectomy less demanding for the average general surgeon. The hand-assisted technique typically does not require a second surgeon as an assistant. In the obese patient, this approach may enable the average surgeon to complete a minimally invasive procedure that otherwise might have been converted. The hand-assisted technique may reduce both the operative time and the conversion rate. In patients with previous surgery (i.e., cholecystectomy), or a bulky tumor, the hand-assisted technique may facilitate the lysis of adhesions and specimen mobilization. Moreover, the author's experience in teaching the hand-assisted laparoscopic surgery is that this technique is adopted more readily by the average surgeon.

There has been debate on whether hand-assisted laparoscopic colectomy is associated with the same short-term benefits compared to the standard laparoscopic operation. For instance, the average surgeon will need an incision of about 7 cm to insert the hand-assisted device. The average specimen extraction excision in the COST and CLASSIC trials, however, was 6 to 7 cm. Some authors have argued that the hand-assisted technique is not as "gentle" as the standard laparoscopic approach; this claim is very difficult to substantiate with hard data. The controlled data that have appeared to date, however, generally supports the notion that hand-assisted laparoscopic colectomy actually does have the same short-term benefits as the standard laparoscopic operation.

OPERATIVE INDICATIONS

The vast majority of right colectomies are performed to manage neoplastic disease, either invasive cancers or endoscopically unresectable polyps. A not infrequent indication for laparoscopic segmental colon resection is a malignant polyp that has been removed colonoscopically. If the polypectomy fails to meet one or more of the accepted criteria for a curative polypectomy, then an oncologic resection is indicated. In these situations, the operation is conducted to remove the area of bowel involved so as to ensure that there is no cancer left within the bowel wall itself and to do a regional lymphadenectomy to remove potentially involved nodes. Less common indications for a laparoscopic right colectomy include right colonic bleeding from a vascular malformation, or inflammatory disease due to right colon diverticulitis. Ileocecal resections may be performed for ileocecal Crohn's disease. For this indication, there is no particular need to take the middle colic vessels.

The oncologic right colectomy involves the following maneuvers: (1) proximal lymphovascular pedicle ligation and complete lymphadenectomy; (2) wide en bloc resection of tumor-bearing bowel segment with adjacent soft tissue and mesentery; (3) avoidance of tumor contamination to the surgical field. An oncologic right colectomy proceeds with proximal ligation of the ileocolic pedicle and the right branch of the middle colic artery for cecal tumors, or the entire middle colic pedicle for tumors in the ascending colon up to the proximal transverse colon. The ileum is divided about 6 inches from the ileocecal valve, which corresponds to a point on the small bowel at which the superior mesenteric artery ends. The transverse colon is divided at its midpoint.

Relative contraindications to a minimally invasive right colectomy include a large inflammatory mass that can be externally palpated, small bowel or cecal dilatation from an obstructing right colon tumor, and perforation with generalized peritonitis. Obesity may or may not be a relative contraindication; some morbidly obese males can have a tremendous amount of intra-abdominal (i.e., mesenteric and omental) fat, which can make a laparoscopic procedure extremely difficult.

PREOPERATIVE EVALUATION, TESTING, AND PREPARATION

For patients being prepared for surgery, a thorough preoperative assessment of cardiac, pulmonary, and nutritional status should be made. Smoking cessation and nebulizer therapy may be required before a patient can safely be brought to the operating room. Patients presenting with significant malnutrition, defined by a loss of more than 10% to 15% of their baseline body weight over a short period of time (3 to 4 months), and with low serum albumin levels (less than 3 g/dL) are at increased risk for infection and fascial/anastomotic dehiscence. Under these circumstances the surgeon should consider, if feasible, the use of preoperative nutritional supplementation.

For patients presenting with a nonobstructing, nonperforated colonic carcinoma, a preoperative colonoscopy is performed to exclude synchronous disease. If the lesion is small, then it should be marked with an India ink tattoo. The author's general rule for right-sided lesions is that all should be marked with an India ink tattoo unless the lesion is adjacent to the ileocecal valve. Ideally, the tattoo should be placed in multiple quadrants near the lesion, which will make subsequent identification easier for the surgeon.

A staging computed tomography (CT) scan of the abdomen and pelvis typically is performed prior to a laparoscopic right colectomy for neoplasia and is helpful for tumor staging. The risk of an infectious complication may be reduced by employing a standard bowel preparation such as 4 L of polyethylene glycol or two doses of an oral sodium phosphate solution on the morning before operation. This mechanical preparation is followed later that day by the oral antibiotic preparation, with three doses of neomycin and either erythromycin or metronidazole taken in the afternoon and evening. Intravenous antibiotics are administered in the preoperative holding area. In addition, most patients may be treated prophylactically with either heparin or a low-molecular-weight heparin derivative.

POSITIONING AND PLACEMENT OF TROCARS

The patient is placed supine on the operating table, intermittent compression devices are placed, a general anesthetic is administered, and a urinary catheter is inserted (Fig. 13-1). Pressure points are padded, and the patient is secured to the table in order that extremes of bed tilt may be utilized. Tucking both arms is more secure for the patient and provides the surgeon with maximal mobility around the table. The patient is prepped from the nipples to the midthigh level, and towels are placed wide on the abdomen and held in position with an adhesive drape.

The hand-assist device is placed in the midline, centered on the umbilicus (Fig. 13-2). The incision size for the device typically is the size of the surgeon's glove in centimeters; sometimes this incision actually can be a centimeter less. In patients who

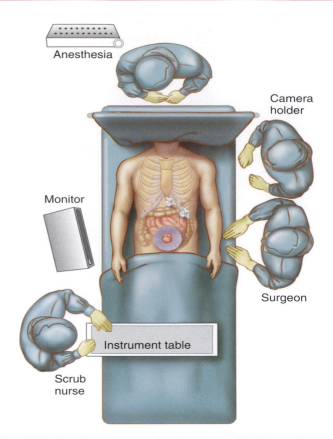

FIGURE 13-1 Operating room set-up for a hand-assisted right hemicolectomy.

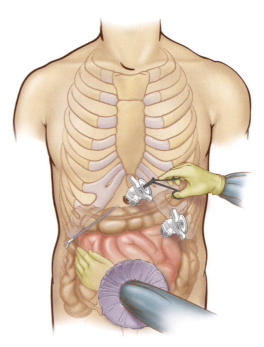

FIGURE 13-2 Trocar and hand port placement for hand-assisted right hemicolectomy.

are long from umbilicus to xiphoid, the incision can be moved slightly up; in patients who are long from pubis to umbilicus, the incision can be moved slightly down. The author uses the GelPort (Applied Medical, Rancho Santa Margarita, CA) hand-assist device. Instruments or staplers may be placed right through this device, even with the hand in place; in addition, the surgeon's hand can be brought in and out of the abdomen without losing pneumoperitoneum.

Pneumoperitoneum then is established through a 5-mm port inserted through the hand-assist device. Two 5-mm ports then are placed, one in the subxiphoid region (for the laparoscope) and one in the left upper quadrant (for the dissecting instrument). The latter port typically is placed in the midclavicular line, about halfway between the costal margin and the upper aspect of the hand-assist incision. When doing hand-assisted laparoscopic surgery, the author uses 5-mm ports exclusively, including a 5-mm, 30-degree laparoscope. If one needs to place a stapling device, then it can be placed through the hand-assist device. For an energy source, the author prefers the 5-mm LigaSure (Valleylab, Boulder, CO) device, which may be used to ligate the named mesenteric vessels; ultrasonic shears also may be used for this purpose.

OPERATIVE TECHNIQUE

The camera operator stands at the patient's left shoulder. The surgeon also is on the left, below the operator. The patient is placed in steep reverse Trendelenburg position, and is rotated to the left. The abdomen is explored visually, and then the liver is palpated. The subsequent minimally invasive right colectomy can be divided into five steps.

Step 1: Hepatic Flexure

The surgeon uses the left hand to grasp the greater omentum along the greater curve of the stomach, and creates a defect just distal to the gastroepiploic vessels. The lesser sac is entered, and the smooth, shiny back of the transverse mesocolon should be visible. This space is developed by taking the greater omentum off the stomach. As the surgeon moves to the right, the anterior surface of the duodenum is exposed, and the hepatic flexure comes into view. The hepatic flexure is mobilized, which should allow Gerota's fascia to be viewed.

Step 2: Right Colon Mesentery

The right colon mesentery is mobilized from the retroperitoneum. In this location there may be a temptation to go directly to the lateral attachments. It usually is easier to mobilize medially first, leaving the lateral attachments for later. The filmy attachments between the third part of the duodenum and the ileal and right colon's mesentery should be divided. This will expose the duodenum over to the ligament of Treitz. This mobilization is helpful for the subsequent transection of the mesentery to the specimen.

Step 3: Ileal Mesentery

With the right colon and ileal mesentery mobilized from the retroperitoneum, the ileal mesentery is draped over the surgeon's hand, and the peritoneum at the base of the mesentery is incised from the right lower quadrant to the duodenum. This maneuver should expose the right retroperitoneum. The duodenum, the head of the pancreas, and Gerota's fascia should be visible. The ureter and gonadal vessels may be seen beneath Toldt's fascia, which covers the right retroperitoneum. The surgeon should avoid the temptation at this point to exteriorized the specimen for transection of the mesentery, because extracorporeal high ligation of the feeding vessels is difficult.

Step 4: Mesenteric Transection

The surgeon grasps the transverse colon in the palm, works a finger down to the base of the transverse mesocolon to the left of the middle colic vessels, and creates a window in this area. The surgeon then moves across the base of the transverse mesocolon from left to right, ligating the middle colic vessels just over the pancreas with the LigaSure or ultrasonic shears. It is advisable to leave a stump of vessel behind in case there is bleeding. After the middle colic vessels have been ligated, there is usually a free space in the mesentery, and the surgeon can feel a decrease in tension on the mesentery. The ileocolic pedicle then is encountered; in about 90% of patients, the right colic artery is a branch of the ileocolic artery or the middle colic artery, so one should not routinely expect to find a right colic artery between the middle colic and ileocolic vessels (Fig. 13-3). The identity of the ileocolic artery may be verified by placing the hepatic flexure back in its place, and then grasping the cecum and pulling it down and to the right. This maneuver will "tent" the ileocolic artery for anatomic confirmation. The hepatic flexure then is pushed back into the left side of the abdomen, and the vessels are ligated with the LigaSure or ultrasonic shears. Similar to the middle colic vessels, a 2-cm stump of the ileocolic vessel should be left on the superior mesenteric artery in case there is bleeding. If the mesenteric vessels are calcified, then it may be advisable to control them with a laparoscopic stapler passed through the hand-assist device alongside the surgeon's hand. After the ileocolic artery has been divided, the mesenteric window between the ileocolic and the superior mesenteric vessels is incised out to the marginal vessel of the ileum.

Step 5: Anastomosis

The pneumoperitoneum is evacuated, the 5-mm ports are removed, and the bowel ends are extracted through the hand-assist device. The marginal vessels along the ileum and the transverse colon are divided, the bowel is divided, and an ileocolic anastomosis is performed. The bowel then is dropped back into the abdomen, the hand-assist device is removed, and the fascia at the umbilicus is closed with a running absorbable suture. The mesenteric defect is generally not closed; the anastomosis should sit comfortably in the right upper quadrant, and the small bowel should lie anterior to this.

POSTOPERATIVE CARE

Postoperative pain is managed with a PCA pump. On postoperative day 1, the nasogastric tube and urinary catheter are removed; the patient is offered clear liquids and is encouraged to ambulate. On postoperative day 2, liquids are continued, the diet is advanced as tolerated, the PCA pump is discontinued, and pain is managed with oral narcotics or an intravenous nonsteroidal anti-inflammatory agent. On postoperative day 3, a soft diet is offered if the patient's abdomen is flat and the patient is tolerating liquids. As soon as the patient can tolerate a diet and is having bowel function (generally passage of stool), he or she can be discharged to home. This usually occurs on postoperative day 3 to 5, depending on the patient's age, home situation, motivation, and anxiety level.

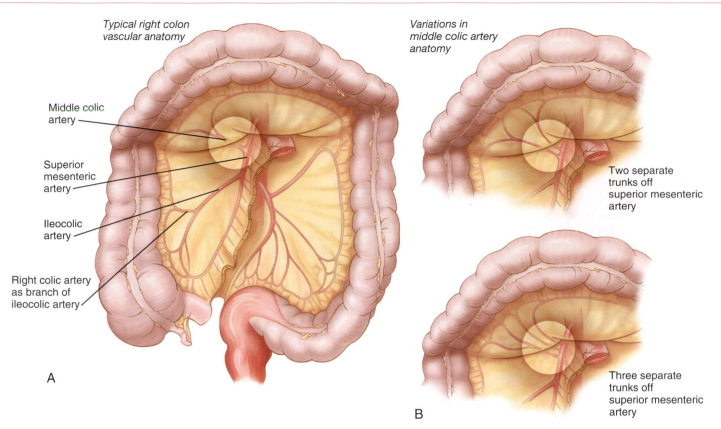

Typical right colon vascular anatomy

Middle colic artery

Superior mesenteric artery

Ileocolic artery

Right colic artery as branch of ileocolic artery

A

Variations in middle colic artery anatomy

Two separate trunks off superior mesenteric artery

Three separate trunks off superior mesenteric artery

B

FIGURE 13-3 **A,** Blood supply to the colon, demonstrating the pertinent arteries in a right hemicolectomy. **B,** Anatomic variations of the blood supply to the right and transverse colon.

PROCEDURE-SPECIFIC COMPLICATIONS

The surgeon should be aware of the well-described complications of colon surgery, including infection, intra-abdominal abscess, anastomotic leak, and bleeding. These complications of colorectal procedures are managed no differently after laparoscopic resection than after open surgery. For management of procedure-specific complications of minimally invasive right colectomy, the reader is referred to the other chapters on laparoscopic colectomy in this book. With regard to conversion, a laparoscopic exploration that results in a conversion to an open operation should not be regarded as a mistake or a complication.

RESULTS AND OUTCOME

Only a limited amount of controlled data on hand-assisted laparoscopic colon surgery has been published. Most studies have grouped multiple types of procedures, or have focused on sigmoid resection for diverticulitis. The conclusions drawn from this limited data are that hand-assisted colon resection is equivalent to standard laparoscopic colon resection in terms of operative time, incision length, conversion rate, complication rate, return of bowel function, and length of stay. In some studies, the operative times and conversion rates have been lower with the hand-assisted technique. Unpublished data (submitted) from the author's institution have indicated that operative times between open surgery and hand-assisted right colectomy were similar, but shorter compared to that of standard laparoscopic right colectomy. Both minimally invasive

approaches to right colon resection had a lower complication rate and shorter length of stay compared to the open approach. Based on the preceding data and personal experience, it has been the author's preference to employ the hand-assisted technique for minimally invasive right colon resection.

Suggested Reading

Abraham NS, Young JM, Solomon MJ: Meta-analysis of short-term outcomes after laparoscopic resection for colorectal cancer. Br J Surg 2004;91:1111–1124.

The Colon Cancer Laparoscopic or Open Resection Study Group: Laparoscopic surgery versus open surgery for colon cancer: Short-term outcomes of a randomized trial. Lancet Oncol 2005;6:477–484.

Fleshman JW, Nelson H, Peters WR, et al: Early results of laparoscopic surgery for colorectal cancer: Retrospective analysis of 372 patients treated by Clinical Outcomes of Surgical Therapy (COST) Study Group. Dis Colon Rectum 1996;39: S53–58.

Guillou, PJ, Quirke P, Thorpe H, et al: Short-term endpoints of conventional versus laparoscopic-assisted surgery in patients with colorectal cancer (MRC CLASSIC trial): Multicenter, randomized controlled trial. Lancet 2005;365:1718–1726.

HALS Study Group: Hand-assisted laparoscopic surgery vs. standard laparoscopic surgery for colorectal disease: A prospective randomized trial. Surg Endosc 2000;14:896–901.

Lacy AM, Garcia-Valdecasas JC, Delgado S, et al: Laparoscopic assisted colectomy vs. open colectomy for treatment of non-metastatic colon cancer: A randomized trial. Lancet 2002;359:2224–2229.

Nakajima K, Lee SW, Cocilovo C: Hand assisted laparoscopic colorectal surgery using GelPort. Surg Endosc 2003;18:102–105.

Nelson H, Sargent D, Fleshman J: Clinical outcomes of surgical therapy study group of the laparoscopic colectomy trial: A comparison of laparoscopically assisted and open colectomy for colon cancer. N Engl J Med 2004;350:2050–2059.

Weeks JC, Nelson H, Gelber S, et al: Short term quality of life outcomes following laparoscopic assisted colectomy versus open colectomy for colon cancer: A randomized trial. JAMA 2002;287:321–328.

CONSTANTINE T. FRANTZIDES, LUIS E. LAGUNA, AND
MARK A. CARLSON

Minimally Invasive Transverse Colectomy

14

Controlled data in the first half of the 2000s demonstrated that the oncologic outcome of minimally invasive colon resection for adenocarcinoma in tertiary centers was not inferior to that of open resection. In fact, in some publications there was the suggestion that oncologic outcome was better with the laparoscopic approach. Prior to the publication of this data, a growing body of evidence indicated that patients who had a minimally invasive colon resection had a better short-term outcome (in terms of pain, wound complications, recovery time, etc.) than patients with the equivalent open operation. So for the most part, the data on colon resection for adenocarcinoma from tertiary centers suggest equivalency or even superiority of the minimally invasive approach over the open approach.

Whether performed for a malignant or a benign indication, transverse colectomy is a relatively uncommon procedure compared to right or left colon resection. Because a transverse colectomy involves mobilization of both the hepatic and splenic flexures, the operative time and difficulty can be greater than for a one-sided resection. In large series of minimally invasive colectomy for both benign and malignant disease, a transverse resection typically accounts for up to 10% of the cases. Thus, transverse colectomy continues to be performed with modest frequency in laparoscopic colon surgery and so belongs in the armamentarium of the laparoscopic surgeon.

OPERATIVE INDICATIONS

In performing a colonic resection for a benign diagnosis, the operator typically resects just the segment of colon that is involved with the disease. There is the theoretical concern that a resection demarcated solely by the extent of benign disease would result in some anastomoses being constructed in a vascular "watershed" region (i.e., an area of the colon that lies between major blood vessels; see Fig. 14-1) and that a colocolostomy in such a region would have an increased risk for ischemia and dehiscence. Currently, it is generally acceptable to construct a colocolostomy during an elective segmental colon resection for a benign diagnosis, the margins of which are based on pathologic extent only. For reference, a transverse colectomy would require an anastomosis between the hepatic and splenic flexures (both hypothetical watershed regions); if this anastomosis can be performed without tension and there are no other extenuating circumstances, then we have no reservations about proceeding with this operation.

The indication for a transverse colectomy for colonic adenocarcinoma is somewhat more complicated. Traditional surgical practice prescribes that the longitudinal extent of resection for colon cancer depends on the location of the tumor with respect to the arterial blood supply (Fig. 14-1). The intent of this strategy is to resect the draining nodal basis en bloc with the tumor, so that at least staging and prognostic information may be obtained. If a tumor resides within a vascular watershed region (e.g., a hepatic flexure lesion), then a resection encompassing the major arteries proximal and distal to the lesion (i.e., an extended right hemicolectomy) would be indicated. For a tumor that overrides the middle colic artery, a transverse colectomy would be ideal. A difficulty may arise in determining to which artery a given tumor has the closest proximity; in cases in which this difficulty arises (such as in the proximal or distal transverse colon), it may be more prudent to perform an extended resection that encompasses both the proximal and distal arteries. For further discussion on the extent of resection for colon cancer, please see Chapter 15, on minimally invasive left colon resection.

The rationale for a transverse colectomy is to preserve colonic length; otherwise, all transverse lesions might as easily be treated with an extended right or subtotal colectomy. If the surgeon finds, however, that the right colonic limb salvaged by a transverse colectomy is unreasonably short (say, 10 cm), then it may be more prudent to perform an extended right hemicolectomy with a transverse ileocolostomy. The ileum usually is easier to mobilize than the right colon, and the former perhaps has the theoretical advantage of increased vascularization over the colon. Regardless of these hypothetical concerns, the extent of resection is a relative choice made by the operating surgeon during the procedure, and clinical guidelines are intended to help the surgeon make this decision.

PREOPERATIVE EVALUATION

The goals of preoperative evaluation for the patient undergoing a colon resection may be organized as follows: (1) obtain a diagnosis for the disease being resected; (2) determine whether the proposed procedure is appropriate; (3) define the segment of colon requiring resection; (4) determine whether there is local involvement of the disease with contiguous organs; (5) if the diagnosis is cancer, determine the clinical stage and whether a concomitant procedure will be necessary; and (6) ensure that the patient will tolerate the proposed procedure.

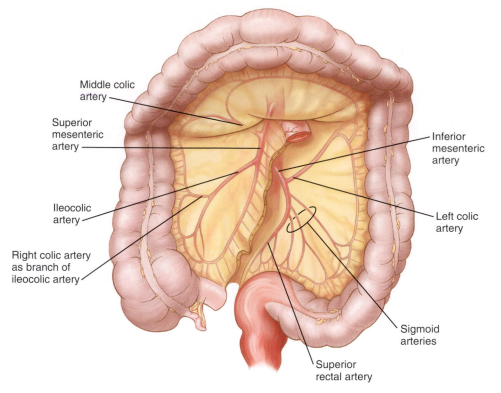

Middle colic
artery

Superior
mesenteric
artery

Ileocolic
artery

Right colic artery
as branch of
ileocolic artery

Inferior
mesenteric
artery

Left colic
artery

Sigmoid
arteries

Superior
rectal artery

Figure 14-1 Colonic blood supply.

For the first five goals, much of the necessary information can be obtained with colonoscopy or barium enema, combined with computed tomography (CT) scanning. Colonoscopy has the advantage of being able to provide tissue for diagnosis, while an air-contrasted barium enema can provide an excellent map of spatial relations. The CT scan can show the lesion dimensions, the presence of invasion, contiguous organ involvement, and distant metastasis (if the diagnosis is cancer). If there is evidence of local invasion by the disease process, then the surgeon should have an intraoperative strategy for dealing with this scenario. For colon cancer, positron emission tomography (PET) scanning may be used to identify or confirm possible nodal or metastatic disease that may not have been seen on a CT scan, and subsequently, these findings may alter surgical therapy. Currently, however, routine PET scanning is not recommended for early-stage colon cancer. In addition, all preoperative patients with colon cancer should have measurement of their carcinoembryonic antigen (CEA) level.

A not uncommon situation arises in which a small lesion of the colon (e.g., a sessile premalignant polyp) is identified for surgical removal, but the lesion is not large enough to be seen with the laparoscope. One method to approach this scenario is to endoscopically tag the lesion with India ink just prior to the minimally invasive resection. Another method is to perform intraoperative colonoscopy; this latter approach can result in intestinal distention, however, which can make laparoscopy difficult. In any event, removal of a small lesion should be confirmed in the operating room by opening the surgical specimen on the back table. If the lesion is not present in the specimen, then a second attempt at localization and resection is indicated while the patient is still anesthetized.

We prefer to perform a bowel preparation on all patients undergoing a colonic resection. Whether or not a bowel preparation is necessary in these patients is an area of controversy. Our regimen consists of a traditional oral gavage with polyethylene glycol, followed by the administration of oral antibiotics (neomycin and erythromycin base) on the day prior to surgery. One-half hour prior to skin incision, a dose of a second-generation cephalosporin and metronidazole is given intravenously (see Chapter 31).

Patient Positioning and Placement of Trocars

For a minimally invasive transverse colectomy, the patient is placed supine and flat with both arms tucked on the operating table. Alternatively, the patient may be placed in the "French" position (supine with the thighs abducted and the knees extended), which allows the surgeon greater operating versatility from one position (i.e., standing between the legs). The upper thighs and upper chest should be belted so that the patient can be placed in extreme rotation ("airplaning"). A footrest will prevent the patient from sliding downward when in extreme head-up (reverse Trendelenburg) position. The goal in positioning the patient for this and many other minimally invasive procedures is to have the anesthetized patient secured to the operating room table with pressure points well padded, so that extremes of table tilting can be performed safely. Prior to the sterile preparation and draping, the operating table may be placed through the extremes of its tilting, so that the adequacy of the patient's belting and padding can be evaluated. The surgeon can stand on either the patient's right or left, depending on the region of the colon being mobilized.

The placement of the trocars for a minimally invasive colectomy needs to allow mobilization of both the right and left colon, especially the hepatic and splenic flexures. This can be done in any number of ways; we prefer a spread of five trocars in an arc across the lower abdomen (Fig. 14-2), all 12 mm in diameter to allow introduction of atraumatic graspers, stapler-cutters, and

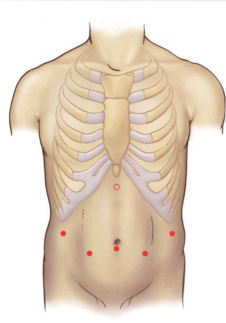

FIGURE 14-2 Trocar placement for minimally invasive transverse colectomy. Five 12-mm trocars are placed in an arc ("smile") across the mid-lower abdomen. An optional sixth trocar (open circle) may be placed in the subxiphoid location to facilitate cephalad retraction of the colon.

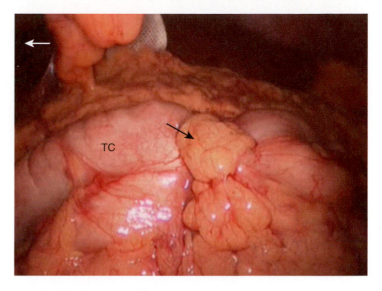

FIGURE 14-3 Transverse colon (TC), with lesion indicated by black arrow. White arrow indicates patient's right.

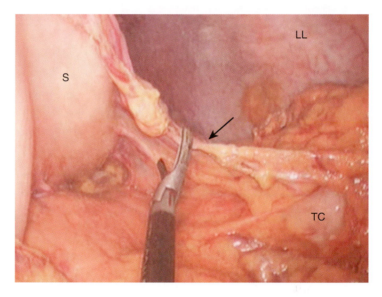

FIGURE 14-4 Entry into the lesser sac through the gastrocolic omentum (arrow). LL, left lateral abdominal wall; S, stomach; TC, transverse colon.

the 10-mm, 30-degree laparoscope. Pneumoperitoneum can be established with either a Veress needle or an optical bladeless trocar (the latter is our preference). As with other laparoscopic procedures, the distance between the trocar sites should be adequate so as to minimize interference between instruments and to improve the ergonometrics of the surgeon's hands and elbows.

OPERATIVE TECHNIQUE

The operating table is rotated so that the patient's right side is elevated. The cecum is grasped and retracted medially, and the right colon is dissected off the lateral abdominal wall with sharp technique, proceeding proximally to the hepatic flexure. If the transverse colon lesion is premalignant or benign, then it would be of benefit to preserve the omentum. With the patient in steep reverse Trendelenburg, the omentum is elevated and the transverse colon is retracted inferiorly. The omentum then is dissected sharply off the transverse colon; the surgeon should stay in the avascular plane between omentum and the colon/mesocolon. This dissection can follow the root of the transverse mesocolon down to the level of the pancreas. The hepatic flexure is swept off the duodenum and right kidney with a combination of blunt and sharp dissection. The dissection of the omentum is taken up to but not including the splenic flexure of the colon.

If the patient has a malignancy of the transverse colon (Fig. 14-3), then it is advisable to remove the omentum with the surgical specimen. We prefer to employ a "no-touch" technique with respect to the malignant lesion, and will mark out the no-touch region with clips prior to commencing the dissection. The gastrocolic omentum then may be incised in an avascular region away from the lesion so that access to the lesser sac is obtained. Starting at this incision, the lesser omentum is transected with the ultrasonic scalpel or similar device along the length of the transverse colon (Fig. 14-4); the surgeon should stay close to the stomach, yet preserve the gastroepiploic arcade.

After the right colon has been mobilized, the operating table is rotated so that the patient's left side is elevated. The proximal sigmoid colon is grasped and retracted medially, and the colon is dissected off the lateral abdominal wall with sharp technique, proceeding proximally to the splenic flexure. The separation of the splenic flexure of the colon from the spleen can be difficult secondary to folding and redundancy of the colon in this region. We prefer to perform this part of the dissection with a combination of the hook electrocautery and the ultrasonic scalpel. Once the splenic flexure has been mobilized, the left colon is swept off the left kidney with a combination of blunt and sharp dissection.

With the right and left colon mobilized, the surgeon can now choose the points of colonic transection (see "Operative Indications"). The mesocolic "wedge" to be resected is marked out with a peritoneal incision from the proximal point of transection to the distal point. If the lesion to be resected is malignant, then it is advisable to proceed with transection of the main vascular trunk supplying the lesion before further dissection (Fig. 14-5). The middle colic artery is taken close to its origin from the superior mesenteric artery with a vascular load of an endoscopic stapler-cutter (Fig. 14-6). After the main vascular trunk has been ligated, the surgeon then can divide the remaining mesocolon and staple across the colon at the proximal and distal margins in whatever order is most convenient.

If the lesion to be resected is benign, then the primacy of vascular trunk ligation is not important. In this case it may be easier for the surgeon first to staple the colon proximally. A window is created in the mesocolon just beneath the mesenteric border of the colon at the proximal point of transection, staying right on the wall of the colon. The colon then is divided with a linear stapler-cutter at a right angle to the bowel axis. The mesocolon is divided between the proximal and distal transection points with the harmonic scalpel or similar device. For a benign lesion, the division of the mesocolon may stay 1 to 2 cm away from the bowel if the surgeon wants to avoid proximity to the mesenteric

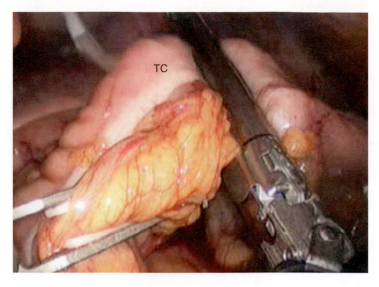

FIGURE 14-7 Division of the distal transverse colon (TC; label is on the specimen side) with a linear stapler-cutter.

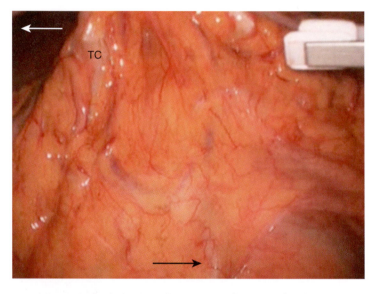

FIGURE 14-5 Demonstration of middle colic artery *(black arrow)* in the transverse mesocolon. *White arrow* indicates patient's right. TC, transverse colon.

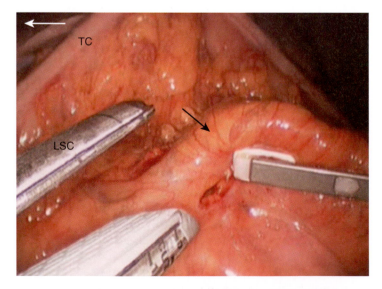

FIGURE 14-6 Division of the middle colic vessels *(black arrow)* with a linear stapler-cutter (LSC). *White arrow* indicates patient's right; laparoscopic grasper is on the proximal (patient) side of the middle colic vessels. TC, transverse colon.

root. The descending colon then is divided at the distal point of transection (Fig. 14-7) similarly to the proximal point of transection. The specimen is placed in a polyethylene bag and placed in the upper abdomen, from where it will be removed at the end of the case.

Prior to creation of the anastomosis, the proximal and distal staple lines are apposed to see if the proposed connection will be under tension; if so, further mobilization of the right and left colon may be needed. The surgeon can fully mobilize the cecum and root of the small bowel, which would bring the right colon past the midline, if necessary. Alternatively, if the segment of right colon is short, then the surgeon could resect this and perform an anastomosis of the terminal ileum to the descending colon. One method used to perform a stapled colocolostomy is to line up the bowel ends in an antiparallel fashion (i.e., with the staple lines adjacent to each other, yielding a "double-barrel" appearance) and place two stay sutures of 2-0 silk along the antimesenteric border to keep the colon ends apposed during the stapling. A colotomy is made at the antimesenteric tip of each of the colon, and the linear stapler-cutter is inserted (Fig. 14-8). The ends of colon are pulled completely over the jaws of the stapler-cutter, and the instrument is fired along the antimesenteric border of each colonic limb. The enjoined colotomy site then can be closed with another load of the stapler-cutter (Fig. 14-9). The "crotch" or bifurcation of the anastomosis then can be reinforced with another 2-0 silk suture. The surgeon should ensure that the second firing of the stapler-cutter, which closes the colotomy, should not narrow the anastomotic lumen. There will be less tendency for this to occur if a 60-mm linear stapler-cutter is utilized for construction of this anastomosis.

Alternatively, the ends of the colon may be aligned in a parallel fashion, with the right colon anterior and the left colon posterior. Two silk stay sutures again are placed along the antimesenteric borders for stabilization. Two colotomies then are made, one in the antimesenteric tip of the right colon, and the second in the antimesenteric border of the left colon, directly adjacent to the first colotomy. The linear stapler-cutter is positioned and fired as described previously. If not performed carefully, a stapled closure of the colotomy in this location can result in narrowing of the left colon at the anastomotic outlet. The surgeon may prefer to close this colotomy manually with

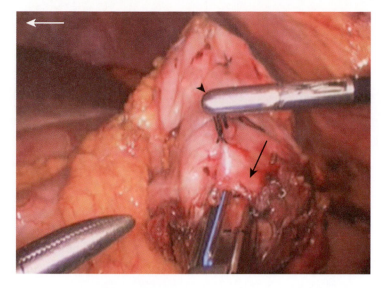

Figure 14-8 Positioning of the laparoscopic linear stapler-cutter through colotomies in the transverse colon *(black arrow)* in preparation of a stapled colocolostomy. Grasper is elevating a stay suture on the future anastomosis *(black arrowhead)*. *White arrow* indicates patient's right.

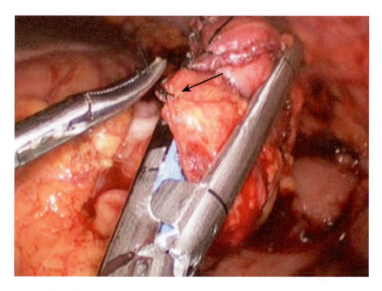

Figure 14-9 The linear stapler-cutter is used to close the colotomy that was created during the stapling of the colocolostomy in Figure 14-8. A Maryland-type grasper is elevating a stay suture on the tip of the colon *(arrow)* that will be excised to close the colotomy.

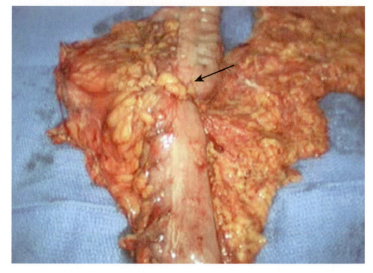

Figure 14-10 Excised specimen. *Arrow* indicates the lesion seen in Figure 14-3.

has been completed, the surgeon can inspect for hemostasis and examine the mesenteric defect that was created. Sometimes this defect is quite huge, and an attempt at closure would cause more problems than not doing anything at all. A small mesenteric defect typically is more problematic and should be closed. The bagged specimen subsequently is retrieved through an enlarged trocar site and then may be examined on a back table (Fig. 14-10). The procedure is finished by evacuating the pneumoperitoneum and closing the fascia of the trocar sites.

POSTOPERATIVE CARE

We do not routinely employ nasogastric tube decompression. A dose of ketorolac tromethamine is given in the operating room; spinal/epidural anesthesia is not utilized. Postoperative analgesia consists of oral propoxyphene and ketorolac. Opioid analgesics are avoided. No further antibiotic doses are given unless the patient has evidence of infection. Clear liquids may be given on postoperative day 1, but a low-residue diet is not initiated until the patient has some sign of resolving ileus (e.g., passing flatus). This diet is maintained for several weeks, and then a regular diet is permitted. A complete blood count is obtained every morning as long as the patient is in the hospital; the length of stay typically is 2 to 4 days. Upon discharge, the patient is given instructions to report fever, abdominal distention, pain, emesis, or wound drainage. Postoperative visits typically are scheduled at 1 week and 1 month. If the patient has a diagnosis of colon cancer, then routine postoperative surveillance is undertaken.

PROCEDURE-SPECIFIC COMPLICATIONS

Primary intraoperative complications include bleeding and enterotomy. Hemorrhage can arise from the spleen during splenic flexure mobilization. As with all other procedures involving perisplenic dissection, the surgeon should utilize meticulous and gentle techniques in the vicinity of the spleen. Enterotomy may be the result of grasper trauma, so the use of atraumatic 10-mm grasping forceps is encouraged. In the presence of multiple dense adhesions, enterotomy should not necessarily be viewed as a complication, as this event sometimes

interrupted sutures of 2-0 silk. If there is sufficient length of the colonic limbs to produce an overlapping region of approximately 10 cm, then a triple-staple technique also can be utilized (see Chapter 6 for a complete description). In brief, after placement of proximal and distal stay sutures, a colotomy is made in the right and left limb at the midpoint of the overlap. The stapler-cutter is fired twice, once in the antegrade direction and once in the retrograde direction; the third fire closes the enjoined colotomy site. This technique produces a widely patent anastomosis.

If the patient is thin and has sufficient mesenteric mobility, then the surgeon may prefer to bring the bowel ends out through a small incision (preferably an enlarged trocar site) and perform an extracorporeal anastomosis. We make no distinctions about how the anastomosis is performed or whether to call the procedure "laparoscopic" or "laparoscopically assisted." The important aspect is that the procedure is minimally invasive. After the anastomosis

cannot be avoided. An enterotomy recognized intraoperatively during a minimally invasive colectomy is closed primarily; if the enterotomy is within several centimeters of one of the staple lines, then it may be more prudent to incorporate the injury within the resected specimen.

Postoperative complications include ileus, internal hernia, anastomotic leak, and intra-abdominal abscess. Unlike other minimally invasive abdominal procedures, colectomy typically produces some period of ileus, which may be prolonged if high doses of opioids are used during anesthesia or postoperatively. Prolonged ileus with fever, peritoneal signs, or elevated white blood cell count should alert the surgeon to the possibility of an anastomotic leak. Occasionally a patient will experience a prolonged ileus (>1 week) that has no discernable cause; this complication should be managed with general supportive care, including parenteral nutrition. A patient who develops signs and symptoms of a postoperative bowel obstruction may have an internal hernia; this complication will be less likely to occur if a small mesenteric defect is closed.

If the patient develops fever, pain, or an elevated white blood cell count in the postoperative period, then the surgeon should obtain a contrast CT scan of the abdomen. Early diagnosis of an anastomotic leak is preferable to a delayed diagnosis; the latter is associated with high morbidity rate. If a noncontained leak is diagnosed early, then a prompt laparoscopic intervention may be able to repair the leak without the need for a colostomy. A delayed diagnosis of a leak may result in the need for a laparotomy with a colostomy. If the patient has a contained leak/intra-abdominal abscess, then this complication may be managed with percutaneous drainage, antibiotics, and close observation. These patients often will not need a reoperation, but they are at risk for anastomotic stenosis or colocutaneous fistula.

RESULTS AND OUTCOME

Transverse colectomy is relatively uncommon procedure. The results of this operation in the literature usually are grouped with the results of other colonic resections. In general, transverse colectomy shares the results of other minimally invasive colon resections. For a more complete discussion, please refer to the chapter on minimally invasive left colon resection (see Chapter 15).

Suggested Reading

Clinical Outcomes of Surgical Therapy Study Group: A comparison of laparoscopically assisted and open colectomy for colon cancer. N Engl J Med 2004;350:2050–2059.

Lacy AM, Garcia-Valdecasas JC, Delgado S, et al: Laparoscopy-assisted colectomy versus open colectomy for treatment of non-metastatic colon cancer: A randomised trial. Lancet 2002;359:2224–2229.

Leung KL, Kwok SP, Lam SC, et al: Laparoscopic resection of rectosigmoid carcinoma: Prospective randomised trial. Lancet 2004;363(9416):1187–1192.

National Comprehensive Cancer Network (NCCN): Clinical practice guidelines in oncology. Colon Cancer 2007;1. Accessed at www.nccn.org.

Schwenk W, Haase O, Neudecker J, Muller JM: Short term benefits for laparoscopic colorectal resection. Cochrane Database Syst Rev 2005(3):CD003145.

Senagore AJ, Dupree HJ, Delaney CP, et al: Results of a standardized technique and postoperative care plan for laparoscopic sigmoid colectomy: A 30-month experience. Dis Colon Rectum 2003;46(4):503–509.

Slim K, Vicaut E, Panis Y, Chipponi J: Meta-analysis of randomized clinical trials of colorectal surgery with or without mechanical bowel preparation. Br J Surg 2004;91(9):1125–1130.

CONSTANTINE T. FRANTZIDES, GEORGE E. POLYMENEAS, AND
MARK A. CARLSON

Minimally Invasive Left Colectomy

Since the earliest descriptions of this technique, minimally invasive colon resection has enjoyed near-universal acceptance as a treatment for benign colon disease. With the publication of data from controlled clinical trials in 2002 and afterward, minimally invasive colon resection also has been increasingly accepted as a treatment modality for colon cancer. In fact, minimally invasive colon resection is now the preferred surgical approach for colorectal malignancy in many tertiary centers. The early concerns about laparoscopic operation on colon cancer, such as incomplete tumor clearance, abdominal wall implants, and so on, have not been borne out in large clinical series nor in randomized trials. Perhaps a pertinent question to ask at this point is how quickly and to what extent will minimally invasive resection become the preferred approach for surgical disease of the colon, regardless of the practice environment.

It is readily apparent that the transition from an open to a minimally invasive operative approach has not happened precipitously with colorectal resection as it did with, say, cholecystectomy. The reasons for this are interesting to discuss and might include the technical demands of a laparoscopic colon operation, controversy regarding the purported patient-related advantages of minimal access over a standard incision, the costs of the laparoscopic equipment, and so on. We will bypass discussion of such controversies and simply state that we place ourselves firmly on the side of the colorectal laparoscopists. It is our opinion that in the patient who requires a colorectal resection, the patient-related advantages of having a minimally invasive operation far outweigh any and all of the supposed disadvantages. We approach all patients with surgical disease of the colon and rectum with the intent to perform a minimally invasive resection.

Does this stance imply that the performance of an open colorectal resection will sink below the so-called "standard of care?" Of course not. For the foreseeable future, the need to perform open colorectal resection will continue to exist, just as the need for open cholecystectomy still exists today for various (though uncommon) indications. Presumably, the future will bring an increase in the number of surgeons who perform minimally invasive colorectal resection; correspondingly, the number of open procedures gradually will decrease. Probably the most important elements to preserve in this gradual transition are patient safety and the preservation of therapeutic efficacy.

In this chapter, we will describe our technique of minimally invasive resection of the left colon. To be specific, this chapter applies to

lesions that are located in the colon from the splenic flexure down to the rectosigmoid junction (or peritoneal reflection). Resection of more distal lesions in the rectum (e.g., low anterior resection) will be described in another chapter. We acknowledge that there are a number of approaches to minimally invasive left colon resection; our preference is to complete this type of resection laparoscopically, that is, without hand-assisted technology.

OPERATIVE INDICATIONS

As discussed for transverse colectomy (see Chapter 14), minimally invasive colon resection now is acceptable for both benign and malignant disease of the colon, and our approach is to consider each colon case as a possible laparoscopic procedure. In Western society, the most common indications for left colon resection are cancer, premalignant polyps, and diverticular disease; the rank order mostly depends on the practice environment. Less common indications for left colon resection in the West include sigmoid volvulus, ischemic colitis, inflammatory bowel disease, and pseudo-obstruction. With the heavy utilization of screening for colorectal cancer, we have experienced a noticeable surge in the percentage of patients with endoscopically unresectable premalignant polyps who are referred for colon resection.

The extent of colon resection is dependent on the diagnosis. Although much has been made of the theoretical limitations of segmental colon resection secondary to limited collateral blood supply, in practice the entire colon is amenable to segmental resection in elective procedures in good-risk patients with little regard to the main feeding vessels. So with a benign or premalignant diagnosis, the extent of resection should be guided by the extent of the disease; that is, just enough colon is resected to remove the offending lesion. With established malignancy, the extent of the longitudinal resection is guided somewhat by the position of the tumor with respect to the draining lymphatics, which parallel the major arteries (see also "Operative Indications" in Chapter 14). The guidelines for the extent of resection in colon cancer have been evolving, however, and radical resections of the mesocolon are not always required.

The sigmoid colon is supplied by an arterial arcade from the inferior mesenteric artery above, which forms an anastomotic network with hemorrhoidal (rectal) arteries from below (see Fig. 14-1). The question arises whether a cancer in the sigmoid colon should be treated with removal of its entire lymphatic basin. That is, should a mid-sigmoid lesion require resection of the entire left/sigmoid colon with high ligation of the inferior mesenteric artery? The prevailing answer is no, as long as there is no gross evidence of positive nodes. Most authorities would agree that high ligation of the inferior mesenteric artery in the absence of gross nodal disease would be excessive and would not improve the patient's survival or staging accuracy.

If the patient does not have gross evidence of nodal disease, then a minimum of 12 nodes in the surgical specimen appear to be adequate for pathologic staging. For example, a clinical T2 N0 lesion of the mid-sigmoid colon may be resected with longitudinal margins of 5 cm, as long as the surgeon is confident that the minimum number of nodes will be present in the specimen. The surgeon may need to extend this minimal longitudinal margin in order to obtain a larger mesenteric wedge that contains enough nodes. If there is gross evidence of nodal disease in a patient with no distant metastasis, then an attempt should be made to clear the involved nodes. If the patient has a clinical T3 or T4 lesion, then the surgeon also should be prepared to perform an en bloc resection of any involved tissue/organ in order to obtain a negative lateral margin. In terms of effecting a surgical cure for a colonic malignancy, the overriding priority is a complete resection (R0, all margins negative).

A patient with stage IV colon cancer still may undergo a limited resection of the primary lesion if the patient is a good operative risk and has a reasonable life expectancy. Such a procedure should be part of a multimodality approach to the patient's cancer, which also might include chemoradiation and metastatectomy. Removal of the primary lesion can prevent local complications, such as bleeding, perforation, and obstruction. Stenting is a treatment alternative for a stage IV colon cancer but is generally less desirable compared to surgical resection.

With regard to colon resection for benign disease, one of the more common debates over operative indications concerns when to perform an elective resection for diverticular disease. Similar to many other nonmalignant diseases that can be treated with surgery, the indication to operate on diverticular disease may be summarized as the point at which medical treatment has failed. This dictum is intentionally vague and allows the physician to individualize care based on the patient's age, comorbidities, social situation, and the like. Our own bias with a patient who has diverticulitis is to offer an elective resection if the patient has had two episodes requiring hospitalization and is a good operative risk.

PREOPERATIVE EVALUATION

The preoperative evaluation of a patient undergoing a colon resection was described in Chapter 14, on minimally invasive transverse colectomy. In addition, a lesion of the left/sigmoid colon occasionally may involve the urinary system, in which case a urologic evaluation (CT scanning, ureterocystoscopy) would be necessary. For tumors involving the rectosigmoid junction, an endorectal ultrasound would be helpful to identify T3 tumors that might be amenable to neoadjuvant chemoradiation (please refer to Chapter 17 on minimally invasive low anterior resection).

PATIENT POSITIONING AND PLACEMENT OF TROCARS

For a laparoscopic left/sigmoid colon resection, the patient is placed in a low lithotomy position with stirrups, which facilitates the per rectal use of the end-to-end anastomotic (EEA) stapler.

A beanbag, viscoelastic cushion, or similar device is used to raise the left hip 20 to 30 degrees off the operating table. The patient then is secured to the operating room table, in stirrups with belts /straps across the upper chest, thighs, and legs. Stirrups that can be adjusted easily during surgery are a helpful accessory; during the laparoscopic dissection, the legs can be maintained in a lower position, but then raised when the EEA stapler needs to be passed per rectum. In addition, we have found it quite useful to have infrared-illuminated ureteral stents (Infravision, Stryker, San Jose, CA) placed by a urologist after induction of anesthesia. These devices permit easier identification of the ureters, which is especially helpful when dealing with a phlegmon in the left lower quadrant.

The surgeon stands on the patient' right and faces a monitor. We prefer to establish a pneumoperitoneum with a Hasson cannula at the umbilicus. Later on, the infraumbilical curvilinear incision which is made for the Hasson can be extended for specimen removal. If the patient has had a previous midline or umbilical incision, it may be prudent to insert an optical bladeless trocar at another trocar site in order to insufflate the abdomen. After the Hasson is placed, two more 12-mm trocars are placed in the right abdomen, superior and inferior to the level of the umbilicus (Fig. 15-1). The precise location of these working trocars will vary depending on the patient's body habitus and the location of the lesion to be resected. We prefer to use 12-mm trocars at all positions for maximal instrument flexibility. Later in the dissection, a fourth trocar may be placed in the left midabdomen along the anterior axillary line; the surgeon should visualize how this trocar will affect the operation prior to placement so that the surgeon can pick the best insertion site. One of the main causes of conversion during minimally invasive colectomy is malpositioning of one of more trocars; unfortunately, there are no absolute rules that will guarantee perfect trocar placement. The surgeon must plan and carefully consider each potential site in relation to the region of dissection and also in relation to the other trocars.

OPERATIVE TECHNIQUE

Prior to initiating the dissection, an abdominal survey is performed to identify and biopsy any metastatic cancer or other concomitant diagnosis. The operating table then is rotated so

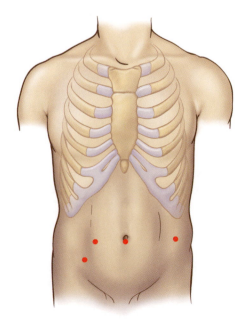

FIGURE 15-1 Trocar placement for a minimally invasive left/sigmoid colectomy.

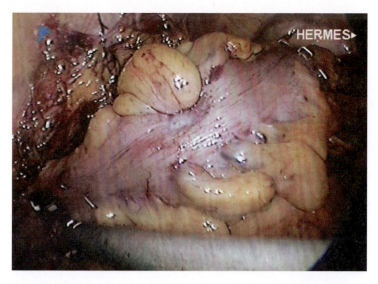

FIGURE 15-2 Placement of clips around a malignant lesion to demarcate the "no-touch" zone.

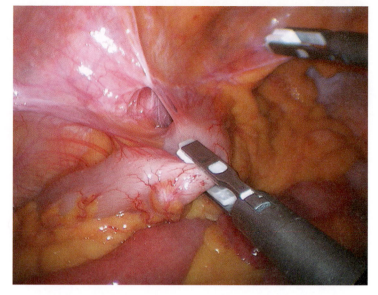

FIGURE 15-4 Medial retraction of the sigmoid colon in a patient with diverticulitis.

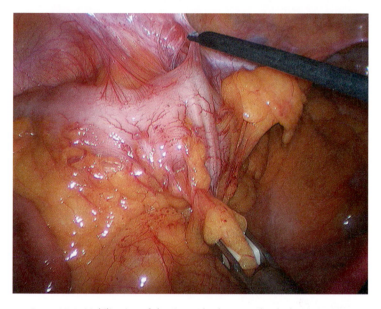

FIGURE 15-5 Mobilization of the sigmoid colon using hook electrocautery.

that the patient's left side is elevated. Because a bolster already has been placed under the patient's left hip for elevation, rotation of the operating room table will bring the patient close to a lateral decubitus position, which facilitates mobilization of the left colon. If there is a malignant lesion in the left/sigmoid colon that has been inked, then clips are placed 5 cm proximal and distal to this area in order to establish the "no-touch" zone (Fig. 15-2). No instrument manipulation of this region of the colon is permitted until the primary vascular trunk has been ligated.

In the presence of diverticular disease or another inflammatory process (Fig. 15-3), the mobilization of the sigmoid colon can be difficult and time-consuming. The proximal left colon is placed on stretch with an atraumatic grasper (Atraugrip, Specialty Surgical Instrumentation, Nashville, TN; Fig. 15-4), and the left colon is dissected away from the lateral abdominal wall using sharp dissection, such as the hook electrocautery, scissors, or ultrasonic scalpel (Figs. 15-5 and 15-6). This is initiated by incising along the line of Toldt. The use of the illuminated ureteral stents is particularly helpful in this circumstance (Fig. 15-7). In addition, we have found that an inflatable balloon retractor (Soft-Wand, Gyrus-ACMI, Southborough, MA) works well to retract, push, or sweep the colon or mesentery. Depending on the redundancy of the sigmoid colon, the location of the lesion, and the nature of the lesion, the splenic flexure may

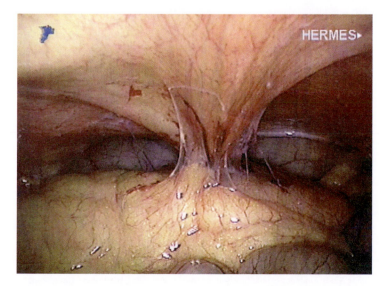

FIGURE 15-3 Intra-abdominal appearance of a patient with a colovesical fistula.

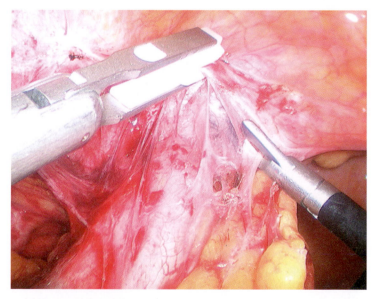

FIGURE 15-6 Sharp dissection of the sigmoid colon from the bladder in a patient with diverticulitis.

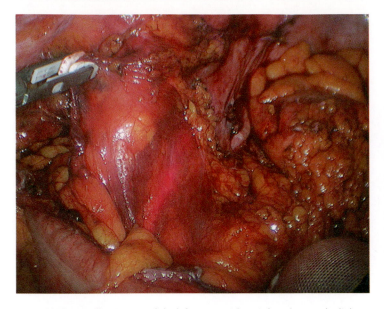

FIGURE 15-7 Transillumination of the left ureter with an infrared stent; the light has been dimmed in order to better appreciate the ureter. The sigmoid colon has been mobilized and is retracted medially with an inflatable balloon retractor.

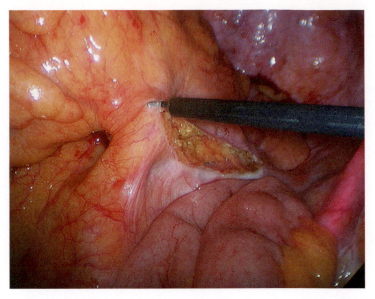

FIGURE 15-8 Incision of the peritoneum on the right side of the sigmoid colon. The transilluminated right ureter is visible in the lower right of the image.

need to be mobilized; this is facilitated by placing the patient in steep reverse Trendelenburg position in addition to the left side up rotation. The splenic flexure then can be taken down with sharp dissection, all the while maintaining gentle stretch on the colon.

If the lesion is in the distal sigmoid, then the mobilization of the sigmoid may continue onto the upper rectum (for lesions involving the rectum, please see Chapter 17, on low anterior resection/abdominal perineal resection). During dissection in the pelvis, the patient may be placed in steep Trendelenburg position with the left side elevated. The small bowel may need to be retracted out of the pelvis with an inflatable balloon retractor, which occasionally may require placement of a fifth trocar. Once the attachments of the colon to the sidewall have been incised, the colon and mesentery can be swept away from the underlying retroperitoneal structures using a combination of blunt and sharp dissection. The presence of a phlegmon, as mentioned previously, will require the continued use of meticulous sharp dissection around the region of inflammation. The ureter may be identified as it crosses the iliac artery close to the external-internal bifurcation. If the gonadal vessels are involved with reaction around the lesion, then these vessels may be sacrificed.

The goal of the left/sigmoid colon mobilization is to have freed the colonic segment to be resected along with its associated mesentery from the lateral abdominal wall, so that the main vascular trunk may be ligated without endangering the underlying retroperitoneal structures (e.g., the left ureter). With this accomplished, the surgeon may mark out a mesenteric "wedge" that encompasses the colonic segment and mesentery to be resected (Fig. 15-8). The left/sigmoid colon is retracted back to the lateral abdominal wall, which exposes the root of the sigmoid mesentery. If the left mesocolon is kept on stretch, then the left colic artery may be seen tenting up the mesocolon. The left colic artery may require ligation if it is in proximity to the disease process; routine ligation of this artery, however, is not necessary (see "Operative Indications"). To delineate the mesenteric wedge of resection, an incision through just the peritoneum of the medial mesocolon is made from the proximal to distal site of colonic transection.

If the patient has a malignancy, then the next step is to ligate the primary vascular trunk to the lesion at the apex of the mesenteric

wedge. Depending on where the lesion is situated in the left/sigmoid colon, this primary vascular trunk may consist of the left colic artery after its take-off from the inferior mesenteric artery, the inferior mesenteric artery after the take-off of the left colic artery, or the inferior mesenteric artery close to its origin from the aorta (see Fig. 14-1). If a high ligation of the inferior mesenteric artery will be performed, then the surgeon should open up the retroperitoneal space on the medial side of the sigmoid colon, and identify the right ureter in the same manner as was done on the left side (see Fig. 15-8). The main vascular trunk then is dissected out and transected with a vascular load of the linear stapler-cutter. The surgeon should visualize the tips of the stapler to ensure that a ureter or other structure has not been caught in the instrument's jaws. The remainder of the mesocolon between the proximal and distal points of transection (i.e., along the peritoneal incision made in the mesocolon) may be divided with additional vascular loads of the linear stapler-cutter (Fig. 15-9). If the mesentery is thick, then

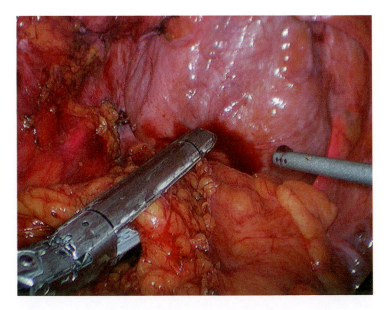

FIGURE 15-9 Transection of the sigmoid mesocolon using the linear stapler-cutter. The left and right ureters are both transilluminated.

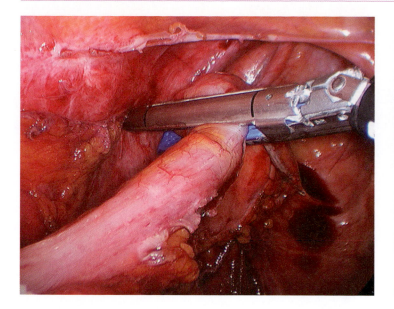

FIGURE 15-10 Distal transection at the rectosigmoid junction using the linear stapler-cutter.

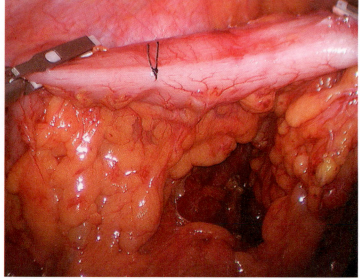

FIGURE 15-11 A stitch has been placed in the distal left colon to mark the beginning of the devascularized sigmoid colon. This stitch will determine the proximal transection point when the specimen is exteriorized.

a blue stapler load, or an ultrasonic/bipolar scalpel device, may be better suited for this step.

If the patient has benign disease, then the order of mesenteric division is not important. The surgeon may elect first to divide the bowel distally (Fig. 15-10). A mesenteric window is bluntly yet gently created just underneath the mesenteric border of the colon at the distal point of transection. The colon is divided here with one or two loads of the linear articulating stapler-cutter, and the mesentery is divided back along the peritoneal score to the proximal point of transection. With benign disease, the surgeon may elect to transect the mesentery within several centimeters of the bowel wall. The colon then is divided at the proximal transection line with the linear stapler-cutter. The resected segment is placed into a polyethylene specimen bag. An atraumatic grasper then is attached to the staple line on the descending colon, and this proximal staple line then is apposed to the distal staple line to ensure that the subsequent anastomosis will not be under tension. After this maneuver, the umbilical trocar incision is extended several centimeters, and the specimen bag is removed through this incision. The proximal staple line then is brought out the umbilical incision with the atraumatic grasper.

Alternatively, the surgeon may place the specimen into a camera bag after the distal transection (see Fig. 15-10) without having performed the proximal transection, and can then secure the bag around the colon with ligature. Prior to exteriorization of the specimen with this technique, a stitch is placed in the colon at the margin between the vascularized and devascularized segments of colon (Fig. 15-11). This bagged specimen then is brought out through the enlarged umbilical trocar incision (Fig. 15-12), and the proximal transection is performed externally with the linear stapler-cutter. About 1 cm of colon adjacent to the proximal staple line then is dissected clean of mesenteric fat in preparation for the anvil of the EEA stapler. A purse-string suture is placed just underneath the proximal staple line, either manually or with an automated purse-string device. The proximal staple line then is trimmed off with scissors, and the proximal colon is dilated with metal sizers in preparation for the anvil head. In this location, the diameter of the EEA stapler typically used is 28, 31, or 34 mm. Generally speaking, the greater the diameter of the stapler that can be used for this anastomosis, the better the functional result.

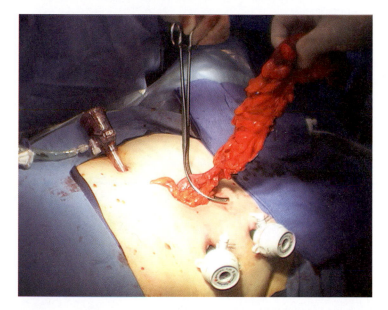

FIGURE 15-12 The specimen has been exteriorized through the umbilical port. This patient had diverticulitis; if the patient had cancer, then the specimen would have been placed into a camera bag prior to exteriorization.

Some surgeons recommend inserting an anvil head one size larger than the largest sizer that could fit in the proximal colon. The surgeon should be careful, however, not to create a full-thickness tear while doing this. If this complication occurs, then this area should be resected for another attempt more proximally.

After sizing of the proximal colon, the appropriate anvil is inserted, the purse-string suture is tied, the colon end is dropped back into the abdomen, the incision is closed, and pneumoperitoneum is reestablished. The surgeon likely will not need use of the umbilical trocar again, so complete closure of this incision should be fine. Prior to transrectal insertion of the EEA stapler, a four-finger anal dilatation is performed. The EEA stapler then is carefully maneuvered into the rectum, and following the curve of the sacrum; the surgeon should visualize the head of the stapler at the staple line of the rectal stump (Fig. 15-13). The spike of the stapler, when ejected, should come directly through the previously placed distal staple line on the distal sigmoid/upper rectum (Fig. 15-14). The anvil is mated to

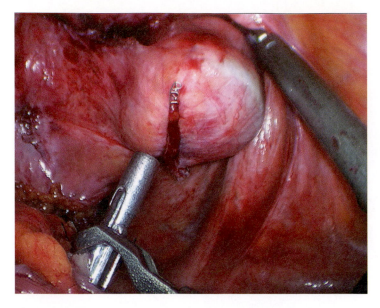

FIGURE 15-13 The circular end-to-end anastomotic (EEA) stapler is placed into the rectal stump so that the surgeon can appreciate the round outline of the stapler head symmetrically applied to the staple line of the rectal stump. This maneuver can be aided by caudad traction on the rectal stump with an atraumatic grasper.

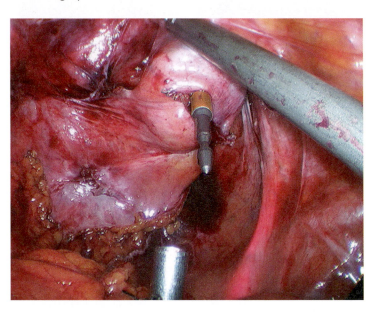

FIGURE 15-14 The spike of the circular stapler is deployed dead-center through the staple line of the rectal stump.

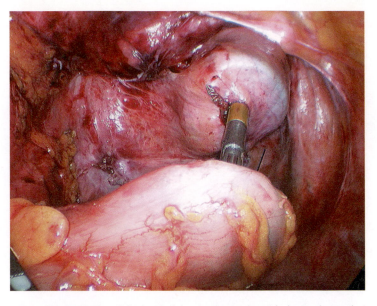

FIGURE 15-15 Mating of the head of the circular stapler with the stapler anvil.

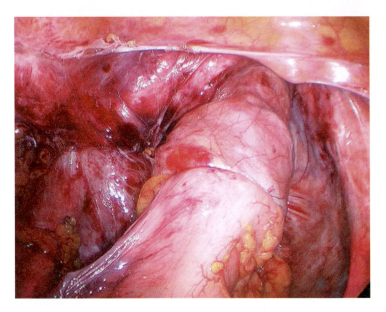

FIGURE 15-16 Firing of the end-to-end anastomotic (EEA) stapler to create the colorectal anastomosis.

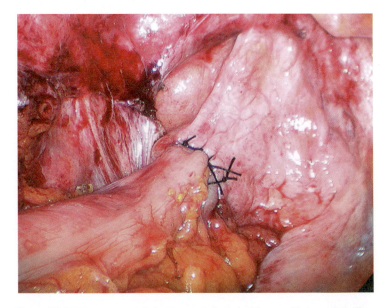

FIGURE 15-17 The anastomosis has been reinforced with several interrupted silk sutures.

the stapler (Fig. 15-15), and the stapler is closed onto the anvil with the roticulator. Prior to firing the stapler, a final check for anastomotic tension is performed and to ensure that the bowel has not been twisted. Pressure is maintained on the firing levers of the EEA stapler for about 10 seconds after firing to ensure that the staples have reached their final configuration (Fig. 15-16). The stapler then is reopened with three half-turns of the roticulator, the stapler gently is rotated 180 degrees within the lumen of bowel, and the stapler is withdrawn from the rectum. The surgeon can reinforce the anterior EEA staple line by manually placing several interrupted sutures of 3-0 silk (Fig. 15-17).

The anastomosis then should be pressure-tested by immersion of the anastomosis in saline followed by insufflation of air into the rectum while the colon proximal to the anastomosis is pinched off with an atraumatic grasper (Fig. 15-18). If there is an air leak (a rare occurrence in a properly performed EEA stapled anastomosis), then interrupted sutures of 2-0 silk are placed until

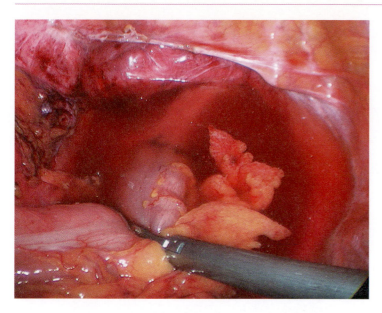

FIGURE 15-18 Pressure testing of the colorectal anastomosis. Air is insufflated transrectally while the colon proximal to the anastomosis is occluded.

the air leak cannot be demonstrated. A final check for hemostasis if performed, the pelvis is reirrigated and aspirated, the pneumoperitoneum is evacuated, and the fascia of the port sites is closed to complete the procedure.

POSTOPERATIVE CARE

The postoperative care after a minimally invasive left/sigmoid colectomy is similar to that described in Chapter 14, on transverse colectomy, and the reader is referred to that section.

PROCEDURE-SPECIFIC COMPLICATIONS

The perioperative complications of minimally invasive left/sigmoid colectomy are somewhat similar to that described in Chapter 14, on transverse colectomy, and the reader again is referred to that section. Because the colocolostomy performed in a left colectomy typically is done with the circular stapler, this anastomosis is at an increased risk of stenosis compared to an anastomosis created with the 60-mm linear stapler. In order to minimize the risk of anastomotic stenosis with the circular stapler, the largest possible diameter EEA stapler should be used. A common cause of leak in an end-to-end anastomosis is technical error. The surgeon should ensure that an end-to-end anastomosis is tension-free, has good blood supply, is performed in the center of rectal stump, encompasses the full-thickness of the bowel wall (i.e., two complete stapler "donuts"), and passes a pressure test. It is our routine to reinforce the anastomosis anteriorly with several interrupted sutures. Sometimes a leak still will occur, however, despite the careful observance of all guidelines. A unique complication of the end-to-end anastomosis is twisting of the proximal colon; the surgeon should carefully check the alignment of the colon prior to firing the circular stapler. Another described intraoperative complication of left colon resection is ureteral injury. In addition to a careful dissection that delineates the ureteral anatomy, the use of lighted ureteral stents may minimize the risk of injury and expedite the procedure, because the surgeon can see the presence of the ureters at all times.

RESULTS AND OUTCOME

As discussed previously, there is now controlled data to support the notion that minimally invasive colon resection for adenocarcinoma is superior to open resection with respect to perioperative complications, immunologic impact, and recovery time. With regard to survival, the studies have shown equivalence or noninferiority of laparoscopic procedures when compared to open colectomy. Initial concern of tumor implantation at trocar sites has not been borne out if the surgeon adheres to oncologic principles. Minimally invasive colectomy has been recognized as a technically demanding procedure, and there has been much discussion in the literature regarding surgeon training and number of cases required for competency. It is beyond the scope of this chapter to enter into this discussion. For the beginner laparoscopic colorectal surgeon, resection of small tumors, as opposed to large tumors or inflammatory disease (e.g., diverticulitis), may be more prudent.

Suggested Reading

The Clinical Outcomes of Surgical Therapy Study Group: A comparison of laparoscopically assisted and open colectomy for colon cancer. N Engl J Med 2004;350:2050–2059.

Lacy AM, Garcia-Valdecasas JC, Delgado S, et al: Laparoscopy-assisted colectomy versus open colectomy for treatment of non-metastatic colon cancer: A randomised trial. Lancet 2002;359:2224–2229.

Leung KL, Kwok SP, Lam SC, et al: Laparoscopic resection of rectosigmoid carcinoma: Prospective randomised trial. Lancet 2004;363(9416):1187–1192.

National Comprehensive Cancer Network (NCCN): Clinical practice guidelines in oncology. Colon Cancer 2007;1. Accessed at www.nccn.org.

Schwenk W, Haase O, Neudecker J, Muller JM: Short term benefits for laparoscopic colorectal resection. Cochrane Database Syst Rev 2005(3):CD003145.

Senagore AJ, Dupree HJ, Delaney CP, et al: Results of a standardized technique and postoperative care plan for laparoscopic sigmoid colectomy: A 30-month experience. Dis Colon Rectum 2003;46(4):503–509.

Slim K, Vicaut E, Panis Y, Chipponi J: Meta-analysis of randomized clinical trials of colorectal surgery with or without mechanical bowel preparation. Br J Surg 2004;91(9):1125–1130.

MORRIS E. FRANKLIN, JR., AND
GUILLERMO PORTILLO

Minimally Invasive Total Colectomy

16

Minimally invasive (or laparoscopic) total colectomy requires mobilization of the entire colon, division of its mesentery, and ligation of all the major vessels of the colon. Vital structures in all four quadrants of the abdomen require exposure and protection. Reports of laparoscopic total colectomy began to appear very soon after reports of laparoscopic segmental colectomy in the early 1990s. The benefits of the latter procedure for benign colorectal disease were almost immediately apparent; with the publication of controlled data in the first decade of 2000, laparoscopic segmental colectomy for malignancy also has been gaining acceptance. Laparoscopic total colectomy, however, has not been accepted as quickly; presumably this has been secondary to technical factors including (1) a difficult anastomosis (often deep in the pelvis), (2) the division of multiple large blood vessels, (3) operation in all four quadrants, and (4) extraction of a bulky specimen.

Total colectomy (also known as total abdominal colectomy, or subtotal colectomy) typically involves resection of the colon from the terminal ileum up to and including a variable length of rectum; the patient then may undergo an ileorectostomy, an end-ileostomy, or other similar procedure. Total proctocolectomy with ileoanal anastomosis involves total colon resection from the abdominal approach, with division of the distal rectum at the level of the *levator ani*, usually 1 to 2 cm proximal to the dentate line. An ileal pouch then is constructed followed by an anastomosis between the ileal pouch and the anal canal. This technique preserves the internal anal sphincter muscle and the anal transitional zone, which reduces the risk of incontinence. This chapter will describe the laparoscopic approach for both total colectomy and proctocolectomy with ileoanal anastomosis.

OPERATIVE INDICATIONS

The most frequent indications for subtotal laparoscopic colectomy and proctocolectomy at our institution have been synchronous colon cancer (30%), familial adenomatous polyposis coli (25%), inflammatory bowel disease (17%), dysmotility/inertia (16%), bleeding arteriovenous malformation (6%), and ischemic colitis (4%); an involved discussion of each of these indications is beyond the scope of this chapter. As implied in the introductory discussion, data from controlled trials have suggested that patient survival after laparoscopic segmental colon resection for malignancy is not worse than that of the open procedure. Although

total colectomy for colon cancer per se has not been tested in a controlled trial, it would be reasonable to assume that this procedure may be performed for synchronous lesions of the colon as segmental resection is done for an isolated lesion that is not advanced, obstructed, or perforated (per National Comprehensive Cancer Network [NCCN] guidelines).

PREOPERATIVE EVALUATION, TESTING, AND PREPARATION

All patients should undergo an extensive review of their past medical history and comorbidities; if a patient is being considered for an ileal pouch–anal anastomosis procedure, then the review of systems also should emphasize anal continence. Physical examination should include digital rectal examination, anoscopy, and proctoscopy. Preoperative testing may include colonoscopy, air-contrast barium enema, chest/abdominal/pelvic computed tomography (CT) scanning, serum carcinoembryonic antigen (CEA) level, and liver function tests as indicated for the particular diagnosis. Although the indication and justification for routine bowel preparation in elective colon surgery has been under increasing debate, it is still our preference for each patient to undergo a 5-day slow colon preparation and, if possible, admission to the hospital the day prior to surgery for administration of oral antibiotics.

PATIENT POSITIONING AND PLACEMENT OF TROCARS

The patient is placed in a modified lithotomy position and secured to the operating table so that extremes of table tilt may be safely applied (Fig. 16-1). Pressure points are well-padded, and a warming blanket is applied. A nasogastric tube and a Foley catheter routinely are placed; arterial and central venous lines are placed as indicated. We prefer to establish pneumoperitoneum with a Veress needle typically in the right or left upper quadrant, well away from any previous incisions. Our trocar placement for a total colectomy is shown in Figure 16-2; typically, four or five 5-mm trocars and one 12-mm trocar (for laparoscopic staplers) are utilized. The operation is viewed with a 5-mm laparoscope through the infraumbilical port.

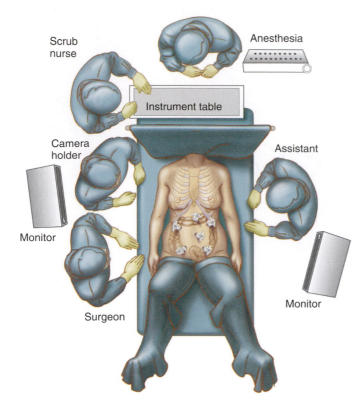

FIGURE 16-1 The modified lithotomy position for a laparoscopic total colectomy.

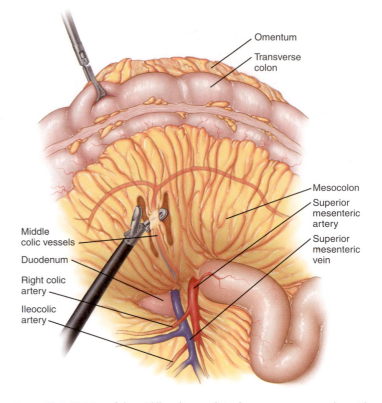

FIGURE 16-3 Division of the middle colic vessels in the transverse mesocolon with a bipolar sealer-cutter.

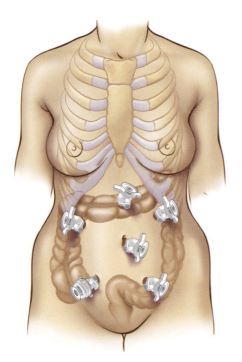

FIGURE 16-2 Placement of trocars for laparoscopic total colectomy.

OPERATIVE TECHNIQUE

The surgeon stands on the patient's right side. The omentum is retracted superiorly over the top of the transverse colon in order to gain access to the transverse mesocolon. The transverse colon then is elevated in order to tent the blood vessels of the mesocolon; sharp dissection is carried out in the midportion of the mesocolon until the middle colic artery and its branches are identified and isolated from surrounding tissue.

Early entry into the lesser sac by peeling the omentum off the transverse colon can facilitate vessel identification and ligation in the mesocolon. The middle colic artery may be divided with the LigaSure (Valleylab, Boulder, CO) device (Fig. 16-3). The mesenteric dissection is continued into the left transverse mesocolon toward the splenic flexure, taking care to identify and control all vessels in the mesentery. The dissection then proceeds to the patient's right, and the hepatic flexure is mobilized away from the duodenum, carefully protecting the duodenum, stomach, and common bile duct.

At this point the surgeon moves to the left side of the patient, and the right colic artery and its associated branches are approached and divided with a medial to lateral dissection (Fig. 16-4). With the duodenum clearly identified, the preperitoneal space is developed in a medial to lateral direction to the white line of Toldt. The dissection then proceeds inferiorly to the ileocolic artery and vein, which are divided. The cecum is elevated in order to identify the terminal ileum, and the mesentery of the small bowel is divided up to a previously determined point of ileal transection. Care should be taken to preserve as much of the blood supply to the terminal ileum as possible. The right colon then is mobilized from lateral to the medial using sharp dissection (Fig. 16-5), thus connecting the medial and lateral planes of dissection.

The surgeon then moves back to the right side of the patient, and the omentum is dissected off the transverse colon by entering the avascular plane between these two structures (Fig. 16-6). The splenic flexure of the colon then is mobilized with sharp and blunt dissection, and the dissection is carried distally along the lateral margin of the proximal left colon. The sigmoid colon is elevated in order to place the inferior mesenteric vessels on stretch. The peritoneum is incised over this pedicle, and a retroperitoneal dissection is performed from medial to lateral, connecting to the space that was developed during the splenic flexure mobilization.

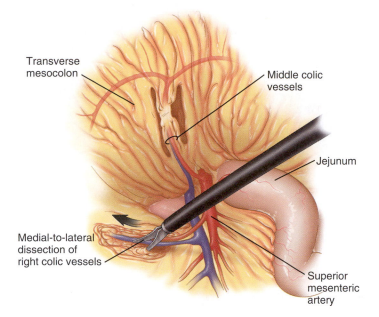

FIGURE 16-4 Dissection of the right colic vessels in the right mesocolon.

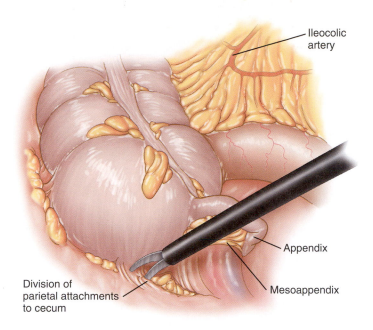

FIGURE 16-5 Mobilization of the cecum and right colon from the abdominal sidewall.

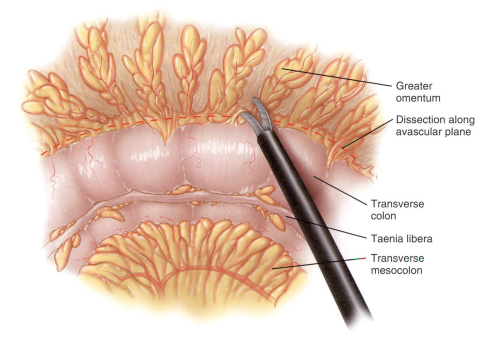

FIGURE 16-6 Dissection of omentum from the transverse colon.

The inferior mesenteric vessels may be divided with the LigaSure device. The lateral pelvic attachments of the descending and sigmoid colon are divided, allowing these structures to move freely to the midline. The left ureter is identified and preserved in the left retroperitoneum where it crosses the iliac artery (Fig. 16-7).

If a proctectomy is to be performed, then a posterior dissection is begun in the avascular plane between the mesorectum and the sacrum. Once a posterior space has been developed, the mesorectal dissection proceeds laterally, alternating between the right and left side, staying in the avascular plane between the mesorectum and the pelvic sidewall while using a combination of sharp and blunt techniques (Fig. 16-8). The dissection is kept close to (but not violating) the mesorectum in order to avoid injury to

a ureter, which is closely applied to the lateral wall. The rectum is elevated, and the posterior dissection is continued to the level of the levator ani. The lateral dissections are continued anteriorly around the rectum, until they meet to create a circumferential mesorectal dissection. Care should be exercised anteriorly to avoid injuring the prostate/urethra in the male or the vagina in the female.

If a subtotal colectomy is to be performed, then adequacy of the distal margin should be confirmed with proctoscopy prior to stapler transection of the rectum. The distal point of transection on the rectum then is cut with scissors or an articulating laparoscopic stapler-cutter. We prefer to irrigate the lumen of the rectal stump with a 3.5% iodine solution. If the

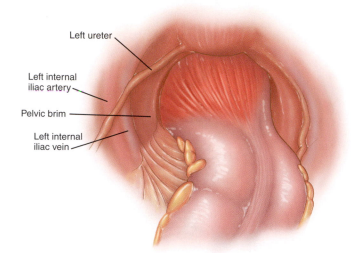

FIGURE 16-7 Identification of left ureter after the sigmoid colon has been mobilized medially.

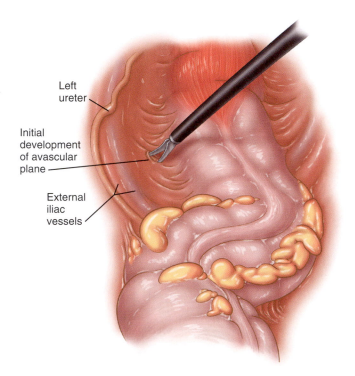

FIGURE 16-8 Mesorectal dissection, left side.

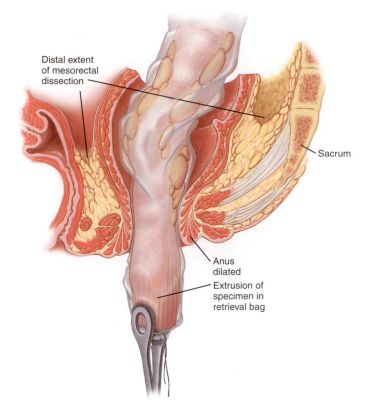

FIGURE 16-9 Transanal extraction of the total colectomy specimen within a plastic retrieval bag.

specimen is to be extracted transanally, then the distal end of the specimen is closed with a laparoscopic suture loop in order to prevent spillage. The distal ileum then is transected with a linear stapler-cutter. A specimen containing colon cancer is deposited into a plastic retrieval bag introduced through the 12-mm trocar or through the anus. The purse-string closure of the plastic retrieval bag is reinforced with a laparoscopic suture loop. The anus is gently dilated, the tails of the suture are grasped with a ring forceps, and the specimen is delivered out of the anus through the bag, using the latter as a sheath to "snake" the specimen out (Fig. 16-9). The specimen and bag should not be extruded as a "bolus." If necessary, an exteriorized portion of the bag can be opened while the rest of the bag resides in the anus, and then the specimen is pulled through the opening in the bag. After the bag has been removed, the anus and pelvis are inspected for tearing and bleeding.

The size of the end-to-end anastomotic (EEA) circular stapler which the ileum can accommodate may be determined by sounding the lumen of the distal ileum with a series of calibrated dilators (passed transanally). We have found that a size 28-mm or 29-mm stapler allows passage of the anvil into the ileum and produces an adequate lumen. If a J-pouch is to be constructed, then we prefer to use a 25-mm stapler. The EEA circular stapler (with the anvil attached) is advanced through the rectum into the abdominal cavity. The anvil then is detached from the stapler, placed into the open end of the terminal ileum, and secured with a suture loop or purse-string suture for the subsequent ileorectal anastomosis. The circular stapler is withdrawn from the rectum, and the rectal stump is closed with a laparoscopic linear stapler-cutter (Fig. 16-10A). We prefer to reinforce both the linear and circular staple lines with a bioabsorbable material (Seamguard, Gore Medical, Flagstaff, AZ). The rectal stump is insufflated with air prior to creating the ileorectal anastomosis to check for leaks. The circular stapler then is reintroduced into the rectum, and the stapler spike is advanced through the rectal stump, adjacent to (not directly through) the center of the staple line (Fig. 16-10B). The spike is removed from the stapler, and the anvil and stapler head are mated (Fig. 16-11A). The circular stapler then is fired per the instructions of its manufacturer, and the anastomosis is completed (Fig. 16-11B).

A careful intraluminal inspection of the anastomosis is performed with a flexible endoscope. The pelvis is flooded with saline, the ileum just proximal to the anastomosis is occluded, and air is insufflated into the rectum in order to check for leaks. If a leak is detected, then this can be repaired with intracorporeal suturing. A protective ileostomy is recommended in high-risk situations (e.g., history of corticosteroid use, pelvic radiation, multiple comorbidities) or if a leak of the ileorectal anastomosis was demonstrated. A diverting loop ileostomy can be created in

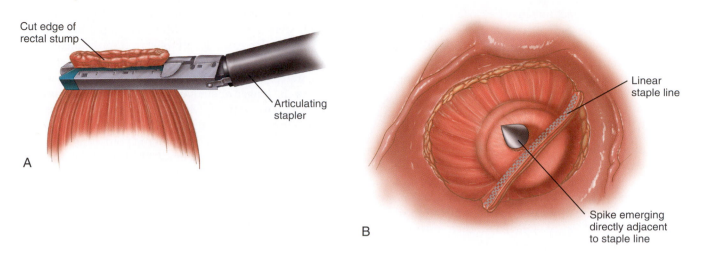

FIGURE 16-10 **A,** Closure of the rectal stump with an articulated stapler-cutter. **B,** Piercing of the rectal stump with the spike of the circular stapler. Note that the spike has been placed directly adjacent to the midportion of the rectal stump staple line.

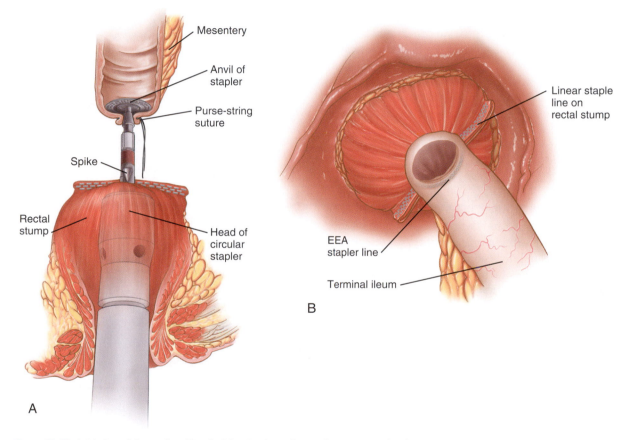

FIGURE 16-11 **A,** Mating of the anvil and head of the circular end-to-end anastomotic (EEA) stapler. **B,** Completed ileorectal anastomosis.

the usual fashion by externalizing a loop of ileum from the right lower quadrant trocar site. The abdominal cavity then is irrigated with saline and suctioned. The trocars are removed under direct vision, the fascia of port sites larger than 5 mm is closed, the pneumoperitoneum is evacuated, and the skin incisions are closed with absorbable monofilament sutures.

POSTOPERATIVE CARE

A nasogastric tube is reserved for the patient who presents with obstruction or perforation, or if a postoperative ileus develops with nausea and vomiting. Otherwise, most patients tolerate a clear liquid diet on postoperative day 1. The diet may be advanced as bowel function returns, as done with other gastrointestinal procedures. Preoperative medications may be resumed on postoperative day 1, or soon thereafter. Perioperative IV antibiotics should not be administered for longer than 24 hours. An epidural catheter may be utilized for analgesia; this seems to decrease the need for oral and injected opioids. The patient typically is discharged around postoperative day 4 or 5, when the patient is tolerating a diet, has normal bladder function, and has pain control with oral analgesics. The patient can resume normal physical activity after 1 month.

If present, a protective ileostomy may be closed at 6 weeks after the colectomy. A colonoscopy or contrast enema is performed prior to stoma closure to evaluate for stricture or other disease. If a patient is undergoing postoperative chemoradiation, then stomal closure is delayed until after this therapy is complete.

PROCEDURE-SPECIFIC COMPLICATIONS

Ureteral injury may be a consequence of a thermal burn, ligation, or laceration; this complication typically is secondary to inadequate exposure of the ureter and poor dissection technique. Preoperative placement of lighted ureteral stents may be beneficial in the intraoperative identification of these structures. If a ureteral injury is incurred, then most often the injury can be managed with primary repair and stenting. An intraoperative urologic consultation may be prudent in this scenario. In regard to tumor recurrence, there is a reasonable body of evidence that indicates that inadequate surgical technique is a risk factor for recurrence after resection of a colorectal cancer, especially if the resected tumor was of advanced stage. Care should be exercised when extracting a specimen through a small incision. A plastic retrieval bag should be used, and the surgeon may consider lavage of the abdominal cavity and incisions with a tumoricidal agent such as iodine solution. Staple line hemorrhage, postoperative small bowel obstruction, urinary retention, and high stomal output are other issues that can arise after this procedure, but they typically respond to conservative care.

Anastomotic leak may be secondary to tension, ischemia, or technical failure. Staple line reinforcement with a bioabsorbable material (see earlier discussion) may reduce the risk of this complication. If a patient has fever, prolonged ileus, unexplained leukocytosis, or abdominal pain, then the anastomosis should be evaluated with a CT or contrast study with gentle rectal instillation of water-soluble medium. The traditional treatment for this complication has been drainage and diversion; however, there have been an increasing number of anecdotal reports of successful treatment with antibiotics, parenteral nutrition, and percutaneous drainage in the minimally symptomatic patient, thus sparing the patient the need for a stoma.

RESULTS AND OUTCOME

Although the advantages of a laparoscopic segmental colon resection over open colon resection were relatively easy to demonstrate, similar advantages of laparoscopic total colectomy initially were not as obvious. More recent publications, however, have shown decreased length of stay, improved cosmesis, and a lower complication rate with the minimally invasive procedure compared to the open procedure. The former approach, however, still has the longer operative time. Our operative time has averaged 3.5 hours, with an average estimated blood loss of 200 mL. Our conversion rate has been 10%, and the mean hospital stay has been 10 days. The most common complications in our practice have been prolonged ileus (10%), bleeding (4%), wound infection (4%), and anastomotic stricture (2%). At the tertiary center where specialization in the described technique is available, the results and outcomes of laparoscopic total colectomy certainly justify its performance.

Suggested Reading

American Society of Colon and Rectal Surgeons: Position statement on laparoscopic colectomy for curable cancer. Dis Colon Rectum 2004;47:A1

Chen HH, Wexner SD, Weiss EG, et al: Laparoscopic colectomy for benign colorectal disease is associated with a significant reduction in disability as compared with laparotomy. Surg Endosc 1998;12:1397–1400.

Clinical Outcomes of Surgical Therapy Study Groups: A comparison of laparoscopically assisted and open colectomy for colon cancer. N Engl J Med 2004;350(20):2050–2059.

Fowler DL, White SA: Laparoscopy-assisted sigmoid resection. Surg Laparosc Endosc 1991;1:183–188.

Franklin ME, Ramos R, Rosenthal D, Schussler W: Laparoscopic colonic procedures. World J Surg 1993;17:51–56.

Franklin ME, Rosenthal D, Abrego-Medina D, et al: Prospective comparison of open vs. laparoscopic colon surgery for carcinoma: Five-year results. Dis Colon Rectum 1996;39:S35–S46.

Jacobs M, Verdeja G, Goldstein D: Minimally invasive colon resection. Surg Laparosc Endosc 1991;1:144–150.

Kockerling F, Reymond MA, Schneider C, et al, The Laparoscopic Colorectal Surgery Study Group: Prospective multicenter study of the quality of oncologic resections in patients undergoing laparoscopic colorectal surgery for cancer. Dis Colon Rectum 1998;41:963–970.

Kockerling F, Schneider C, Reymond MA, et al, Laparoscopic Colorectal Surgery Study Group (LCSSG): Early results of a prospective multicenter study on 500 consecutive cases of laparoscopic colorectal surgery. Surg Endosc 1998;12:37–41.

MacRae HM, McLeod RS: Handsewn vs. stapled anastomoses in colon and rectal surgery: A meta-analysis. Dis Colon Rectum 1998;41:180–189.

Monson JRT, Darzi A, Carey PD, Guillou PJ: Prospective evaluation of laparoscopic-assisted colectomy in an unselected group of patients. Lancet 1992;340:831a–833a.

NCCN: Clinical practice guidelines in oncology. Colon Cancer 2007;1. Accessed at www.nccn.org.

Phillips EH, Franklin M, Carroll BJ, et al: Laparoscopic colectomy. Ann Surg 1992;216:703–707.

HUBERT A. PRINS AND
ANTONIO M. LACY

Minimally Invasive Low Anterior Resection and Abdominal Perineal Resection

17

The prognosis of rectal cancer is in part related to (1) the invasiveness of the tumor (T) into the bowel wall, (2) the presence of tumor in lymph nodes (N), and (3) the presence of metastatic disease (M). For classification of rectal cancers, the tumor–node–metastasis (TNM) system commonly is used (Table 17-1). Other prognostic factors of colorectal cancer are related to the biologic behavior of the tumor, but they are not included in the TNM system. Curative treatment of rectal cancer requires a multimodality approach in which surgery currently is an essential component. In tumors with a TNM stage of T3 N0 M0 or T1–T3 N1–N2, preoperative or postoperative chemoradiotherapy or chemotherapy alone typically is a component of curative treatment (see the National Comprehensive Cancer Network [NCCN] Guidelines in "Suggested Reading"). A locally invasive lesion (T4 N0–2 M0) may undergo induction chemoradiation in order to increase the chance of resectability.

OPERATIVE INDICATIONS

The traditional indication for an abdominal perineal resection has been an adenocarcinoma located in the distal one third of the rectum; a tumor in the proximal two thirds of the rectum has been an indication for a low anterior resection. These indications have been in flux recently, and currently it appears that an oncologically sound resection with coloanal anastomosis may be possible for a tumor close to the anal verge (i.e., within several centimeters). A discussion of this issue, however, is beyond the scope of this chapter. Regardless of the exact procedure, the goal of the resection is to achieve a circumferential tumor-free margin within the surgical specimen and to remove all tumor-bearing lymphatic tissue. This typically is accomplished with a total mesorectal excision (see "Suggested Reading"). For advanced/unresectable rectal cancer, nonsurgical options for symptomatic control may be considered, such as palliative chemotherapy, radiotherapy, stenting, or laser therapy. In select cases (such as an elderly patient with multiple comorbidities who has a T1–T2 N0 M0 lesion), a full-thickness excision with transanal endoscopic microsurgery (TEM) might be considered. There has been controversy, however, over whether the rate of local recurrence after a TEM procedure is higher than after a traditional total mesorectal excision.

PREOPERATIVE EVALUATION

The diagnosis of rectal cancer should be established with the pathologic examination of a colonoscopic biopsy specimen. A full colonoscopy should be done to look for synchronous lesions. Further preoperative evaluation then should assess the extent of the disease and the patient's comorbidities. Local extent (i.e., T stage) and position of the tumor may be delineated with endorectal ultrasound or high-resolution computed tomography (CT) or magnetic resonance imaging (MRI) scanning of the pelvis. The distance of the tumor from the anal verge should be estimated with a combination of digital examination and proctoscopy/rigid sigmoidoscopy, as performed by the surgeon. This latter evaluation will help the surgeon decide whether to perform an abdominal perineal or a low anterior resection. A CT scan of the chest and abdomen should indicate whether the patient has M1 disease. In addition, positron emission tomography (PET) may be helpful in detecting metastatic disease, but currently this study is not routinely recommended. Hematologic tests should include a complete blood count, liver function tests, and a carcinoembryonic antigen (CEA). If there is a possibility that the patient may receive a colostomy, then a preoperative consultation with an enterostomal therapist would be appropriate. As always, an appropriate cardiopulmonary evaluation with the necessary consultations should be performed as indicated for this and all other major abdominal procedures.

PATIENT POSITIONING AND PLACEMENT OF TROCARS

The patient is placed in the Lloyd-Davies position, as shown in Figure 17-1. A urinary catheter is inserted, and the entire abdomen is prepared and draped. The positions of the operating team also are shown in Figure 17-1. The surgeon stands next to the camera operator on the patient's right side; the first assistant stands on the patient's left side. The trocars are placed as shown in Figure 17-2. The supraumbilical site (5 mm) is used as the camera port throughout the procedure. A 12-mm trocar is placed in the left lower quadrant, and is used for the LigaSure (Valleylab, Boulder, CO) device and graspers. Another 12-mm trocar is placed in the right lower quadrant for the same devices and also for the stapler-cutter; in addition, a temporary ileostomy

Table 17-1 Five-Year Survival Rates for Rectal Cancer in Relation to TNM Stage

Stage	TNM Classification	Five-Year Survival Rate
I	T1–T2 N0 M0	60%
II	T3–T4 N0 M0	40%
III	T1–T4 N1–N2 M0	25%
IV	T1–T4 N1–N2 M1	0–5%

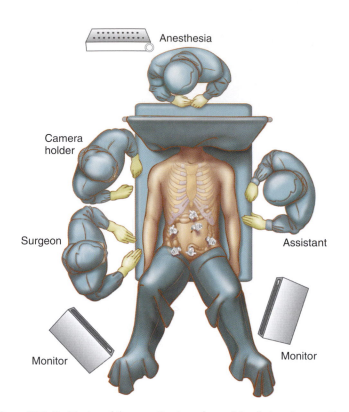

FIGURE 17-1 Positioning of the operating team for a minimally invasive resection of the rectum.

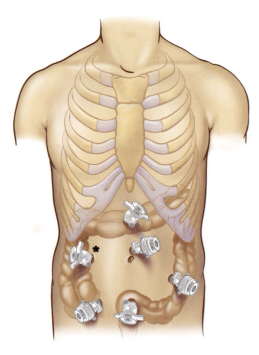

FIGURE 17-2 Trocar positions for a minimally invasive resection of the rectum. The trocar marked with an *asterisk* is optional and, if needed, may be placed wherever the surgeon deems appropriate.

(if needed) may be positioned at this site. A 5-mm port is placed in the suprapubic midline, and primarily is used during the anterior dissection of the mesorectum. Another 5-mm port is placed midway between the xiphoid process and the umbilicus, and primarily is used for mobilization of the splenic flexure. On occasion, an extra 5- or 12-mm port (making a total of six) may be introduced if the surgeon desires an additional site for retraction or dissection; in Figure 17-2, an extra 5-mm port is shown positioned in the right midabdomen.

OPERATIVE TECHNIQUE

Low Anterior Resection

An exploratory laparoscopy is performed first to determine if the patient has peritoneal seeding or liver metastases that were not visualized with the preoperative imaging. The finding of metastatic disease does not alter the need to resect the primary tumor; such a finding, however, may justify a decrease in the extent of the resection. The splenic flexure and the descending colon then are mobilized from the lateral abdominal wall. The patient is placed into reverse Trendelenburg position, and the table is rotated so that the patient's left side is elevated. The first assistant elevates the omentum cephalad in order to expose the distal transverse colon. We like to employ a combination of the LigaSure device and the hook electrocautery to mobilize the splenic flexure. This dissection is carried out until the splenic flexure can be brought below the umbilicus.

Prior to initiating the pelvic dissection in a woman, it may be beneficial to suspend the uterus to the supraumbilical region with a stitch. While the first assistant retracts the descending colon cephalad and lateral, the peritoneum on the medial side of the descending and sigmoid colon is incised. The inferior mesenteric artery and vein then are identified as they cross the pelvic brim. The left/sigmoid colon then is reflected medially, and the surgeon identifies and preserves the left ureter. At this point the surgeon can safely ligate the inferior mesenteric artery and vein; we prefer to ligate them separately. The artery is clipped 1 to 2 cm from its aortic origin in order to minimize the risk of injury to autonomic nerves. The vein is divided similarly, at a level just inferior to the pancreas.

After the inferior mesenteric vessels have been ligated, the abdominal dissection of the rectosigmoid is continued into the pelvis. The first assistant continues to retract the sigmoid colon medially and cephalad, and the surgeon resumes incising the peritoneal reflection along the white line of Toldt, using the hook electrocautery. The sigmoid is kept under tension, and the avascular plane that separates the mesorectum from the pelvic sidewall is identified. The surgeon should identify and preserve the hypogastric nerves, which originate just above the pelvic brim close to the posterior midline, then bifurcate into right and left branches and follow a posterolateral course between the pelvic sidewall and the mesorectum. The surgeon also should identify and preserve the nervi erigentes (pelvic splanchnic nerves), which emerge from sacral foramina and join presacral nerves to form the neurovascular bundle at the lateral edges of the seminal vessels. On the anterior portion of the mesorectum, the surgeon should enter the plane of the ill-defined Denonvilliers' fascia, which separates the anteriorly positioned bladder, prostate, and seminal vesicles from the posteriorly positioned mesorectum.

As the dissection of the mesorectum progresses, the surgeon should determine if a low anterior resection with primary anastomosis will be feasible. If we can obtain a 2-cm distal longitudinal margin, then we will proceed with the low anterior resection. The region of the rectum to be transected is circumferentially cleaned of tissue using the hook electrocautery or the LigaSure device. The rectum then is transected with the articulated linear stapler-cutter, using 3.5-mm cartridges. The specimen is placed into a protective polyethylene bag, and then it is exteriorized through a lateral extension of either the suprapubic or the supraumbilical port site. The proximal transection of the left colon is performed with a linear stapler-cutter, and the specimen is removed from the field.

The exteriorized proximal staple line is dissected clean, and then a purse-string suture is applied with an automated device. Once the purse-string has been placed, the staple line is opened and the proximal colon is sized for the anvil of the end-to-end anastomotic (EEA) stapler. The largest size anvil that can be inserted safely is placed into the proximal colon, and the purse-string suture is tied. The proximal colonic end with anvil is dropped back into the abdomen, the incision is sutured, and pneumoperitoneum is reestablished. The EEA stapler then is inserted transanally. In order to avoid the construction of an ischemic anastomosis, the spike of the stapler is brought through or directly adjacent to the previous staple line. The anvil is mated to the stapler, the stapler is closed and fired, and the anastomosis is created. The anastomotic integrity then is checked with transanal insufflation of air while the suture line is submerged in saline.

Abdominal Perineal Resection

If a 2-cm distal longitudinal margin cannot be obtained, then we will perform an abdominal perineal resection. The initial part of this procedure (up to the rectal transection) is the same as for the low anterior resection. Instead of cleaning off an area of rectum for transection, the surgeon should continue the mesorectal dissection down to the levator muscles. Using an angled laparoscope, the view of surgical field during this part of the procedure typically is better than what is seen during an open resection. The more complete the mesorectal dissection during the abdominal portion of this procedure, the easier will be the subsequent perineal portion of the procedure.

Upon completion of the mesorectal dissection, the surgeon can perform the colostomy. The proximal transection of the colon is performed intracorporeally using the linear stapler-cutter with 3.5-mm cartridges. A 3-cm skin disk on the patient's left abdomen, which has been previously marked by the enterostomal therapist, is excised. A cruciate incision is made in the anterior rectus sheath; the muscle is split, and the peritoneum is entered. The proximal colon is exteriorized through this colostomy site, and the colostomy is matured using interrupted everting seromuscular-cutaneous sutures, after the method of Brooke.

After the colostomy has been created, we like to place the patient in the prone jack-knife position, as shown in Figure 17-3. Although some extra anesthesia time is required for the repositioning, the prone position provides excellent exposure of the anus and reasonably comfortable operating position for the surgeon. Alternatively, the patient may be maintained in the Lloyd-Davies position for the perineal portion of the procedure; this allows for laparoscopic monitoring of the perineal dissection. In the prone position, the buttocks can be retracted laterally with wide heavy-duty tape. The anus is sewn shut with a silk purse-string suture. An elliptical incision is made around the anus (maintaining a minimal distance of 2–3 cm). Most of the subsequent dissection is performed with the hand electrocautery device. The perineal incision is carried through the ishiorectal fat down to the levators. The levators then are incised in the line of the incision; vigorous use of the cautery or application of ligatures often is necessary to control vessels in the muscular layers.

The perineal dissection typically is easiest in the lateral and posterior regions. Once the levators have been incised, a finger can be inserted underneath the remaining muscle layers, thereby allowing them to be pulled up into view for transection by the cautery. A properly performed perineal dissection will leave a cuff of levator muscles attached to the specimen. A landmark for the posterior dissection is the tip of the coccyx, which can be palpated directed in the midline above the specimen. The surgeon should be able to enter the dissection plane that was created during the abdominal portion of the procedure. Once this has been done, completion of the posterior and lateral dissection of the perineal portion of the procedure should soon follow.

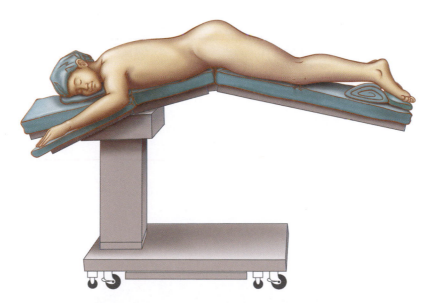

FIGURE 17-3 Prone jack-knife position is used during the perineal portion of an abdominal perineal resection. The colostomy should be created during the abdominal portion prior to repositioning the patient into the prone position.

The anterior dissection can be more difficult and time-consuming. In a woman, the posterior vagina may be preserved if there is no evidence of tumor invasion, and the anterior plane of the dissection is maintained between the posterior vagina and the specimen. In a man, the anterior dissection will stay between prostate/urethra and the specimen; this dissection should be performed carefully to avoid urethral injury (especially in an irradiated field). Palpation of the urinary catheter can facilitate a difficult dissection in this location. In some cases the specimen can be exteriorized out of the perineum through the channel that was created posteriorly; this may facilitate the remainder of the anterior dissection. After the specimen has been removed, a closed-suction drain is placed into the hollow of the sacrum and is brought out through a stab incision posterolateral to the main incision. The pelvic floor then is closed in three layers (levator muscles, subcutaneous tissue, and dermis) with absorbable sutures.

POSTOPERATIVE CARE

The patient is maintained on intravenous fluids, and the nasogastric tube is removed within 12 to 24 hours after the operation. The diet is advanced as tolerated by the patient after removal of the nasogastric tube. Mobilization of the patient should start no later than 24 hours after the procedure. If a pelvic drain has been placed, then it can be removed on postoperative day 2 or 3.

PROCEDURE-SPECIFIC COMPLICATIONS

Perioperative complications of minimally invasive resection of the rectum include ureteral injury, anastomotic leak, and intra-abdominal abscess; these complications were discussed in Chapters 14 and 15, on transverse and left/sigmoid colon resection. One aspect of anastomotic leak particular to very low anterior resections is the need for a protective colostomy. A traditional guideline that has been used is that if a colorectal anastomosis is within 5 cm of the anal verge, then the surgeon might consider creating temporary protective ostomy. Whether this guideline is appropriate for minimally invasive low anterior resections is not clear. A complication that can affect the male patient is impotence, presumably secondary to injury to the pelvic nerves. This potential complication emphasizes the importance of identifying and preserving the nerve plexuses during a total mesorectal excision. In addition, very low anterior resections with a coloanal anastomosis can result in a various degree of fecal incontinence, especially in the older patient. This potential complication should be discussed preoperatively, and the surgeon should carefully weigh the risk of performing a sphincter-preserving procedure in each case.

RESULTS AND OUTCOME

The prognosis of a patient who undergoes a curative resection of a rectal cancer largely depends on the TNM classification, as indicated in Table 17-1. Local-regional control has improved since emphasis has been placed on total mesorectal excision; in addition, the utilization of preoperative radiotherapy in select cases can reduce the local recurrence rate. The utilization of the minimally invasive approach for the resection of rectal adenocarcinoma does not appear to have had a negative impact on the long-term survival of these patients. Indeed, there may be a positive impact on survival with the use of minimally invasive technique. With respect to follow-up after resection of a colorectal malignancy, careful monitoring of the patient with CT scanning, CEA level, and colonoscopy during the first 5 years may improve survival, although this is somewhat controversial.

Suggested Reading

The Clinical Outcomes of Surgical Therapy Study Group: A comparison of laparoscopically assisted and open colectomy for colon cancer. N Engl J Med 2004;350:2050–2059.

Heald RJ, Moran BJ, Ryall RD, et al: Rectal cancer: The Basingstoke experience of total mesorectal excision, 1978–1997. Arch Surg 1998;133:894–899.

Kapiteijn E, Marijnen CA, Nagtegaal ID, et al: Preoperative radiotherapy combined with total mesorectal excision for resectable rectal cancer. N Engl J Med 2001;345:638–646.

Lacy AM, Garcia-Valdecasas JC, Delgado S, et al: Laparoscopy-assisted colectomy versus open colectomy for treatment of non-metastatic colon cancer: A randomised trial. Lancet 2002;359:2224–2229.

Leung KL, Kwok SP, Lam SC, et al: Laparoscopic resection of rectosigmoid carcinoma: Prospective randomised trial. Lancet 2004;363(9416):1187–1192.

Middleton PF, Sutherland LM, Maddern GJ: Transanal endoscopic microsurgery: A systematic review. Dis Colon Rectum 2005;48:270–284.

NCCN: Clinical practice guidelines in oncology. Colon Cancer 2007;1. Accessed at www.nccn.org.

Sauer R, Becker H, Hohenberger W, et al: Preoperative versus postoperative chemoradiotherapy for rectal cancer. N Engl J Med 2004;351:1731–1740.

Schwenk W, Haase O, Neudecker J, Muller JM: Short term benefits for laparoscopic colorectal resection. Cochrane Database Syst Rev 2005(3):CD003145.

Slim K, Vicaut E, Panis Y, Chipponi J: Meta-analysis of randomized clinical trials of colorectal surgery with or without mechanical bowel preparation. Br J Surg 2004;91(9):1125–1130.

DANIEL A. LAWES AND
TONIA M. YOUNG-FADOK

Minimally Invasive Proctocolectomy and Ileal Pouch–Anal Anastomosis

18

Proctocolectomy with ileal pouch–anal anastomosis (IPAA) has become the treatment of choice for patients requiring operative intervention for ulcerative colitis or inherited conditions, such as familial adenomatous polyposis, that predispose to the development of colorectal cancer. The main advantage of IPAA over alternative surgical procedures is that it involves complete removal of diseased tissue while avoiding a permanent stoma, allowing fecal continence to be maintained. This improves postoperative quality of life and leads to greater patient satisfaction. First described by Parks over 25 years ago, the technique of IPAA has evolved through a number of technical controversies, ranging from the configuration and size of the ileal pouch, the need for anal canal mucosectomy, the relative merits of hand-sewn versus stapled pouch–anal anastomosis, and the need for a temporary defunctioning stoma. All of these variations of the IPAA procedure have been performed via a midline laparotomy to obtain access to the abdomen.

Over the past decade, however, the advantages of laparoscopic compared to open colorectal surgery have become widely accepted. Nevertheless, laparoscopic colorectal surgery is technically difficult, and IPAA is one of the more challenging colorectal procedures to perform. This procedure is complicated further in the patients with inflamed bowel, malnutrition, and immunosuppression. Although initial results for laparoscopic IPAA (LIPAA) were disappointing because of longer operative time, postoperative ileus, and length of hospital stay compared to the open approach, more recent studies have demonstrated the feasibility and improved outcomes of LIPAA. A variety of techniques have been employed in these studies, including (1) laparoscopic mobilization of the abdominal colon followed by open rectal dissection through a Pfannenstiel incision; (2) laparoscopic hand-assisted surgery; and (3) laparoscopic mobilization of both the colon and rectum with intra- or extracorporeal division of the blood vessels and extracorporeal pouch formation. More recent data have suggested that although LIPAA takes longer to perform than its open equivalent, the advantages of laparoscopic surgery seen with other colonic procedures appear to be maintained, including improved recovery time, shorter hospital stay, and improved cosmesis. In addition, the complication rates and long-term functional results are comparable between LIPAA and open surgery groups.

We have simplified the technique of LIPAA, dividing it into five reproducible steps, allowing the colon and rectum to be exteriorized and the pouch to be constructed through a small periumbilical incision, which maintains the postoperative benefits of laparoscopic colorectal surgery. Herein we describe the most simplified version of this procedure.

OPERATIVE INDICATIONS

The indications for LIPAA are identical to the open procedure. The most common indication is ulcerative colitis associated with one of the following factors: symptomatic disease refractory to medical therapy; side effects of medical therapy; inability to wean from steroids; desire to avoid specific medications; presence of cancer or dysplasia; and, in children, growth retardation. These tend to be criteria for an elective procedure. LIPAA also may be appropriate for those with a known genetic predisposition to develop colorectal cancer, such as familial adenomatous polyposis (FAP) or hereditary nonpolyposis colon cancer (HNPCC), if the polyps or cancer involves the rectum. LIPAA usually is performed in two stages, with laparoscopic proctocolectomy, IPAA, and formation of a defunctioning ileostomy performed in the first stage, followed by closure of the ileostomy in the second stage. The ileostomy closure usually is done 3 months after the initial procedure, when the patient has been weaned from steroid therapy and is well nourished.

In the emergency setting in a patient with fulminant colitis, toxic megacolon, perforation, or hemorrhage, proctocolectomy and creation of an ileal pouch is contraindicated. The procedure of choice is total abdominal colectomy/subtotal colectomy with an end-ileostomy; the rectum is left as a stump. The feasibility and safety of laparoscopic subtotal colectomy in the emergency setting has been demonstrated. Given the reduction in adhesions often seen with a laparoscopic approach, it may be possible to perform the subsequent completion proctectomy and IPAA laparoscopically.

PREOPERATIVE EVALUATION

Preoperative evaluation remains the same as for the open procedure. Patients should undergo standard history, physical examination, and laboratory tests, including blood typing and screening, with further evaluation as appropriate. All patients undergo preoperative consultation with an enterostomal thera-pist, both for educational purposes and to mark the most appro-priate site for the planned diverting loop ileostomy. Patients with a malignancy should undergo a standard staging proto-col and appropriate preoperative oncologic management of the tumor. Chemoradiation for rectal cancer should be adminis-tered as needed, and does not interfere with subsequent laparo-scopic rectal dissection. Radiation therapy, if indicated, should be given preoperatively to avoid radiating the pouch and pro-ducing a poor functional outcome. Prior to reversal of a defunc-tioning ileostomy, it is our practice to perform a water-soluble contrast pouchogram.

PATIENT POSITIONING IN THE OPERATING SUITE

The patient lies on the operating table on foam "egg-crate" pad-ding that is taped to the table; this helps prevent the patient from slipping during steep changes of table position. It is essential that the operating table can change position easily and allow a wide range of movements; this will facilitate access to different areas of the abdomen by using gravity to move the small intestine from the operative field. The patient's distal sacrum is positioned at the end of the table in order to gain access for mucosectomy or a stapled anastomosis. Knee or thigh length pneumatic com-pression devices are applied to the legs, which are placed in pad-ded Lloyd-Davies stirrups (Fig. 18-1). The patient's thighs must be parallel to the abdomen to prevent interference with instru-ments in the lower quadrant ports. The patient's hands are pro-tected with further foam padding and the arms secured with a sheet, wrapped around the arms and folded beneath the torso. Additional "egg-crate" padding is laid on the patient's chest before securing the upper body with a chest strap, which also reduces the risk that the patient will slip during position changes.

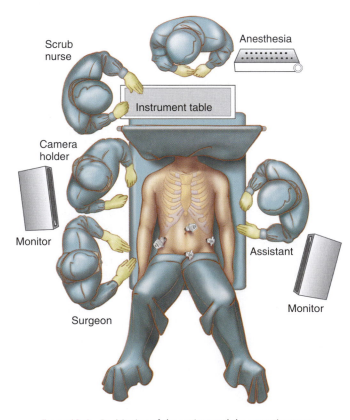

FIGURE 18-1   Positioning of the patient and the operating team.

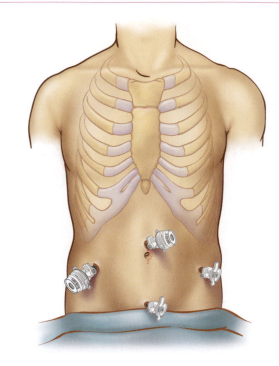

FIGURE 18-2   Port placement for the ileal pouch–anal anastomosis procedure.

The bladder is catheterized, an orogastric tube placed, and following the skin preparation, the patient is draped in a standard sterile manner with leggings and adhesive drapes to expose the abdomen. The laparoscopic tubing and leads are placed on the OR table and checked. The laparoscopic "stack" containing the light source, camera, and insuffla-tor are positioned on either the right or left side to produce minimum interference with table changes and surgeon move-ment, depending on configuration of the operating room. A 30-degree, 10-mm laparoscope is used throughout the pro-cedure. Two video screens are utilized, one on either side of the patient, with the ability to move them between the patient's ankles and shoulders, which will allow the surgeon, assistant, and scrub nurse each quadrant during the operation. Other instruments that we routinely use are two 5-mm Babcock graspers, laparoscopic scissors with a finger-operated cautery switch, a vessel-sealing device, a laparoscopic articulated sta-pler with 30- and 45-mm cartridges, suction irrigation, and a smoke evacuator. After port placement, both the surgeon and assistant stand on the patient's right side and face the left colon so that eyes, hands, and operative site are aligned.

POSITIONING AND PLACEMENT OF PORTS

We routinely use one 12-mm blunt port, one 12-mm standard port, and two 5-mm ports (Fig. 18-2). The first port inserted is a 12-mm supraumbilical blunt trocar. A 3- to 4-cm skin incision is cre-ated, skirting the umbilicus (this will ultimately be used for exterior-ization and, in heavier patients, facilitates access to the fascia for the initial cut-down), and the port is inserted by cut-down method. We find that creating the planned skin incision at the start of the opera-tion facilitates the insertion of the first trocar without any subsequent adverse effect on cosmesis or incision size, since this incision will be used for colonic extraction and pouch creation. Following insuffla-tion to 13 mm Hg, the camera is introduced and the abdominal cavity inspected. The umbilical port remains the camera port throughout the procedure. Subsequent ports are inserted under direct vision in a diamond shape configuration. A 5-mm port is inserted in the left lower quadrant (LLQ), a second 5-mm port is placed in the suprapubic region and a 12-mm port inserted in the right lower quadrant (RLQ). It is our practice to place the RLQ port through the planned temporary ileostomy site (marked by the enterostomal therapist preoperatively), which may need to be moved further laterally to avoid interference with the other ports. A disk of skin and subcutaneous fat is excised prior to the insertion of this port to facilitate creation of the loop ileostomy at the end of the operation. A 5-mm reducer is used with this port for most of the dissection, but this port ultimately is used for the linear stapler to transect the rectum at the level of the pelvic floor. We utilize this standard diamond port configuration for all laparoscopic colorectal cases and find that it allows excellent access to the entire abdominal cavity. On occasion, in a particularly difficult case, a further 5-mm port is introduced, its position being dictated by the specific requirements of the case.

OPERATIVE TECHNIQUE

We divide the operation into five distinct steps: (1) mobilization of the left colon and splenic flexure; (2) mobilization of the right colon and hepatic flexure; (3) rectal dissection and transection; (4) exteriorization of the colon and ileal pouch formation; and (5) ileal pouch–anal anastomosis and formation of loop ileostomy (Table 18-1).

Mobilization of the Left Colon and Splenic Flexure

The patient is positioned in steep Trendelenburg position with the left side of the operating table elevated. The surgeon and assistant stand on the right side of the patient. The surgeon holds a grasper in the left hand through the RLQ port and cautery scissors in the right hand via the suprapubic port.

Table 18-1 Laparoscopic Proctocolectomy and Ileal Pouch–Anal Anastomosis: Steps and Key Points

Step 1: Mobilization of Left Colon and Splenic Flexure
Left colon
  Trendelenburg position, left side inclined up
  Identify ureter
Splenic flexure
  Reverse Trendelenburg position, left side inclined up
  Mobilization of the omentum
  Mobilization to the midline and level of umbilicus

Step 2: Mobilization of the Right Colon and Hepatic Flexure
Right colon
  Trendelenburg position, right side inclined up
  Identify ureter, duodenum, and inferior vena cava
Hepatic flexure
  Reverse Trendelenburg position, right side inclined up
  Mobilization to the midline and level of umbilicus

Step 3: Pelvic Dissection
Trendelenburg position
Suspend uterus
Transection of rectum at level of pelvic floor

Step 4: Exteriorization, Resection, and Pouch Formation
Exteriorization via 4–5 cm periumbilical incision
Extracorporeal transection of mesentery
Extracorporeal evaluation of small bowel
Creation of ileal J-pouch
Replace small bowel: Trendelenburg, right side tilted up

Step 5: Ileal Pouch–Anal Anastomosis
Check alignment of pouch mesentery
Check posterior vaginal wall is clear of stapler

The first maneuver is to ensure that the small bowel is swept out of the pelvis toward the patient's right shoulder. It usually is unnecessary to grasp the bowel, as gravity usually moves the small bowel and maintains its position. The sigmoid colon is identified and retracted medially to expose the left lateral peritoneal reflection or white line of Toldt. The peritoneum directly medial to this line is scored with the cautery scissors (Fig. 18-3). We prefer the use of cautery for mobilization of the colon, since this technique mimics the open procedure, allows the operation to proceed more expeditiously, and ensures that the correct bloodless dissection plane is maintained. Dissection is continued cephalad between the sigmoid mesocolon and retroperitoneum. Medial traction is maintained on the colon, creating gentle tension and allowing the correct plane to be opened with combination of blunt dissection and cautery. It is important at this point to identify the left ureter, which usually is visible running medial to the gonadal vessels and over the left iliac vessels. With the ureter identified, dissection continues toward the splenic flexure along the left lateral peritoneal reflection. Traction is important to allow the correct plane to be identified; this may be facilitated by the assistant, who can retract the colon with a grasper in the right hand via the RLQ port, while the surgeon uses the cautery scissors through the LLQ port, and a grasper through the suprapubic port. With appropriate traction and identification of the correct plane, one avoids dissecting in a plane lateral to the true peritoneal reflection, which runs the risk of mobilization of the kidney or pancreas.

When the descending colon has been mobilized to the level of the spleen, the greater omentum then is mobilized from the colon. The patient is repositioned in reverse Trendelenburg position, with the left side of the operating table elevated. The surgeon stands between the patient's legs to facilitate splenic mobilization. The assistant uses a grasper placed via the RLQ port to elevate the omentum cephalad, so that it hangs down to form a cape of fatty tissue, thus exposing the distal transverse colon. The surgeon retracts the transverse colon caudad, and the peritoneum joining the colon and omentum is divided to gain entry into the lesser sac. Dissection continues along the superior border of the colon until the spleen is reached; all of the distal transverse colon is freed from omentum. In the obese patient or in the patient who has severe colonic inflammation, this plane may be difficult to identify; in these cases, the splenocolic attachments may be divided using an energy device to enter the lesser sac from above. The assistant retracts the omentum inferiorly, and the fatty attachments between the stomach and colon to the left of the midline can then be identified and safely divided until the lesser sac is entered. Dissection proceeds toward the spleen, with the assistant grasping the superior cut edge of the omentum, while the surgeon provides countertraction on the inferior edge using a grasper via the LLQ port, and with the power source via the suprapubic port. Once the omentum has been divided, the splenic flexure is retracted inferiorly, and any further retroperitoneal adhesions are divided. Mobilization is considered to be satisfactory when the splenic flexure can easily be brought down to a point below the level of the umbilicus. Complete mobilization of the transverse/left colon at this point will make it easier to exteriorize the colon later in the procedure.

Mobilization of the Right Colon and Hepatic Flexure

The patient is then placed in steep Trendelenburg position with the right side of the operating table elevated. Both surgeon and assistant move to the left side of the patient. The grasper is held

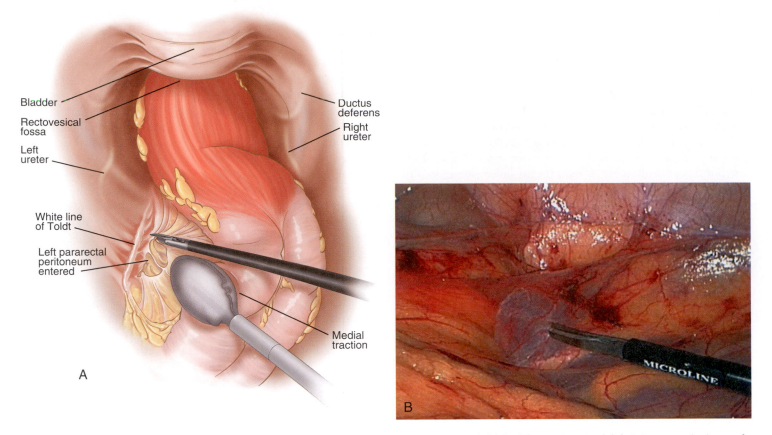

FIGURE 18-3 **A,** Incision of the left lateral peritoneal reflection of the sigmoid colon. Top of drawing is caudad; left of drawing is patient's left. **B,** Intraoperative image of the same, except that view is directed to the patient's right. Ultrasonic scalpel indicates point of incision into peritoneum between the sigmoid mesocolon (to the left of the instrument) and the lateral abdominal wall (to the right of the instrument).

in the surgeon's right hand via LLQ port, and cautery scissors are held in the left hand via the suprapubic port, which should prevent crossing of the instruments. The peritoneum inferior to the junction of the cecum and terminal ileum is lifted anteriorly and cephalad (i.e., toward 2 or 3 o'clock on the screen). This exposes the "valley" where the mesentery of the colon meets the retroperitoneum, and runs roughly parallel to the iliac artery (Fig. 18-4). In a patient with normal body mass index (BMI), the right ureter can be seen through the peritoneum; in a heavier patient, however, the ureter must be identified after opening the peritoneum. The peritoneum is scored along this valley, allowing gas

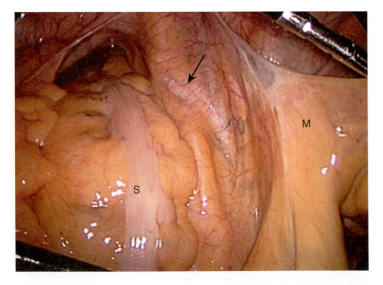

FIGURE 18-4 Exposure of the base of the ileocecal region. Top of the photograph is caudad, and the *arrow* indicates the right ureter. M, mesentery of ileocecal region; S, sigmoid colon.

to enter the tissues, which should identify a layer of filmy connective tissue that delineates the correct bloodless plane. This plane is developed both medially and superiorly while traction is maintained on the cecum. Once the cecum and terminal ileum are mobilized, the right lateral peritoneal reflection alongside the ascending colon is opened, and the colon is mobilized medially (Fig. 18-5). The surgeon should follow the correct plane of dissection as it turns medially and obliquely between the posterior aspect of the ascending colon mesentery and the retroperitoneum, in order to avoid inadvertent posterior mobilization of the right kidney. Adequate mobilization for this step has been achieved when the duodenum, inferior vena cava, and right ureter have all been exposed, identified, and protected.

The patient then is moved to reverse Trendelenburg position (still with the right side of the table elevated), and mobilization of the hepatic flexure is commenced. The instruments are switched so that the cautery scissors are now in the surgeon's right hand via the LLQ port, and the grasper is in the left hand through the suprapubic port. The gastrocolic attachments may be divided with cautery or another energy device, depending on the surgeon's preference and patient's BMI. The gastrocolic attachments are grasped just cephalad to the colon and the correct plane is sought by elevating the tissues and looking for the area where the tissues can be seen to slide over the retroperitoneum (Fig. 18-6). This plane is developed until it meets with the dissection which was performed inferiorly and laterally. Again, the duodenum should be exposed and protected. At this point, the entire right colon can be pulled across to the left side of the abdominal cavity, ensuring that full mobilization has been performed to the midline. Any remaining attachments to the retroperitoneum or duodenum are divided at this time. As with the left colon, mobilization is considered adequate when the hepatic flexure can be brought below the level of the umbilicus.

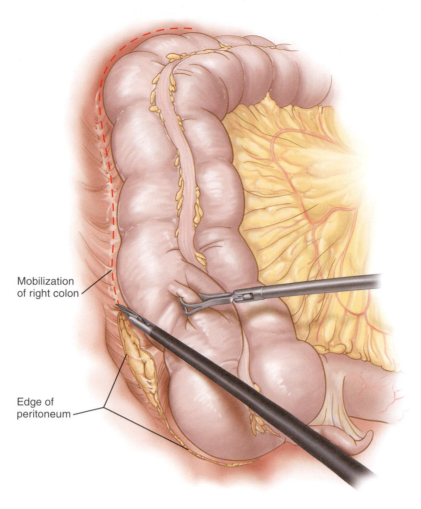

FIGURE 18-5 Incision of the peritoneal reflection lateral to the right colon. Top of drawing is cephalad.

Rectal Dissection and Transection

The patient's position is altered to steep Trendelenburg with the table in a neutral position. The surgeon remains on the left side of the patient, while the assistant moves to the right side. The small bowel is moved from the pelvis into the upper abdomen. The surgeon holds the cautery scissors in the left hand via the LLQ port and a grasper in the right hand via the suprapubic port. The assistant holds a grasper in the right hand via the RLQ port. The posi-

tion of both ureters is confirmed, and the assistant retracts the sigmoid cephalad and toward the right side of the patient. The surgeon retracts the rectum upward toward the anterior abdominal wall, and continues the dissection from the distal aspect of the sigmoid mobilization, along the left lateral peritoneal reflection. This dissection is extended along the left pararectal peritoneum, thus entering the lateral aspect of the presacral space (Fig. 18-7). Once the

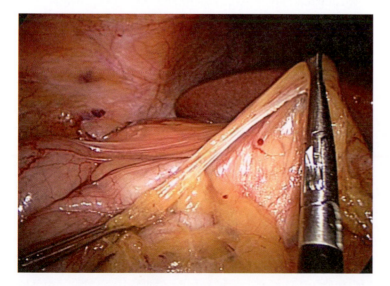

FIGURE 18-6 The grasper on the right is elevating a portion of the gastrocolic ligaments away from the hepatic flexure of the colon. View is directed toward the patient's right; the right lobe of the liver is visible in the background.

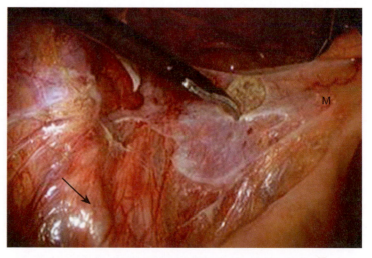

FIGURE 18-7 Entry into presacral space beneath the mesorectum (M). *Arrow* indicates the left iliac artery. Top of the photograph is caudad.

filmy connective tissue behind the mesorectum is identified, the surgeon moves the grasper into this plane and retracts the rectum superiorly, which facilitates gas entry into the tissues. Cautery dissection is continued lateral and posterior to the rectum as far as possible. As dissection proceeds toward the pelvic floor, it should be remembered that the mesorectum begins to curve anteriorly, following the curve of the sacrum; this plane should be followed in order to avoid inadvertent damage to the presacral venous plexus.

For dissection on the right side of the rectum, the surgeon and assistant may change places. The sigmoid is retracted out of the pelvis and toward the left side by the assistant, and the rectum then is lifted toward the anterior abdominal wall by the surgeon. The right pararectal peritoneum is scored at the level of the sacral promontory to enter the presacral space (Fig. 18-8), and the dissection is joined with the previous dissection on the left, taking care to identify and preserve the presacral nerves. The right pararectal tissues and pararectal peritoneum are divided. When the posterior and both lateral sides of the rectum are mobilized to the pelvic floor, the peritoneum anterior to the rectum is divided. The assistant again retracts the sigmoid out of the pelvis, while the surgeon retracts the rectum toward the sacrum. In the female patient, the uterus may need to be retracted through an additional port, or by placing two sutures through the anterior abdominal wall and then through the avascular area of the broad ligament, or by using a uterine manipulator. Dissection continues in the rectovaginal or rectoprostatic plane until the entire rectum has been mobilized circumferentially down to the level of the pelvic floor. This may be facilitated in the female patient by placing a sponge stick in the vagina in order to retract it away from the rectum. The distance from the anal verge can be confirmed with a digital rectal examination while a grasper is positioned at the distal limit of dissection. If the dissection is sufficiently distal, then an articulated, laparoscopic linear stapler-cutter is inserted via the RLQ port, and the rectum is transected at the level of the pelvic floor. Several stapler firings may be required for this to be completed.

Exteriorization of the Colon and Ileal Pouch Formation

Prior to exteriorization of the colon, the operating table should be in a neutral position. The colon should be in its correct anatomic position without any small bowel lying over it, as this may hinder exteriorization. A grasper is placed on the cut edge of the rectum, and all other instruments are removed. The pneumoperitoneum is released, the umbilical port is removed, and the periumbilical incision is extended to 4 to 5 cm. The grasper is passed up to the incision so that the rectum may be delivered. With gentle manipulation, the entire colon and rectum can be brought out through this incision (Fig. 18-9). Due to the position of the incision, intracorporeal division of the vessels is not necessary; provided the hepatic and splenic flexures have been adequately mobilized, extracorporeal work is possible. After exteriorization, the omentum either may be dissected from the transverse colon and returned to the abdomen, or removed with the specimen. The colonic mesentery and its blood supply are divided and ligated in a standard manner. The terminal ileum is transected with a linear stapler so that the ileocolic artery is preserved. The small intestine is fully exteriorized (the base of the small bowel mesentery lies beneath this incision) and inspected for any signs of Crohn's disease; any remaining attachments of the small bowel mesentery to the duodenum are lysed. A 15-cm stapled J-pouch, our preferred reservoir, is created with two firings of the 80- or 100-mm linear stapler. The anvil of a circular stapling device is secured in the apex of the pouch with a purse-string suture. With the patient in Trendelenburg position and the right side of the table elevated, the small bowel and pouch are returned to the abdominal cavity, and the pouch is placed in the pelvis. The peritoneal cavity is irrigated with warm saline, which then is aspirated. The periumbilical incision is closed with interrupted absorbable sutures. Two adjacent sutures at the cephalic end of the incision are left untied and are used to resecure the blunt 12-mm port in the fascial incision. Pneumoperitoneum then is reestablished.

Ileal Pouch–Anal Anastomosis and Formation of Loop Ileostomy

The peritoneal cavity is inspected for hemostasis. The pouch is brought down to the pelvis, ensuring that the mesentery is not twisted. This is confirmed by visualizing the cut edge of the small bowel mesentery and tracing it from the top of the pouch to the duodenum. An assistant is deployed to the perineum to insert the circular stapler into the anal canal, and the spike is brought out adjacent to the staple line at the top of the rectal stump. The anvil is coupled to the stapler, the stapler components are approximated under direct vision, and the stapler then is fired

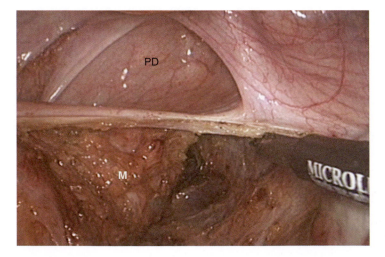

FIGURE 18-8 Right side of rectal dissection. Top of the photograph is caudad. M, mesorectum; PD, pouch of Douglas.

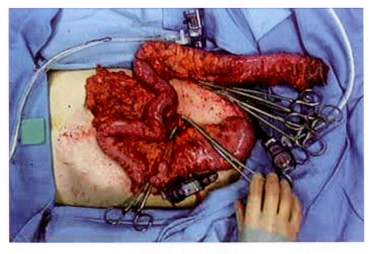

FIGURE 18-9 Exteriorization of colonic specimen through the umbilical port incision. Left of photograph is cephalad.

and removed. The surgeon should exercise care in women in order to avoid incorporating the posterior wall of the vagina into the staple line.

A drain is placed adjacent to the pouch via the suprapubic port. To create the ileostomy, an appropriate loop of small bowel that comfortably will reach the anterior abdominal wall at the site of the intended ileostomy is identified and held with a grasper. The pneumoperitoneum is evacuated, and the anterior and posterior rectus fasciae are opened in a cruciate fashion. The grasper is then used to pass the small bowel loop through the trephine, and a loop ileostomy is made in the standard fashion. The pneumoperitoneum is reestablished, the remaining trocars are removed under direct vision, and closure of the midline incision is completed with the two untied sutures (Fig. 18-10).

Laparoscopic Proctocolectomy and IPAA—More Complex Approaches

The preceding approach avoids intracorporeal division of the mesentery and blood vessels and is feasible in patients with normal body mass index. In the obese patient, or in the patient in whom an oncologic resection is indicated, intracorporeal division may not be feasible or appropriate, so intracorporeal transection of the mesentery would be indicated. In such cases, the intra-abdominal colon and rectum are mobilized and the rectum is transected at the pelvic floor as described. The mesentery then is sequentially divided with an energy device such as the ultrasonic or bipolar shears, starting at the base of the inferior mesenteric artery or superior rectal vessels, and working toward the ileocolic pedicle, which is preserved. By mobilizing the colon and rectum first and transecting the vessels afterward, there is no prolonged period of colon ischemia. Following this step, the colon and rectum may be exteriorized through a periumbilical incision, or even via the ileostomy site, which avoids the need to enlarge the supraumbilical port site incision.

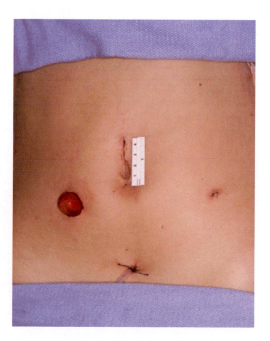

FIGURE 18-10 Appearance of abdomen upon completion of procedure. Top of photograph is cephalad.

POSTOPERATIVE CARE

On completion of the operation, the orogastric tube is removed. On postoperative day 1, the patient is given limited clear liquids and encouraged to ambulate, provided he is not nauseated and the abdomen not distended. If liquids are tolerated, then on postoperative day 2 a low-fiber diet is commenced, intravenous fluid replacement is stopped, analgesia is converted to an oral formulation, the urinary catheter is removed, and patient mobilization is increased. The enterostomal therapist commences training by postoperative day 3. Provided that the patient is comfortable and tolerating a full diet, he may be discharged at this time.

PROCEDURE-SPECIFIC COMPLICATIONS

Proctocolectomy and IPAA is complex and technically challenging. In addition to complications that can occur in most major abdominal operations (i.e., postoperative hemorrhage, intraabdominal abscess, and small bowel obstruction), complications specific to this procedure may include the following:

Pouch Torsion

Twisting of the pouch at the anastomosis is a catastrophic complication; those undergoing a laparoscopic procedure may be at greater risk. Twisting can be avoided by checking the orientation of the pouch prior to coupling the anvil to the stapler. This is best done by tracing the cut edge of the pouch mesentery from the apex up to the duodenum and ensuring that it lies straight without any twisting. This procedure then can be repeated following engagement of the anvil with the circular stapler.

Continued Proctitis

Patients may continue to have symptoms of proctitis if an excessively long rectal stump has been left in situ. This risk can be minimized by ensuring that the rectum has been mobilized all the way down to the pelvic floor. A digital rectal examination performed in conjunction with the assistant placing an atraumatic grasper at the distal limit of dissection should confirm the distance of the dissection from the anal verge. Once the dissection has reached a satisfactory level, the surgeon should ensure that the stapler is applied at the level of the pelvic floor. This can be challenging, particularly in a narrow male pelvis, and we recommend the use of an articulating stapler to obtain a staple line that lies flush with the pelvic floor. We have found that deploying this stapler via the RLQ port provides the easiest means of placing the staple line in the correct position. The length of staple cartridge is of less importance than the ability to place the stapler in the correct anatomic position; a shorter cartridge may be reapplied several times in order to divide the distal rectum/upper anal canal. Placing the stapler may be facilitated by an assistant placing a fist on the perineum and pushing up into the pelvis. Care should be taken to avoid damaging other structures, particularly the vagina, while transecting the rectum. If stapling is impossible, or if there are other considerations such as cancer or dysplasia within the rectum, then a mucosectomy with a hand-sewn pouch–anal anastomosis can be performed at this stage.

Ileal Pouch–Anal Anastomosis Leaks and Strictures

Leaks and strictures of the ileal pouch–anal anastomosis often are the result of tension or ischemia. Although the use of a defunctioning ileostomy reduces the clinical impact of an anastomotic leak, the subsequent function of the pouch may be poor. It is essential that the pouch is not under tension and that full mobilization of the small bowel mesentery is performed. This should be achieved during the mobilization of the terminal ileal mesentery; any remaining attachments can be divided via the periumbilical incision which overlies the root of the small bowel mesentery. Additional techniques that can increase pouch mesenteric length include releasing incisions on the peritoneum of the small bowel mesentery; division of one of the vessels in the mesentery (e.g., either the ileocolic or ileal branch of the superior mesenteric artery); and altering the pouch to an S configuration, which can yield several additional centimeters of length. Our goal is to mobilize the small bowel so that the apex of the pouch can reach the pubic symphysis.

Pouch–Vaginal Fistula

A pouch–vaginal fistula may result from pelvic sepsis, anastomotic dehiscence, unsuspected Crohn's disease, or a technical error at the time of surgery. It is essential to rule out Crohn's disease prior to undertaking a proctocolectomy and IPAA. If there is doubt over this issue, then the surgeon may perform a laparoscopic subtotal colectomy for further histologic evaluation of the specimen, with the intention to perform a laparoscopic proctectomy and IPAA if the appropriate pathologic findings are confirmed. During the circular stapling of the ileal pouch to the anal canal, the surgeon should ensure that the posterior vaginal wall has not been caught in the stapler. This may be checked by performing a vaginal examination after the stapler has been closed, but prior to firing.

Pouchitis

Pouchitis is nonspecific inflammation of the ileal pouch and may occur in up to 60% of patients. Its incidence tends to increase with time. Pouchitis is more common in patients with ulcerative colitis than with other conditions such as FAP. The patient with pouchitis presents with fever, malaise, abdominal discomfort, and bloody diarrhea. The diagnosis can be confirmed with pouchoscopy and biopsy. Most patients will respond to a short course of oral or topical antibiotic therapy, such as metronidazole or ciprofloxacin. Topical steroid therapy or probiotic dietary supplementation may have some benefit. Surgery does not have any role in the prevention or management of pouchitis, other than for pouch diversion or excision in those with severe, refractory disease.

RESULTS AND OUTCOME

The operative technique for LIPAA often varies from center to center. The three most commonly reported approaches are (1) laparoscopic mobilization of the colon followed by proctectomy and pouch formation via a Pfannensteil incision; (2) hand-assisted laparoscopic IPAA; and (3) totally laparoscopic dissection with exteriorization via a midline wound just large enough to extract the specimen (as described in this chapter). The variability in operative technique has rendered direct comparison between published reports difficult. Hand-assisted procedures may facilitate intracorporeal dissection and acquisition of skills, especially for practicing surgeons without prior laparoscopic experience. The use of a hand device or Pfannensteil incision necessitates a larger incision, though; the impact of this is unknown.

The earliest series of the laparoscopic pouch procedure confirmed its feasibility, but suggested that the laparoscopic approach had a longer operative time than the open procedure, with an increased length of hospital stay and a prolonged postoperative ileus. More recent studies have confirmed that the time of operation tends to be longer with the laparoscopic approach, but it is now apparent that the length of stay and duration of postoperative ileus are shorter with the laparoscopic procedure compared to the open approach. In addition, there does not appear to be any difference in perioperative morbidity rate between these two approaches, and the longer term (1 year) function and quality of life indicators also appear to be equal. LIPAA also has a clear advantage over open surgery in terms of cosmesis, which may be quite important in the patients who are young and body conscious, and who may be undergoing prophylactic surgery because of a genetic predisposition to cancer. LIPAA remains, however, a challenging procedure and should be undertaken only by experienced laparoscopic colorectal surgeons who are familiar with the open procedure.

Suggested Reading

Antolovic D, Kienle P, Knaebel H-P, et al: Totally laparoscopic versus conventional ileoanal pouch procedure—Design of a single-centre, expertise based randomised controlled trial to compare the laparoscopic and conventional surgical approach in patients undergoing primary elective restorative proctocolectomy—LapConPouch Trial. BMC Surg 2006;6:13.

Dunker MS, Bemelman WA, Slors JF, et al: Functional outcome, quality of life, body image, and cosmesis in patients after laparoscopic-assisted and conventional restorative proctocolectomy: a comparative study. Dis Colon Rectum 2001;44:1800–1807.

Kessler H, Hohenberger W: Multimedia article: Laparoscopic restorative proctocolectomy for ulcerative colitis. Surg Endosc 2006;20:166.

Larson DW, Dozois EJ, Piotrowicz K, et al: Laparoscopic-assisted vs. open ileal pouch–anal anastomosis: Functional outcome in a case-matched series. Dis Colon Rectum 2005;48(10):1845–1850.

Wexner SD, Johansen OB, Nogueras JJ, Jagelman DG: Laparoscopic total abdominal colectomy: A prospective trial. Dis Colon Rectum 1992;35:651–655.

JOHN G. ZOGRAFAKIS

Laparoscopic Appendectomy

Each year an estimated 250,000 appendectomies are performed in the United States. The advantages of minimally invasive surgery that have been applied to most intra-abdominal procedures have been applied to appendectomy. With the advancement of laparoscopic equipment and techniques over the last 10 years, more procedures are performed laparoscopically for simple acute appendicitis as well as complicated appendicitis, including retrocecal and perforated appendicitis. The first appendectomy was performed by gynecologist Kurt Semm in 1980 for an organ that had endometrial implants. Removal of the appendix is well suited for laparoscopy, as it incorporates most of the fundamental laparoscopic skills, including division of the appendix with a linear stapler, control of the vascular pedicle, and abdominal irrigation. In addition, if the patient is found to have a normal appendix, another advantage that laparoscopy confers is the ability to survey the abdominal and pelvic organs for other disease processes, such as pelvic inflammatory disease or diverticulitis.

OPERATIVE INDICATIONS

Classically, appendicitis begins with periumbilical pain that subsequently migrates to the right lower quadrant. In addition to abdominal pain, the patient can have anorexia, low-grade fever, and leukocytosis. Unfortunately, this classical presentation of appendicitis has variable expression, and some or even all of the symptoms can be absent. Conversely, a patient may have all of these symptoms and signs but not have appendicitis. Not surprisingly, appendicitis has been labeled as "the great pretender." Although it has been documented that nonoperative treatment of appendicitis is feasible in carefully selected patients, appendicitis without abscess still is considered a surgical disease that can be treated successfully with an appendectomy in the vast majority of patients.

If surgical intervention is undertaken for the diagnosis of right lower quadrant pain, then laparoscopy offers advantages over a standard McBurney-type open incision. If the appendix is found to be normal at the time of exploration, then the surgeon can perform a diagnostic laparoscopy in order to identify confounding disease processes involving the ovaries, fallopian tubes, stomach, intestine, gallbladder, and so forth. Relative contraindications to laparoscopic appendectomy are similar to those for general laparoscopy. Although laparoscopic appendectomy has been performed safely throughout all trimesters of pregnancy, abdominal insufflation

may induce labor during the latter stages of pregnancy. Access to the abdominal cavity must be performed safely so as to not injure the gravid uterus. Cirrhosis and portal venous hypertension are relative contraindications for laparoscopy.

PREOPERATIVE EVALUATION, TESTING, AND PREPARATION

The preoperative work-up of the patient with right lower quadrant pain should be completed at the discretion of the surgeon. With the almost immediate availability of computer tomography (CT) scan, this imaging modality may be considered and used as an adjunct to assist in the work-up of the patient with atypical right lower quadrant pain. The sensitivity of abdominal CT scan in demonstrating findings consistent with appendicitis approaches 95%. Mesenteric streaking in the surrounding adipose tissue, a dilated or "full" appearing appendix greater than 1 cm, the presence of an appendiceal fecolith, and free fluid noted in the right paracolic gutter and pelvis may be diagnostic of acute appendicitis in the appropriate clinical setting.

In addition to medical risk stratification and basic laboratory testing, women of childbearing age should have a pregnancy test. The possibility of conversion to an open procedure should be discussed with the patient. Administration of intravenous fluids is begun immediately and with antibiotics. For simple acute appendicitis, a second-generation cephalosporin should be administered preoperatively (with one dose being given 30 minutes before skin incision); combination regimens (e.g., aminoglycoside plus a cephalosporin) are used for suspected complex or perforated appendicitis (see Chapter 31).

PATIENT POSITIONING AND PLACEMENT OF TROCARS

The patient is placed in the supine position, with the left arm tucked at the patient's side. Care should be taken to pad the exposed bony prominences. The main monitor should be placed on the patient's right side, opposite the surgeon who is positioned with the first assistant on the patient's left side. The electrocautery generator and suction canisters may be placed above the patient's extended right upper extremity. The scrub nurse is positioned to the right of the monitor, at the patient's lower right side.

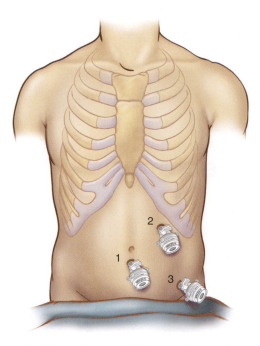

Figure 19-1 Trocar placement for laparoscopic appendectomy.

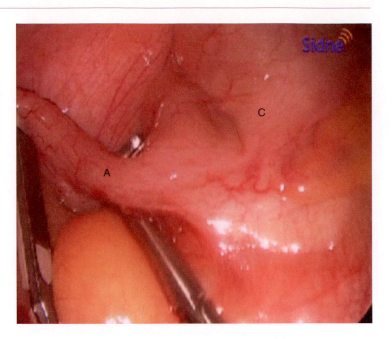

Figure 19-2 Isolation of the base of the appendix (A). C, cecum.

Alternatively, the patient may be positioned in a lithotomy position, keeping the same room and personnel set-up. The patient should be secured to the table using padded lower leg and chest straps. After induction of general anesthesia, an orogastric tube and Foley catheter should be placed to decompress the stomach and bladder, respectively.

Pneumoperitoneum can be established with insertion of a Hasson cannula (i.e., open technique) in the infraumbilical position. The inflamed appendix later may be extracted through this site, extending the incision as necessary. Other options for gaining abdominal access include the Veress needle and an optical bladeless trocar. A 30-degree, 10-mm laparoscope is inserted through the umbilical trocar port (trocar 1), and two left-sided trocars are placed: trocar 2 (12 mm) in the left upper quadrant and trocar 3 (5 mm) in the left lower quadrant (Fig. 19-1). Both left-sided trocars are placed lateral to the rectus abdominus muscle, at least 4 inches apart in the midclavicular line. This allows for triangulation of the trocars with the point at the umbilical incision, pointing toward the appendix in the right lower quadrant. After initiation of pneumoperitoneum (15 mm Hg) and trocar placement, the patient is placed in a slight Trendelenburg position and rotated to the patient's left.

OPERATIVE TECHNIQUE

A diagnostic laparoscopy is performed. The greater omentum can be reflected into the upper abdomen, exposing the right lower quadrant. The small intestine can be retracted out of the operative field with the aid of gravity. An atraumatic grasper is used to identify the cecum, appendix, and terminal ileum.

Division of the Appendix and Mesoappendix

If inflammation is identified around the distal half of the appendix, dissection is best begun at the base of the appendix. The base may be grasped and elevated toward the anterior abdominal wall. The avascular plane of the mesoappendix at the appendicocecal junction can be dissected bluntly using a curved forceps (Fig. 19-2). After creating a window at the base of the appendix, a laparoscopic

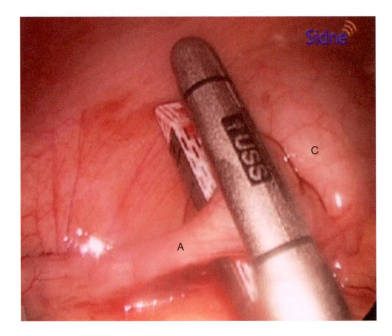

Figure 19-3 Laparoscopic linear stapler used to divide the appendix (A), including a "cap" of cecum (C).

linear stapler (2.5-mm staples, white load) is utilized to transect the appendix (Fig. 19-3). After dividing the appendix, the mesoappendix also can be controlled with a laparoscopic linear stapler. The peritoneum overlying the mesoappendix can be scored either by hook electrocautery or by sharp dissection. Care should be taken to identify and protect the terminal ileum and cecum. The mesoappendix then can be divided, which occasionally will require multiple firings of the stapler. Although the author's preference is to divide the appendix prior to the mesoappendix, some surgeons may begin their dissection by dividing the mesoappendix. This technique is illustrated further in Figure 19-4A to E.

Removal of the Appendix and Closure

In order to minimize the risk of wound infection, the inflamed appendix should be removed using a wound protection device.

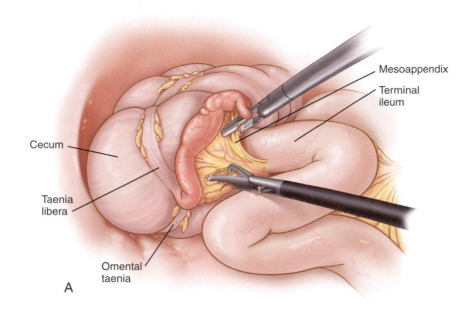

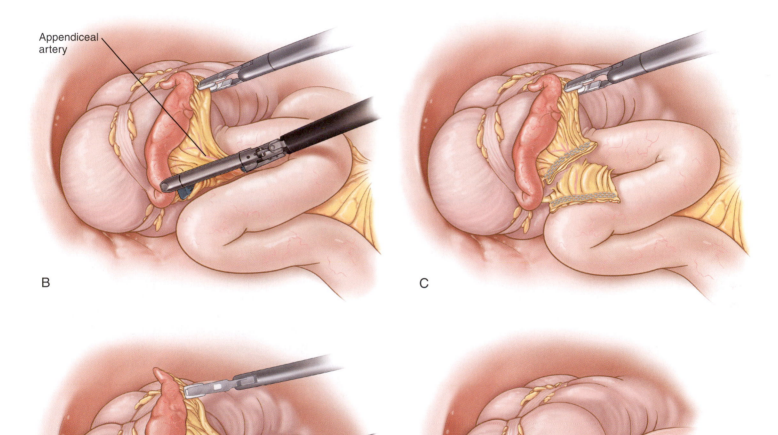

FIGURE 19-4 **A,** A curved dissector is used to create a window in the mesoappendix and isolate the appendiceal artery. **B,** A laparoscopic linear stapler (vascular load) is placed across the mesoappendix. **C,** Successful division of the mesoappendix. **D,** Laparoscopic linear stapler placed across the base of the appendix. **E,** Completed appendectomy. Intact staple lines are identified on the base of the cecum and mesoappendix.

The appendix is placed in a polyethylene specimen retrieval bag, and then can be removed through the 10 mm umbilical trocar position. After the appendix is removed, the right lower quadrant, paracolic gutter, and pelvis should be irrigated with saline, and the staple lines on the base of the cecum and mesoappendix are evaluated for integrity and hemostasis. After the appendectomy is completed, routine abdominal evaluation may be performed. The distal small bowel can be mobilized to look for any other abnormalities that may be present, such as Meckel's diverticulum or inflammatory bowel disease. Abdominal wall or inguinal hernia defects also may be documented. A fascial closure device then should be used to close any trocar sites greater than 5 mm with heavy absorbable suture. The wounds should also be irrigated prior to completing a intracuticular closure with suture.

Complex Appendicitis

In the case of retrocecal appendicitis, laparoscopic mobilization of the cecum and ascending colon is necessary in order to expose the tip and base of the appendix. Using a blunt atraumatic grasper, the cecum is grasped along the tenia coli and retracted superior and medial. This allows division of the colonic attachments to the right lateral side wall. The avascular plane along the white line of Toldt can be entered using hook cautery, scissors, or other sharp dissection. This will facilitate mobilization of the colon, which then can be completed bluntly. Once the appendix is identified, the base can be divided as described earlier, using a laparoscopic linear stapler. The mesoappendix frequently is adherent to the base of the cecum, and care should be taken in order to prevent injury to the adjacent bowel during dissection of the mesoappendix. If the appendix is necrotic, then the linear stapler still may be utilized to transect the base. If needed, the surgeon then may perform a partial cecectomy, removing a "cap" of cecum at the former location of the appendiceal base. This staple line may be oversewn using absorbable suture if there is a concern about the integrity of the closure. When amputating a piece of the cecum, identification of the ileocecal valve is necessary in order to prevent injury to the small intestine. For complicated appendicitis with a preoperatively identified pelvic abscess, CT-guided aspiration with delayed laparoscopic appendectomy is appropriate therapy. Identification of an intra-abdominal or pelvic abscess at the time of surgery can be managed laparoscopically, though. After removal of the appendix, the abscess cavity should be drained and debrided. Copious irrigation should be performed until the effluent is clear.

Alternative Techniques

The described stapler technique is reliable and reproducible. There are other techniques, however, for division of both the appendix and mesoappendix. Analogous to the open appendectomy, multiple sequential suture endoloops may be placed laparoscopically to divide the appendiceal organ. It is better, however, to divide the mesoappendix first (with hemoclips or an ultrasonic scalpel), which isolates the specimen at the base of the appendix. After the mesoappendix is divided, sequential endoloops may be placed over the base of the appendix. The specimen then is divided between the endoloops and removed.

Negative Appendectomy

In about 15% of patients operated on for appendicitis, the appendix is not the cause of the patient's pain. If a normal appendix is found, then an appendectomy should be performed in order to avoid a future diagnostic dilemma. A careful evaluation of the abdominal cavity should be performed to look for other signs of pathology, such as salpingitis, cholecystitis, diverticulitis (both colonic or from a Meckel's diverticulum), duodenal or gastric perforation, or mesenteric adenitis. If active inflammatory bowel disease is identified in the pericecal region (i.e., possible Crohn's disease), the appendix should not be removed because of the risk of a stump complication. Such a patient should undergo medical evaluation and treatment for the inflammatory bowel disease.

POSTOPERATIVE CARE

The management of the postsurgical laparoscopic appendectomy patient will vary depending on the severity of the illness. One dose of preoperative antibiotics is sufficient for simple appendicitis, whereas a longer postoperative course may be necessary for complicated appendicitis. Pain control is obtained using scheduled intravenous ketorolac with intermittent intravenous morphine/oral narcotic administration. A clear liquid diet may be initiated immediately after surgery in uncomplicated cases. Earlier return of bowel function and decreased rate of venous thromboembolism has been described with early ambulation, which should begin immediately after surgery. Once the patient is tolerating liquids, has appropriate pain control, and is hemodynamically stable, he may be discharged to home; this often occurs in less than 24 hours. Routine follow-up 7 to 10 days after surgery is indicated for dressing removal and wound assessment.

PROCEDURE-SPECIFIC COMPLICATIONS

Well-described procedure-specific complications of appendectomy, whether open or laparoscopic, include paralytic ileus, superficial wound infection, intra-abdominal abscess, enterocutaneous fistula, and perirectal abscess. The occurrence of paralytic ileus is somewhat unpredictable but would be expected to some degree in a patient with purulent, perforated appendicitis. The management remains supportive, although novel pharmacologic treatments are on the horizon. The incidence of superficial wound infection appears to be decreased in laparoscopic appendectomy compared to the open approach; again, treatment is the time-honored method of wound drainage with or without antibiotics. Recent meta-analytic data suggest that the incidence of intra-abdominal abscess may be higher after laparoscopic appendectomy compared to the open procedure. This interesting observation requires careful study. Minimizing the amount of widespread intra-abdominal irrigation may decrease this postoperative complication. The standard treatment of an intra-abdominal abscess (i.e., percutaneous drainage with antibiotics) is applied to this complication of appendectomy. A perirectal abscess has a similar pathogenesis to intra-abdominal abscess (i.e., inadequate clearance of bacteria and associated debris), but in the former case the material drains into the pelvis and into the retroperitoneum and is treated with incision and drainage. The development of an enterocutaneous fistula is managed with a standard nonoperative protocol, which has variable descriptions but basically includes resuscitation and stabilization; establishment of adequate drainage; diagnostic testing to delineate the fistula anatomy; a period of nutritional support with observation; and operative intervention for patients who fail nonoperative treatment.

RESULTS AND OUTCOME

A number of meta-analyses have documented the safety and efficacy of laparoscopic appendectomy compared to the open procedure. All the advantages of minimally invasive surgery apply to laparoscopic appendectomy; the typical patient has (1) decreased pain, (2) a decreased narcotic requirement, (3) a better cosmetic result, (4) a shorter length of stay, and (5) fewer wound-related complications. As mentioned earlier, there appears to be a higher incidence of intra-abdominal abscess after the laparoscopic approach than after the open approach to appendectomy. The understanding of this observation is not yet complete; the pathologic cause may be related to possible spread of infected material by less than careful laparoscopic technique. Another criticism of laparoscopic appendectomy compared to its open counterpart has been the increased expense of the laparoscopic procedure. This increased expense may be partially offset with the use of reusable instrumentation; in addition, operative time for the typical surgeon should decrease with increased experience, which also should reduce the cost of the procedure.

Suggested Reading

Cothren CC, Moore EE, Johnson JL, et al: Can we afford to do laparoscopic appendectomy in an academic hospital? Am J Surg 2005;190(6):950–954.

Curet M, Allen D, Josloff R, et al: Laparoscopy during pregnancy. Arch Surg 1996;131:546–551.

Frazee R, Bohannon W: Laparoscopic appendectomy for complicated appendicitis. Arch Surg 1996;131:509–513.

Lukish J, Powell D, Morrow S, et al: Laparoscopic appendectomy in children: The use of the endoloop vs. the endostapler. Arch Surg 2007;142(1):58–61.

Ortega AE, Hunter JG, Peters JH, et al: A prospective, randomized comparison of laparoscopic with open appendectomy. Laparoscopic Appendectomy Study Group. Am J Surg 1995;169(2):208–212.

Wehrman WE, Tangren CM, Inge TH: Cost analysis of ligature versus stapling techniques of laparoscopic appendectomy in children. J Laparoendosc Adv Surg Tech A 2007;17(3):371–374.

Wu JM, Chen KH, Lin HF, et al: Laparocopic appendectomy in pregnancy. J Laparoendosc Adv Surg Tech A 2005;15(5):447–450.

Yau KK, Siu WT, Tang CN, et al: Laparoscopic versus open appendectomy for complicated appendicitis. J Am Coll Surg 2007;205(1):60–65.

Hepatobiliary System

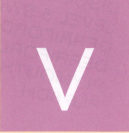

Laparoscopic Cholecystectomy

CONSTANTINE T. FRANTZIDES, MARK A. CARLSON, AND MINH LUU

20

In terms of raw numbers, there probably are more experts on the performance of laparoscopic cholecystectomy than on any other minimally invasive procedure. Just about every general surgeon does this procedure, does it a lot, and most do it very well. So we will not make an obnoxious claim that we are the *übermensch* of laparoscopic cholecystectomy. What we can provide in this chapter is our perspective, which has been generated after performing many of these procedures ourselves, and by reading and listening to what others have said and written about the technical aspects of laparoscopic cholecystectomy.

The transition from open to laparoscopic cholecystectomy that occurred during the early 1990s stands as a glaring example of how *not* to introduce a new technology. The proliferation of ductal injuries that ensued from this transition was overshadowed only by the eagerness of the media and medicolegal elements to publicize and prosecute these events. We in the surgical community have no one to blame but ourselves for this unfortunate chapter in the history of minimally invasive surgery. The rush to embrace the new technology simply was too hasty and ill conceived. Be that as it may, the transition to laparoscopic cholecystectomy was completed quickly, and the issue of common bile duct injury now is under somewhat better control, although not eliminated.

We believe that a safe dissection is paramount in the performance of laparoscopic cholecystectomy, and we will describe in detail the technical maneuvers we perform to accomplish such a dissection. Other surgeons may emphasize reliance on intraoperative cholangiography to attain the same information that we like to obtain with dissection. This issue of routine versus selective intraoperative cholangiography has been debated over and over again in the literature. We will not regurgitate this debate in this chapter, but simply acknowledge that it exists and that there are multiple approaches to the performance of a safe laparoscopic cholecystectomy.

OPERATIVE INDICATIONS

The indication for cholecystectomy in the vast majority of patients is symptomatic gallstones. This indication covers a spectrum of clinical manifestations, from occasional attacks of biliary colic to gangrenous cholecystitis to gallstone pancreatitis. If the patient has symptoms from gallstones and has no absolute contraindications to an operation under general anesthesia, then laparoscopic cholecystectomy generally is indicated. Nonoperative treatment of gallstones (e.g., oral bile acids or shock wave lithotripsy) has limited efficacy. Routine removal of a gallbladder for asymptomatic cholelithiasis is more controversial, but may be a reasonable treatment alternative in a patient with one or more of the following characteristics: "porcelain" (i.e., calcified) gallbladder; gallbladder mass or polyp; young age; diabetes mellitus; organ transplant; sickle cell anemia; and others (the list is growing). Incidental cholecystectomy for asymptomatic cholelithiasis also may be a reasonable option during a bariatric or other gastrointestinal procedure.

The timing of cholecystectomy to treat acute cholecystitis is controversial; there is a wealth of retrospective data to support immediate cholecystectomy, delayed operation months later, and everything in between. There is no doubt that removal of an acutely inflamed gallbladder is more difficult than removal of a noninflamed gallbladder, but as many authors have demonstrated, this can be accomplished without an increased incidence of complications. Our own preference is to treat a patient with acute cholecystitis medically (IV fluids, antibiotics, bowel rest, pain relief) for up to 1 week, and then remove the gallbladder under "subacute" conditions. If the patient worsens during the first 24 to 48 hours of this treatment, then an emergency cholecystectomy would be indicated. If a patient has gangrenous cholecystitis with severe inflammation that has made dissection in the region of the porta hepatis particularly hazardous, then laparoscopic partial cholecystectomy with drainage is a treatment option.

The timing of cholecystectomy in association with gallstone pancreatitis also is somewhat controversial. For the critically ill patient who has extensive pancreatic necrosis, early laparoscopic cholecystectomy generally is dangerous and not useful; the damage already has been done. For the patient with mild, mostly laboratory-based pancreatitis, early cholecystectomy is more reasonable. The difficulty in timing the gallbladder removal is with the patients who fall in between these two extremes. In general, we guide our decision based on the clinical stability of the patient; we prefer to perform laparoscopic cholecystectomy for gallstone pancreatitis electively on a patient whose disease status is quiescent or markedly improved.

Occasionally a patient is referred for treatment of biliary colic, but the patient has no gallstones. In this situation a careful evaluation for other sources of the patient's symptoms should be carried out (see "Preoperative Evaluation"); if the results of this evaluation rule out other causative diagnoses (e.g., peptic ulcer disease, sphincter of Oddi dysfunction), or if a decreased gallbladder ejection fraction without sphincter dysfunction is noted, then cholecystectomy may relieve the patient's symptoms. The diagnosis in this situation might be "acalculous cholecystitis." This particular entity classically has been described in critically ill patients in whom the clinical manifestations typically are much more severe.

PREOPERATIVE EVALUATION

The goals of the preoperative evaluation for laparoscopic cholecystectomy may be organized as follows: (1) confirm the clinical diagnosis with objective data; (2) evaluate the status of the common bile duct; (3) determine whether preoperative endoscopic retrograde cholangiopancreatography (ERCP) will be necessary; and (4) determine the appropriateness and urgency for the procedure in relation to the patient's health and history. Routine tests should include a broad chemistry panel (including liver function tests, amylase, lipase), a complete blood count, and an abdominal ultrasound. If the patient has evidence of biliary obstruction, then one option would be to perform a preoperative ERCP, which generally is what we prefer. With this strategy the common duct can be cleared prior to laparoscopic cholecystectomy; if clearance is not possible, then the surgeon should prepare a strategy to deal with this scenario (please refer to Chapter 21, on cholangiography and common bile duct exploration).

For the patient with acute cholecystitis, an abdominal computed tomography (CT) scan can help delineate the severity of the process. If the diagnosis of cholecystitis is not clear, then a nuclear medicine gallbladder emptying study (cholescintigraphy or hepatobiliary iminodiacetic acid [HIDA] scan) may help solve the problem by demonstrating nonfilling of the gallbladder. If gallstones are not present in a patient who is having biliary colic, then an extensive evaluation using the preceding tests and possibly including an upper gastrointestinal (GI) series, magnetic resonance imaging (MRI) scan, esophagogastroduodenoscopy (EGD), and ERCP with sphincter of Oddi manometry may determine the cause of the patient's pain. Cholecystectomy often is performed for vague symptoms in patients who have no gallstones; in order to prevent unnecessary gallbladder removal, the surgeon should ensure that there are no remedial causes for the patient's symptoms.

PATIENT POSITIONING AND PLACEMENT OF TROCARS

The patient is placed supine on the operating room table with the right arm tucked. The operating table should be compatible with a C-arm apparatus if intraoperative cholangiography/fluoroscopy is necessary. If there is a likelihood of open conversion, then it may be helpful to have the patient positioned over a flex point on the operating room table, so that "cracking" the operating room table will help splay open the subcostal region. The surgeon stands on the patient's left and faces the monitor; and the assistant stands on the right.

We prefer to establish pneumoperitoneum by inserting a Hasson cannula at the umbilicus (Fig. 20-1). If there is an old incision in this location, then intra-abdominal access may be obtained with a Veress needle or optical bladeless trocar

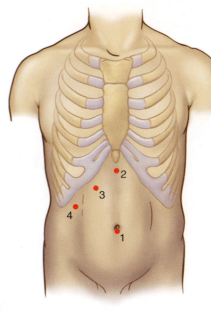

FIGURE 20-1 Trocar positions for a laparoscopic cholecystectomy. Positions 1 and 2 represent 10-mm trocars; 3 and 4 represent 5-mm trocars.

elsewhere. After insufflation, the gallbladder region is inspected, and a 5-mm trocar is inserted subcostally in the right midclavicular line; approximately over the gallbladder. A 10-mm port then is inserted in the subxiphoid region just to the right of the falciform ligament. The table is rotated to elevate the right side, and reverse Trendelenburg (head up) position is applied. The gallbladder is grasped and elevated, and the second 5-mm trocar is inserted in a position such that it can grasp the fundus without causing interference with the other trocars (typically lower than the other 5-mm trocar and in the right anterior axillary line).

OPERATIVE TECHNIQUE

Frequently adhesions from the gallbladder to the omentum, transverse colon, or duodenum need to be lysed so that the gallbladder can be visualized. In the presence of acute inflammation, these adhesions sometimes can be peeled away bluntly; if the adhesions have been present chronically, then it may be best to take them down sharply to avoid tissue tearing and bleeding. We prefer to perform careful dissection with the hook cautery for most of this procedure. Some authors have warned against the use of electrocautery, particularly in the triangle of Calot region, out of concern for electrothermal proximity injury to biliary or vascular structures. If the hook cautery is used improperly, then these injuries certainly can happen. Our definition of "proper use" of the hook electrocautery is, when applying energy, always to have to the hook's tip in sight, always to have the hook pulled away from the tissue, never to push the hook into the tissue, and always to take tissue in thin layers in order to avoid hooking into a vital structure. Energy should be applied in short bursts of less than 1 second, particularly inside the triangle of Calot; a tissue strand requiring a longer application for hemostasis likely should not have been handled with the hook but rather clipped. Electrocautery scissors also is an option for this procedure, but we prefer the hook because it also has excellent function as a right-angle dissector.

After the omental adhesion is taken down, the surgeon may find that the gallbladder is too tense with fluid to allow a grasper

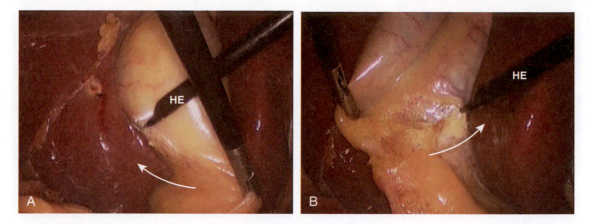

FIGURE 20-2 **A,** Lateral incision of the peritoneum. **B,** Medial incision of the peritoneum. *Arrows* indicate direction of peritoneal incision.

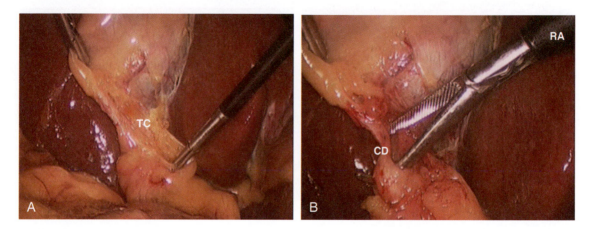

FIGURE 20-3 **A,** Peritoneum overlying the junction of the infundibulum with the cystic duct is gently peeled down with a grasper. **B,** A right-angle dissector (RA) creates a window posterior to the cystic duct (CD). TC, region of the triangle of Calot.

to obtain purchase on the organ. In this case we prefer to puncture the dome of the gallbladder with a laparoscopic needle-aspirator, and decompress the organ. The needle entry site then should be closed either with clips or a suture. If the gallbladder still cannot be grasped with a 5-mm instrument, a right lateral 5-mm port can be upsized to a 10-mm port to allow use of a 10-mm atraumatic grasper or Babcock forceps. At this point the fundus of the gallbladder is elevated over the liver by the first assistant working through the right lateral port.

We prefer to begin the gallbladder dissection by the infundibulum; we have not been impressed with the "top-down" approach, even in the presence of severe acute inflammation. A V-shaped incision is made in the peritoneum (only) overlying the infundibulum, using the hook electrocautery. Each arm of the V extends up on its respective side of the gallbladder (Fig. 20-2). It is important to follow "proper use" rules of the electrocautery during this and subsequent dissection to avoid injury to underlying structures. Some surgeons prefer to grab the peritoneum overlying the infundibulum and simply rip it downward to expose the underlying vital structures. We find this technique to be esthetically displeasing and potentially rough and dangerous to the underlying ducts and vessels.

After the V has been made, the peritoneum is swept downward with gentle blunt dissection (Fig. 20-3A). The goal of the dissection at this point is to identify the junction of the gallbladder neck (infundibulum) with the cystic duct. We accomplish

this with a wide and thorough dissection of the triangle of Calot; we do not employ routine cholangiography. Our indication for cholangiography primarily has been for suspected choledocholithiasis, which typically represents only 10% to 20% of our cases (please refer to Chapter 21, on intraoperative cholangiography and common bile duct exploration). Occasionally the infundibulum is somewhat redundant, and overrides the junction of the cystic duct with the common bile duct. If this region is not dissected out, then the surgeon may miss a short cystic duct and clip/transect the common bile duct instead.

The junction of the gallbladder infundibulum with the cystic duct should be dissected clean circumferentially (Fig. 20-3B). This means that the space between the posterior gallbladder and the liver bed needs be opened up. We will routinely mobilize the lower one third to one half of the gallbladder off the liver bed prior to clipping and cutting any tubular structures in the triangle of Calot. If the gallbladder is completely free of the liver bed in this location and the posterior wall of the gallbladder is plainly visible, then the surgeon can be certain that the common bile duct is not adherent to the gallbladder's back wall (a common scenario in catastrophic ductal injuries in which a segment of the common bile duct gets resected). The other advantage to this early mobilization of the gallbladder off the liver bed is to identify any ductal or vascular aberrancy.

During the dissection in the triangle of Calot, the surgeon should not be fixated on a single view of the dissection. The

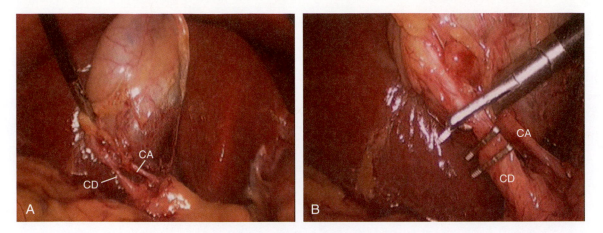

FIGURE 20-4 **A,** Completed dissection of the triangle of Calot region, demonstrating the cystic duct (CD) and cystic artery (CA). **B,** The cystic duct has been doubly clipped and now is cut with the hook scissors.

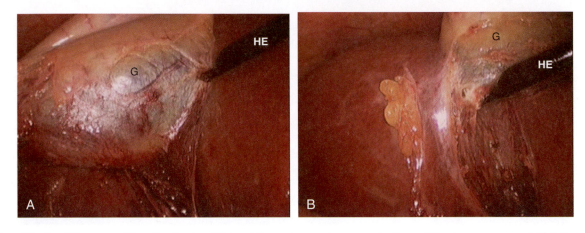

FIGURE 20-5 **A,** The gallbladder (G) is retracted laterally, allowing division of the medial attachments to the liver with hook electrocautery (HE). **B,** The gallbladder is retracted medially, allowing similar division of the lateral attachments with hook electrocautery.

surgeon should frequently alter the angle of the view, move the gallbladder around, and approach from the infundibulum from both a lateral and medial direction. Lateral stretch on the gallbladder is particularly important, as this tends to splay out the gallbladder, infundibulum, and cystic duct away from the liver bed and common duct. There should be frequent reassessments of the anatomic arrangements as the dissection proceeds, and the surgeon should constantly question any assumptions that she or he has made about the anatomy and rely on a healthy skepticism of the structures as they unfold into view.

Most commonly, the cystic artery is positioned medially and slightly posterior to the cystic duct (Fig. 20-4A). The artery's identity can be verified by tracing it superiorly into the body of the gallbladder, where it will form an arcade. In addition, if traction is reduced on the gallbladder, the surgeon may be able to see the artery pulsate. Another landmark of cystic artery location is the presence of a lymph node anterior to the artery along its midpoint. Once the junction of the infundibulum and the cystic duct has been delineated, the surgeon may clip and transect the cystic duct and cystic artery with confidence (Fig. 20-4B). Typically, two clips are placed on the patient side of both the duct and artery, and one clip is placed on the specimen side. A common error that a surgeon-in-training will make is to leave inadequate space between the clips to cut the structure with a scissors. The clip on the specimen side can be buried with impunity into the specimen to allow space for the scissors. The surgeon should not cut

a vessel or duct flush with the patient-side clip, because this clip then will be at risk to slide off. Following the preceding technique of complete dissection of the triangle of Calot prior to clipping and cutting, the authors have yet to incur any common bile duct injury in their combined practice.

Once the dissection has been accomplished and the cystic duct and artery have been controlled, the superior portion of the gallbladder is removed from the liver bed using hook electrocautery (Fig. 20-5). The surgeon should dissect close to the gallbladder wall by keeping it on stretch with respect to the liver. We suspect that some of the high ductal injuries (at the confluence or above) that have been inflicted, but not necessarily recognized, during laparoscopic cholecystectomy have been secondary to electrical energy injudiciously applied to the liver bed during the latter part of the procedure. After removal from the liver bed, the gallbladder then is placed into a polyethylene specimen bag and removed from the abdomen through either the subxiphoid or umbilical port. We like to inspect the gallbladder specimen on the back table to verify the correctness of the anatomy and to evaluate for any unsuspected masses. The liver bed is inspected for hemostasis, and the right upper quadrant is washed with saline. If the dissection has been particularly difficult or bloody, then the surgeon may leave a closed suction drain in gallbladder fossa and exiting out one of the 5-mm trocar sites. The pneumoperitoneum is evacuated, the fascia of the 10-mm ports is closed, and the procedure is terminated.

POSTOPERATIVE CARE

The typical cholecystectomy can be done as an outpatient procedure or a 23-hour stay; older or more infirm patients may require a longer period of observation. If a patient in good health is not ready for discharge on postoperative day 1, then this should raise the suspicion that the patient may have a complication. A clear liquid diet is given the evening of surgery, and a regular diet may be given the next day. Routine lifting restrictions are given upon discharge, and the patient may be seen in follow-up at 1 week and 1 month postoperatively. The patient also is instructed to report any occurrence of fever, abdominal distention, obstipation, diffuse abdominal pain, jaundice, or incisional drainage.

PROCEDURE-SPECIFIC COMPLICATIONS

Intraoperative complications include gallbladder perforation with stone spillage, hemorrhage, enterotomy, and common bile duct injury. A perforation of the gallbladder is a relatively benign complication; the most expedient solution is simply to aspirate the gallbladder empty with the pool sucker, and remove any spilled stones. At the end of the procedure, the right upper quadrant should be irrigated with a large volume of saline until there is a clear return. Hemorrhage from the liver bed usually can be controlled with electrocautery. More severe hemorrhage can occur from injuries to porta hepatis structures such as the portal vein or, more commonly, the cystic artery. These injuries can be avoided by staying close to the gallbladder infundibulum rather than close to the porta hepatis. It should be acknowledged that an infected and inflamed gallbladder with vascular adhesions in the porta hepatis region will increase the risk of hemorrhage. It is not clear that open conversion in the presence of a severe inflammation will decrease the risk of a hemorrhagic complication.

Common bile duct injury can occur secondary to multiple mechanisms, and a full discussion of this complication is beyond the scope of this chapter. The best way to avoid a ductal injury is to perform a careful dissection supplemented by cholangiography as needed (see earlier discussion). Despite the best application of preventive measures, a common bile duct injury still may occur and does not necessarily indicate a deviation from the standard of care. A partial transection of the common duct that is recognized intraoperatively may be managed laparoscopically by placement of a T-tube, depending on the experience of the surgeon. A complete transection (or, more commonly, a segmental resection) of the common duct may be managed by a Roux-en-Y choledochojejunostomy, performed by a surgeon who is experienced with this procedure. Intraoperative recognition of an enterotomy (either in the duodenum or secondary to trocar injury to other portions of the bowel) should be managed by primary closure. The management of retained common bile duct stones is extensively discussed in Chapter 21, on cholangiography and common bile duct exploration.

Postoperative complications of laparoscopic cholecystectomy include cystic stump leak, retained stone, unrecognized common bile duct injury, and unrecognized intestinal perforation. A cystic stump leak typically presents as a fluid collection (biloma) in the right upper quadrant. The patient may have isolated hyperbilirubinemia (conjugated). An investigation including a CT scan (to diagnose the biloma) and an ERCP (to determine the biloma's source) should be performed. A biloma resulting from a liver bed leak can be percutaneously drained and is self-limiting. A cystic stump leak will require a percutaneous drain and an endoscopically placed common bile duct stent. If the bile leak is from an unrecognized bile duct injury, then this should be managed as described earlier. Unrecognized intestinal perforation most commonly occurs secondary to trocar placement and less commonly with duodenal injuries; this complication may go undetected for several days. This complication has a high morbidity risk if it remains unrecognized beyond the first 3 to 4 days postoperatively. In the present era of outpatient surgery, it is extremely important for the patient to be able to recognize symptoms that may be associated with an intestinal perforation; thus, patient education is critical.

RESULTS AND OUTCOME

When performed for symptomatic cholelithiasis, patient satisfaction after a laparoscopic cholecystectomy is remarkably high (95% or greater). If the gallbladder is removed for other diagnoses (e.g., biliary dyskinesia), then overall patient satisfaction drops into the 70% to 80% range. With regard to common bile duct injury, the true incidence in the general community is difficult to know; recent large meta-analyses of published retrospective data place this incidence at less than 0.5%. This injury rate represents an improvement over the rates reported in the early 1990s, but the nature of this data makes it subject to publication bias. More important, however, laparoscopic cholecystectomy is widely regarded as the procedure that heralded a major change in the approach to abdominal surgery. This change continues to the present day, as more and more procedures are being performed with minimally invasive technique. Furthermore, the morbidity associated with a major incision is receiving (appropriately so) an increased amount of attention. Laparoscopic cholecystectomy was the core component of this systemic change.

Suggested Reading

Adamsen S, Hansen OH, Funch-Jensen P, et al: Bile duct injury during laparoscopic cholecystectomy: A prospective nationwide series. J Am Coll Surg 1997;184:571–578.

Carlson MA, Frantzides CT, Ludwig KA, et al: Routine of selective use of intraoperative cholangiography in laparoscopic cholecystectomy. J Laparoendosc Surg 1993;3:31–37.

Davidoff AM, Pappas TN, Murray EA, et al: Mechanisms of major biliary injury during laparoscopic cholecystectomy. Ann Surg 1992;215:196–202.

Frantzides CT, Sykes A: A re-evaluation of antibiotic prophylaxis in laparoscopic cholecystectomy. J Laparoendosc Surg 1994;4:375–378.

Ludwig K, Bernhardt J, Steffen H, Lorenz D: Contribution of intraoperative cholangiography to incidence and outcome of common bile duct injuries during laparoscopic cholecystectomy. Surg Endosc 2002;16:1098–1104.

Shea JA, Healey MJ, Berlin JA, et al: Mortality and complications associated with laparoscopic cholecystectomy: A meta-analysis. Ann Surg 1996;224:609–620.

Strasberg SM, Hertl M, Soper NJ: An analysis of the problem of biliary injury during laparoscopic cholecystectomy. J Am Coll Surg 1995;180:101–125.

JOSEPH B. PETELIN

Laparoscopic Common Bile Duct Exploration and Intraoperative Cholangiography

Nearly 8 years after Langenbuch performed the first cholecystectomy in 1882, Courvoisier performed the first successful common bile duct exploration (CBDE) in 1890. In the 1930s, Mirizzi introduced intraoperative cholangiography, and in the early 1940s Royer in Argentina first performed and reported laparoscopic cholangiography. This was followed by reports of laparoscopic cholangiography in Europe by Calamé in the 1950s. What happened to the innovative work of these laparoscopic pioneers is a mystery. However, in a personal conversation with the author, Calamé indicated that his chief suggested that he move on to more "productive" pursuits. Over a century later, in 1985, Eric Muhe in Boblingen, Germany, performed the first laparoscopic cholecystectomy. This subsequently became the standard of care for treatment of symptomatic gallbladder disease. This was soon followed by the reintroduction of laparoscopic cholangiography and several minimally invasive surgery (MIS) techniques to treat choledocholithiasis. These maneuvers include glucagon administration, flushing the ductal system, dilatation of the distal common bile duct/sphincter, balloon catheter manipulation, basket extraction—with or without fluoroscopic guidance, and choledochoscopic extraction. Choledocholithiasis is present in approximately 10% of those patients who present for cholecystectomy. Definitive treatment of these patients includes cholecystectomy and clearance of the entire ductal system or, if the duct cannot be cleared, then reestablishment of unobstructed hepatic-enteric continuity with bypass or a prosthesis.

OPERATIVE INDICATIONS

The most common indication for laparoscopic common bile duct (CBD) exploration is an abnormal intraoperative cholangiogram or sonogram. Preoperative studies, including unexplained elevated liver function tests; a dilated ductal system; sonographic evidence of bile duct stones; scintigraphic, endoscopic, or radiographic evidence of common bile duct obstruction; history of biliary pancreatitis; or surgeon suspicion of CBD disease may also warrant laparoscopic common bile duct exploration. The most common relative contraindications to laparoscopic common bile duct exploration (LCBDE) are lack of surgical skill and training to perform the maneuvers required for LCBDE, absence of any of the preceding indications, severe uncorrectable coagulopathy, and local conditions in the porta hepatis that would make exploration impossible.

CBD stones may be found in three distinct clinical situations: preoperatively, intraoperatively, and postoperatively. In the first situation, the clinician has two choices: (1) endoscopic retrograde cholangiography and extraction with or without sphincterotomy (ERC ± S) before operation or (2) laparoscopic cholecystectomy (LC) and LCBDE. Both modalities are successful in clearing the common duct in over 90% of cases. However preoperative ERC ± S often yields a normal examination in up to 40% to 60% of cases. Moreover, these patients are exposed to the added morbidity and mortality risks for ERC ± S. Numerous authors have suggested that the choice of clearance method should be based on the surgeon's expertise in laparoscopic surgery, the local availability of expert endoscopists, and the general condition of the patient.

Some authors have suggested strategies that are dependent on the preoperative likelihood of choledocholithiasis: high risk (jaundice, cholangitis, documented CBD stones, dilated CBD), medium risk (elevated bilirubin, alkaline phosphatase, and amylase; small stones; pancreatitis), and low risk (absence of any of the above). Although there is considerable discussion about how patients are classified in the scheme, there is some value to this approach. For high-risk patients in institutions where LCBDE expertise is not available, preoperative ERC ± S should be considered. For medium-risk patients in these institutions, preoperative noninvasive biliary tract imaging with magnetic resonance cholangiopancreatography (MRCP) or somewhat more invasive endoscopic ultrasound (EUS) may be considered. Intraoperative imaging with laparoscopic cholangiography (LIOC) or laparoscopic ultrasound (LUS) is also appropriate in this group of patients undergoing LC, especially in institutions where LCBDE expertise is available. For low-risk patients, decisions regarding routine versus selective LIOC are usually determined by the surgeon, although the author strongly recommends the use of routine LIOC for all LC patients.

When common bile duct stones are discovered intraoperatively, the surgeon either proceeds with LCBDE, converts the case to "open" common duct exploration, or leaves the stones in place for subsequent ERC ± S. Although any of these alternatives is acceptable and associated with success rates of 90% or more, the latter two are more costly and are associated with increased morbidity. If LCBDE is unsuccessful or not attempted, then the decision regarding conversion to "open" common duct exploration versus postoperative ERC ± S depends on the local availability of expert endoscopists. The third situation, in which retained CBD

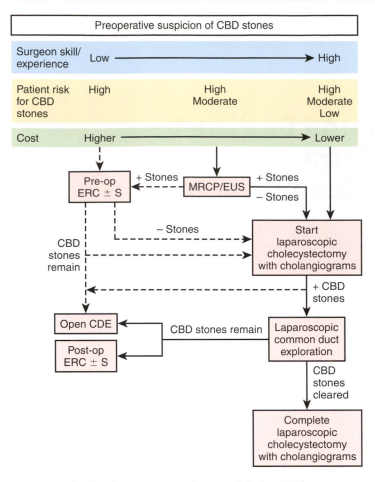

FIGURE 21-1 Algorithm for management of common bile duct (CBD) stones suspected prior to cholecystectomy. CDE, common duct exploration; ERC ± S, endoscopic retrograde cholangiography and extraction with or without sphincterotomy; EUS, endoscopic ultrasound; MRCP, magnetic resonance cholangiopancreatography.

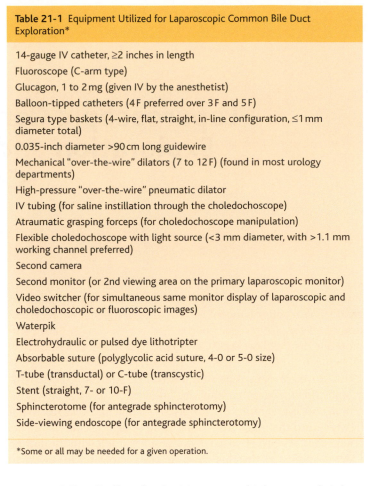

Table 21-1 Equipment Utilized for Laparoscopic Common Bile Duct Exploration*
14-gauge IV catheter, ≥2 inches in length
Fluoroscope (C-arm type)
Glucagon, 1 to 2 mg (given IV by the anesthetist)
Balloon-tipped catheters (4 F preferred over 3 F and 5 F)
Segura type baskets (4-wire, flat, straight, in-line configuration, ≤1 mm diameter total)
0.035-inch diameter >90 cm long guidewire
Mechanical "over-the-wire" dilators (7 to 12 F) (found in most urology departments)
High-pressure "over-the-wire" pneumatic dilator
IV tubing (for saline instillation through the choledochoscope)
Atraumatic grasping forceps (for choledochoscope manipulation)
Flexible choledochoscope with light source (<3 mm diameter, with >1.1 mm working channel preferred)
Second camera
Second monitor (or 2nd viewing area on the primary laparoscopic monitor)
Video switcher (for simultaneous same monitor display of laparoscopic and choledochoscopic or fluoroscopic images)
Waterpik
Electrohydraulic or pulsed dye lithotripter
Absorbable suture (polyglycolic acid suture, 4-0 or 5-0 size)
T-tube (transductal) or C-tube (transcystic)
Stent (straight, 7- or 10-F)
Sphincterotome (for antegrade sphincterotomy)
Side-viewing endoscope (for antegrade sphincterotomy)

*Some or all may be needed for a given operation.

stones are encountered postoperatively, usually is best treated with ERC ± S. These considerations are illustrated in the algorithm of Figure 21-1.

PATIENT POSITIONING AND TROCAR PLACEMENT

In addition to the basic equipment used to perform laparoscopic cholecystectomy, a number of other instruments, listed in Table 21-1, may be required to facilitate LCBDE. For maximum efficiency these tools should be organized in a central location—preferably a common bile duct exploration cart—that may be moved from room to room as necessary. The operating room set-up for LCBDE is shown in Figure 21-2. It is helpful to use a separate Mayo stand for the LCBDE instruments. Port placement (Fig. 21-3) is quite similar to that utilized for laparoscopic cholecystectomy.

OPERATIVE TECHNIQUE

Surgical Approaches to the Common Bile Duct

Laparoscopic common bile duct exploration may be accomplished through the cystic duct or through a choledochotomy. Stone characteristics, ductal diameters, the anatomic layout of the triangle of Calot (including the location of the cystic duct/common duct junction and the course of the cystic duct), and

surgeon skill will affect the decision as to which approach is best in a particular case. If a transcystic approach appears feasible, it usually is attempted before choledochotomy because it is less invasive and is associated with lower morbidity rate and higher patient satisfaction. Factors that influence the route of choice

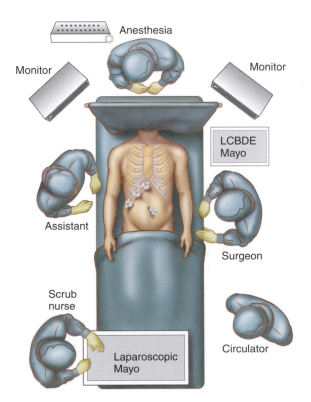

FIGURE 21-2 Operating room set-up for a laparoscopic common bile duct exploration (LCBDE).

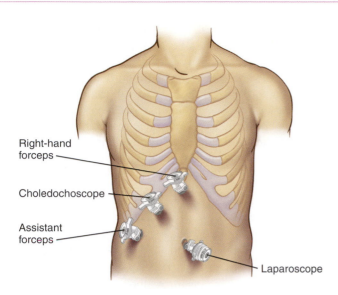

Right-hand forceps

Choledochoscope

Assistant forceps

Laparoscope

FIGURE 21-3 Port placement and utilization for a laparoscopic common bile duct exploration.

are listed in Table 21-2. Negative influences listed in this chart have a more profound impact on selection of the access route than positive or neutral ones. It is difficult to access the proximal ductal system when a cystic duct approach is employed, unless the cystic duct is very short or patulous and oriented at about 90 degrees to the common duct. When a choledochotomy is used, the scope may be directed into either the proximal system or the distal bile duct.

Ductal Imaging

The surgeon should be facile with his or her favorite method of intraoperative imaging of the ductal system: percutaneous cholangiography, portal cholangiography, or intraoperative LUS. Although some surgeons prefer sonography, most surgeons favor fluoroscopic imaging. It has become preferred over static x-rays

because it is faster and more detailed and allows surgeon interaction with the images in real time, meaning that the surgeon can scan the ductal system by moving the C-arm while injecting contrast material.

Percutaneous Cholangiography

In this technique a 14-gauge IV needle/catheter is inserted somewhat tangentially toward the triangle of Calot through the abdominal wall approximately 3 cm medial to the midclavicular port. The needle is removed and the catheter is used as a sleeve for introduction of the cholangiogram catheter. This sleeve also acts as a "mini-port" which may be used for introduction of balloons and baskets during common bile duct exploration. The catheter is grasped with forceps introduced through the medial epigastric port and placed into the cystic duct. It is fixed into position with a clip applied transversely across the axis of the catheter at its insertion point into the cystic duct. Fluoroscopy then is performed.

Portal Cholangiography

This method requires removal of an instrument from one of the ports, usually the midclavicular port. The catheter is introduced through this port freely or with an instrument that directs it into the cystic duct. Some instrument models also fix the catheter into the cystic duct. The major disadvantage of this technique is that it uses an existing port that would otherwise be occupied by an instrument providing exposure in the porta hepatis. Additionally, the instrument's radiopacity may obscure parts of the duct system during fluoroscopy.

Laparoscopic Ultrasonography

With this technique a 10-mm diameter, 7.5-MHz ultrasound transducer is inserted through a 10-mm port and is placed in direct contact with the tissues to obtain real-time sonographic images. Proponents of LUS suggest that it is faster and more accurate than cholangiography in their hands. Critics argue that fluoroscopic imaging is faster than LUS and doesn't require additional equipment expense. Whereas cholangiograms may be used as "maps" of the ductal anatomy in cases in which intense inflammation obscures visual cues, this is not possible with sonography. Interest in LUS for ductal evaluation has increased but widespread use has not.

Preparation of the Access Route: Dilatation of the Cystic Duct

When choledochoscopic maneuvers are needed, the duct will need to accept a 9- or 10-F scope. This is not a problem with a choledochotomy, but if a transcystic route is planned, and if the duct is not already large enough for scope insertion, it may be dilated either with over-the-wire mechanical graduated dilators or pneumatic dilators. A guidewire (0.028- or 0.035-inch) is inserted through the midclavicular port, through the cystic duct, and into the common duct. If graduated dilators are used, a 9-F size usually is the first to be advanced over the wire into the duct. Each successively larger dilator is advanced over the wire, until the duct is patulous enough to accept the scope. I have found that if a 9-F dilator will not easily enter the cystic duct initially, then it is unlikely that dilatation to a large enough diameter (11 or 12 F) will occur. More costly pneumatic dilators may also be advanced over the wire into the cystic duct. The dilatation balloon is filled while observing both the video monitor and the pressure gauge on the screw-type syringe attached to the dilator. After dilatation,

Factor	Transcystic Approach	Choledochotomy
Stone Characteristics		
One stone	+	+
Multiple stones	+	+
Stones ≤ 6 mm diameter	+	+
Stones > 6 mm diameter	–	+
Intrahepatic stones	–	+
Duct Diameters		
Diameter of cystic duct < 4 mm	–	+
Diameter of cystic duct > 4 mm	+	+
Diameter of common duct < 6 mm	+	–
Diameter of common duct > 6 mm	+	+
Cystic Duct Location		
Cystic duct entrance, lateral	+	+
Cystic duct entrance, posterior	–	+
Cystic duct entrance, distal	–	+
Local Conditions		
Inflammation, mild	+	+
Inflammation, marked	+	–
Surgeon Skill Set		
Suturing ability, poor	+	–
Suturing ability, good	+	+

Table 21-2 Factors That Influence the Choice of Approach (Transcystic or Choledochotomy) for a Laparoscopic Common Bile Duct Exploration

+, positive or neutral effect; –, negative effect.

the guidewire may be removed or left in place for subsequent guidance of the choledochoscope. In the latter case, the wire is loaded into the distal end of the working channel of the scope, which then is advanced into the ductal system over the wire.

Choledochotomy

Some authors routinely prefer common duct access through a choledochotomy. Others use this approach when the cystic duct cannot be dilated enough to accept passage of the scope or the largest common duct stone, or if intrahepatic disease is suspected. Choledochotomy may be accomplished with a laparoscopic scalpel or scissors inserted through the medial epigastric port. Most authors prefer a longitudinal incision, avoiding the 3 and 9 o'clock axial CBD blood supply, although one group from Italy routinely uses a transverse incision. The author prefers to start with a 1-cm incision and extend it if necessary to accommodate removal of the largest stone. This limits the amount of time that will be spent later in closing the choledochotomy. Stay sutures, which are commonly used in open common duct exploration, are not necessary for LCBDE, and are potentially harmful; if they are accidentally torn out of the duct, CBD closure may be difficult or incomplete, or may result in a stricture.

Irrigation Technique

When very small stones (<3 mm diameter), sludge, or sphincter spasm is suspected to be responsible for lack of flow of contrast material into the duodenum, transcystic flushing of the duct with saline or contrast material following IV administration of glucagon (1–2 mg) may force the debris into the duodenum. The process is monitored fluoroscopically. This technique often works well for 1- to 2-mm stones, but surgeons should not expect this method to be successful in clearing stones 4 mm and larger from the duct.

Balloon Techniques

In this technique a 4-F Fogarty balloon catheter is inserted into the abdomen through the 14-gauge sleeve used to perform the percutaneous cholangiograms. Forceps introduced through the medial epigastric port guide the catheter into the common duct through the cystic duct. The catheter is gently advanced into the duodenum if possible. I have found that if the Fogarty is easily advanced past the 10-cm mark, then its tip and balloon are usually in the duodenum. The balloon is inflated and the catheter is withdrawn in a cephalad direction parallel to the CBD until resistance is met at the sphincter; the duodenum is observed to move with the catheter at this point. The balloon is deflated, the catheter is withdrawn about 1 cm, and the balloon is reinflated. This should position it in the most distal portion of the duct, just proximal to the sphincter. The catheter is then withdrawn through the cystic duct, using the forceps from the medial epigastric port. Stones expressed from the cystic duct usually are removed through one of the larger ports. In the unusual event of displacement of the stone into the proximal hepatic duct, irrigation of the duct combined with operating table position changes usually will return the stone to the distal duct.

The combined use of the choledochoscope and a balloon catheter is particularly useful for stones that defy capture with a basket, even under direct vision through the choledochoscope. The balloon is inserted alongside the scope (not in the scope channel). The balloon is advanced past the stone, inflated, and withdrawn toward the scope. The entire scope-stone-balloon ensemble then is withdrawn through the ductal orifice. This technique is especially useful when dealing with intrahepatic stones.

Basket Techniques

Stone retrieval baskets may be inserted without the choledochoscope through the 14-gauge sleeve used for cholangiography. The basket is advanced into the common duct through the cystic duct, using forceps introduced through the medial epigastric port. The basket is opened immediately after it is advanced into the common bile duct. The deployed wires offer not only a "soft" distal end to the catheter, but also provide increased resistance when the catheter reaches the distal end of the bile duct. When the basket is located in the distal common duct, it is moved back and forth in small increments while slowly withdrawing it as the wires of the basket are being closed. Stone capture is identified when the basket fails to close completely. The captured stone is removed through the cystic duct, and the stones are delivered from the abdomen as described previously. Great care must be exercised with this method so that accidental "capture" of the papilla of Vater does not occur. A fluoroscope may be used to more accurately localize the stone(s) and basket tip. This technique, however, requires positioning of the fluoroscope in such a way as to avoid interference with movements of the forceps in the medial epigastric port. In some individuals, especially the obese, adequate fluoroscope position cannot be achieved. If a choledochotomy approach is used, then the free basket may be inserted directly into the CBD from its 14-gauge abdominal wall sleeve access point using the same technique described above. However, with this approach the basket may be inserted in either direction into the CBD, thereby allowing access to hepatic duct and intrahepatic stones. Additionally, the choledochoscope may be inserted alongside the basket for visualization of the capture process. Alternatively, the basket may be inserted through the working channel of the scope as described next.

Choledochoscopic Techniques

Choledochoscopic techniques are used when the preceding conservative measures fail to clear the common duct. The choledochoscope is inserted in the most direct route toward the CBD (usually via the midclavicular port) and, with or without wire guidance, into the cystic duct or the choledochotomy. At the level of the skin, the surgeon initially uses an atraumatic forceps inserted through the medial epigastric port to help guide the scope into the common duct. Saline is instilled through the working channel of the scope to dilate the duct and provide better visualization. Further manipulations require the surgeon to use both hands on the scope in most cases. One hand controls twisting maneuvers on the body of the scope at the cannula site, while the other holds the scope head and directs the tip of the scope with the deflection lever. It is best to keep the choledochoscopic and laparoscopic images in view simultaneously, either on separate monitors or preferably on the same screen with a video switcher during duct exploration and stone capture. The surgeon manipulates the scope so that a stone is in direct view. The surgeon inserts the basket into the working channel of the scope and captures the stone(s) as described earlier, while the assistant controls the scope at the port site. If the scope will not traverse the cystic duct/common duct junction, further dissection along the lateral border of the cystic and common bile duct (or a Kocher maneuver) may allow the junction to "unwrap" and "roll" anteriorly, thereby providing a less convoluted path into the common duct. In addition, it is important for the assistant to displace the gallbladder in a cephalad direction. This stretches the CBD to its full length and moves it anteriorly, allowing easier scope passage and manipulation. If this not consistently done, then the CBD collapses in an "accordion" fashion, and both visualization and scope manipulation are inhibited.

Lithotripsy

Intraoperative electrohydraulic or laser lithotripsy techniques have seen limited use since the introduction of LCBDE. Intraoperative lithotripsy may be indicated for an impacted stone that defies less aggressive removal techniques or a stone that is too large to be captured and removed through the cystic duct or the choledochotomy. Electrohydraulic lithotripters (EHL) are much less expensive than laser models, and consequently have been used somewhat more frequently but still not often. EHL devices must be used with great caution because they may cause unwanted ductal damage if the tip of the EHL probe is not applied accurately to the stone. A pulsatile saline jet (e.g., Waterpik, Water Pik, Inc., Fort Collins, CO) may be used through the working channel of the scope to free stones or debris from the duct wall. The surgeon will have to configure his or her own adapter to connect the device to the scope, because there are no ready-made adapters for this application.

Sphincterotomy and Drainage Procedures

Laparoscopic antegrade sphincterotomy is accomplished by passing a sphincterotome through the working channel of the choledochoscope and through the sphincter of Oddi. The cutting action of the device is monitored by simultaneous side-viewing endoscopy of the duodenum. This technique achieves excellent results as a drainage procedure, but it is logistically difficult to accomplish. It requires more equipment and an additional endoscopic team to be present in an already crowded operating room. Laparoscopic antegrade sphincterotomy has not gained widespread acceptance. Others have employed endoscopic retrograde sphincterotomy at the same time as the LCBDE, but again, this combination has not gained widespread acceptance.

Surgical biliary bypass may be indicated in the patient with a dramatically dilated common bile duct, multiple common duct stones, nonremovable impacted distal common duct stones, retained common duct stones not amenable to ERC ± S, and obstruction secondary to tumor. Four laparoscopic operations have proved feasible: CBD stent placement, cholecystoenterostomy, choledochoduodenostomy, and choledochoenterostomy. Stent placement also may be used in lieu of a T-tube after LCBDE, but requires subsequent upper GI endoscopy for its removal. Plastic removable stents generally are used for treatment of benign disease (such as a perforated or strictured CBD), while metal nonremovable stents usually are inserted in cases of malignant nonresectable disease. Cholecystoenterostomy requires patency of the cystic duct. In skilled hands the patency rates and morbidity/mortality rates of all these options compare favorably with open techniques. These procedures require advanced technical skills including laparoscopic suturing and knotting. Therefore, they only should be attempted by surgeons with proficiency in these techniques.

Completion Cholangiography and Cystic Stump Closure

A cholangiogram is repeated after the ductal exploration is complete. If the cholangiogram reveals residual stones, the surgeon must decide whether to proceed with further LCBDE, convert to open CBDE, perform a biliary bypass, or leave the stones in place for subsequent ERC ± S. The cystic duct stump should be secured either during the common duct exploration (when a choledochotomy is made) or after the completion cholangiogram. If the cystic duct is dilated greater than 5 mm, or if subsequent ERC ± S is planned, then ligatures (instead of or in addition to clips) should be considered to secure the duct in order to prevent subsequent leak.

T-Tube or C-Tube Placement

A choledochotomy may be closed either primarily or around a T-tube. T-tubes are used for three reasons: (1) for decompression of the duct, in the case of residual distal obstruction, (2) for access for ductal imaging in the postoperative period, and (3) for access and removal of residual common duct stones, should they be left after common bile duct exploration. Potential disadvantages of T-tubes include bacteremia, dislodgement, obstruction, or fracture of the tube. Some authors recommend broad-spectrum antibiotic coverage while the T-tube is in situ. T-tube cholangiography should be performed before removal of the tube. Removal of T-tubes postoperatively has been suggested as early as 4 days and as long as 6 weeks. The most appropriate management plan lies somewhere between these two extremes. Complications of T-tube removal include bile leaks, peritonitis, and the need for reoperation.

If a T-tube is used, then a 14-F tube is prepared by removing the back wall of the T portion. The entire T-tube is placed into the abdomen through a 10-mm port; then the T is inserted into the common duct. After the tube is in the duct, the outlying portion is temporarily occluded at its tip with a hemoclip or ligature; this prevents bile drainage into the peritoneal cavity while the remainder of the cholecystectomy is completed. This clip is later removed just prior to delivery of the tube through the abdominal wall. The common duct closure is completed with either 4-0 or 5-0 polyglycolic acid suture in either a continuous or interrupted fashion. The magnification afforded by the laparoscope and camera allows more precise placement of the sutures than in open surgery. The suture is secured with intracorporeal ligation techniques rather than extracorporeal techniques because of the fragility of the duct. The security of the closure is tested by temporarily advancing the tube out of one of the 5-mm right upper quadrant ports and injecting saline through the tube. If there is a leak, the common duct closure may be reinforced or resutured and then tested again. During the remainder of the case, while the tube is completely inside the peritoneal cavity, its tip should remain occluded with a clip or ligature. The tube ultimately should exit the abdominal cavity through the port with the most direct route to the CBD. Alternatively, the choledochotomy may be closed and a transcystic C-tube may be inserted to decompress the common bile duct, and provide access for subsequent cholangiography. This tube usually is loosely secured to the cystic duct so that it stays in place but allows subsequent percutaneous removal.

Primary Closure of the Choledochotomy

Despite the advantages of T-tube drainage, and because of the potential complications of T-tube placement, primary closure of the common bile duct without a T-tube or a C-tube has been advocated by some authors in open biliary tract surgery. Shorter operative times and length of hospital stay have been observed with primary closure. No increase in bile leak or peritonitis has been noted with primary closure in the literature on open procedures. This same technique has been employed in 33% of the author's patients who underwent choledochotomy; no complications were encountered in this group. Higher patient satisfaction has been associated with primary closure.

Drain Placement

After completion of the common bile duct exploration and subsequent cholangiography, the cystic duct and choledochotomy are secured and the cholecystectomy is performed. Drains are not routinely used after transcystic LCBDE. A drain may be indicated, however, if intense inflammation, infection, or contamination is present, a choledochotomy has been performed, or tissue integrity is questionable. If used, a closed-system suction drain is inserted through a 10-mm port into the porta hepatis and usually is brought out the abdominal wall through one of the 5-mm port sites.

PROCEDURE-SPECIFIC COMPLICATIONS

Failure to Clear the Common Duct

Inability to clear the common duct may be related to intense inflammation in the porta hepatis, obesity, intrahepatic stones, impacted stones, multiple stones, stones distal to a stricture, inadequate equipment, and surgeon inexperience. Surgeon inexperience is the most important factor here. For most surgeons who perform an average of 50 laparoscopic cholecystectomies per year, approximately 5 patients (10%) with common bile duct stones will be identified. This suggests that a surgeon may have an opportunity to hone his or her LCBDE skills only once every 2 months or so—and a learning curve of approximately 20 years. Surgeons may shorten this learning curve to some extent by performing routine intraoperative cholangiography, which employs many of the same maneuvers that are used for transcystic ductal exploration, such as catheter and basket insertion into the ductal system. Participation in a LCBDE course or laparoscopic fellowship also is extremely valuable in providing the training needed to perform successful LCBDE. After the duct has been explored, completion cholangiography is essential to document the status of the ductal system. Intraluminal opacities or failure of contrast agent to pass into the duodenum is usually indicative of retained intraductal material, mass, or stricture. If attempts to remove these blocks are unsuccessful, then the surgeon must decide whether to convert to open common bile duct exploration or resort to postoperative endoscopic retrograde techniques for stone removal; however, this is expensive. Therefore, it behooves the laparoscopic biliary surgeon to become proficient in LCBDE techniques.

Common Duct Injury

Improper identification of the anatomy is the most common cause of common duct injury and may be more likely when there is intense inflammation in the porta hepatis. One common scenario begins with less than optimal camera work, which leads to poor visualization or distortion of the porta hepatis. This complication may be avoided by having a thorough knowledge of the anatomy and its multiple variants, as seen laparoscopically with good camera work. In a second common scenario, the case may be fairly well controlled until bleeding is encountered in the triangle of Calot. If it is controlled with electrocautery and if too much energy is transmitted to the CBD, then the patient may develop jaundice secondary to a stricture of the common bile duct or the common hepatic duct.

Intraoperative cholangiography via the cystic duct, or the gallbladder if necessary, may provide clues as to the location of the common bile duct and delineate the local anatomy. This should allow the surgeon to avoid maneuvers that might injure the duct. During the ductal exploration itself, aggressive manipulation of instruments or the duct itself may lead to ductal injury. Introduction of instruments into the common bile duct must be done gently. This is especially true when using baskets in the ductal system because they may puncture the duct more easily than larger, more blunt instruments. Similarly, application of electrohydraulic lithotripsy to stones in the duct must be done accurately and under direct vision in order to avoid injury to the duct wall.

The best time to recognize CBD injury is at the time of its occurrence, when it can be either repaired primarily or bypassed. Unfortunately, most injuries are not recognized at the index procedure but present later with fever, tachycardia, abdominal pain, ileus, and jaundice. At that point, the patient should be stabilized and then referred to a center specializing in biliary tract surgery. Roux-en-Y hepaticojejunostomy usually is the procedure of choice for most severe common duct injuries.

Bile Leak

Bile may leak from the gallbladder bed, the cystic duct orifice, the cystic duct/common duct junction, or the common duct itself. This may be the result of dissection and manipulation of these structures during LC or LCBDE. Good visualization and gentle tissue handling techniques may help reduce the incidence of this problem. Additionally, the cystic duct should be adequately secured. This may require suture ligation if the cystic duct is large, thickened, or short; if significant distal common duct manipulation was used; and if recent pancreatitis caused distal ductal hypertension. Suture ligation or "loop" ligation of the cystic duct stump should be considered when the surgeon suspects that postoperative endoscopic retrograde cholangiopancreatography (ERCP) may be required. The diagnosis of a bile leak may be suggested by postoperative fever, excessive bilious drain output, ileus, generalized abdominal pain, and elevated liver function studies. A radionuclide scan may confirm the presence of a leak and the possibility of a distal bile duct obstruction. Sonography or CT scanning of the abdomen may help localize a bile collection, if there is one. If a drain is already in place, and if there is no evidence of distal obstruction of the common bile duct, then observation, intravenous fluids, and antibiotic coverage may be all that is necessary. If no drain is in place, and if a bile collection is localized, then radiographically directed placement of a drain with a period of observation may be adequate. Postoperative ERCP with stent placement across the sphincter of Oddi may be necessary to relieve a relative distal obstruction caused by spasm, edema, or debris. Surgical intervention may be warranted if the leak will not seal itself, or if generalized peritonitis develops.

Abscess

Patients requiring LCBDE often are older with more intense gallbladder inflammation than those requiring a simple LC. So, they may be more prone to the development of postoperative infectious problems at the surgical site. Although prophylactic antibiotics typically are used in these cases, the finding of acute or gangrenous cholecystitis or cholangitis usually indicates the need for therapeutic antibiotic coverage. The perihepatic space should also be thoroughly freed of debris and stones as completely as possible prior to the procedure. Placement of a closed system suction drain may be prudent. Postoperative fever, tachycardia, ileus, and abdominal pain may signal the presence of a problem at the surgical site. Sonography or CT scanning may confirm the presence of an abscess, and provide guidance for percutaneous drain placement. If this is not successful, surgical intervention may be warranted.

Pancreatitis

Pancreatitis may be caused preoperatively by passage of common duct stones; or it may be caused intraoperatively by manipulations in the distal duct or passage of stones through the distal duct. Baskets, balloons, and the choledochoscope must be gently manipulated in order to avoid such injury. High-pressure balloon dilatation of the sphincter of Oddi has been used by some authors but may cause hyperamylasemia or frank pancreatitis. Although this technique occasionally may be successful, it is not widely recommended. Passage of the choledochoscope into the duodenum similarly is a potentially hazardous practice and should be used only when necessary to gently push debris into the duodenum, or when the orifice into the duodenum is widely patent, such as after preoperative sphincterotomy or intraoperative intravenous glucagon administration. Pancreatitis may present postoperatively with excessive abdominal or back pain, fever, ileus, anorexia, or failure to thrive. The diagnosis may be confirmed with amylase and lipase measurements. CT scanning of the abdomen may be necessary if the patient does not improve with intravenous fluids, NPO status, and nasogastric suction. Antibiotics may be required if pancreatic abscess is suspected or confirmed with imaging studies.

RESULTS AND OUTCOME

Thousands of successful laparoscopic common bile duct explorations have been reported since the introduction of laparoscopic cholecystectomy in the late 1980s. In experienced hands successful ductal clearance rates exceed 90%. Morbidity (8–10%) and mortality (<1%) rates have been low in these series and are comparable to those of open CBDE. Generally speaking, it is believed that the incidence of complications is lower with the laparoscopic approach to common bile duct stones than with the open approach. Most laparoscopic surgeons have preferred the transcystic route for ductal exploration when feasible; in most series, it is successful in 80% to 90% of cases. Some authors prefer a transductal approach, however, and this is successful in 90% of cases as well. As discussed earlier, there are well-defined criteria that should lead a surgeon to one or the other approach.

Laparoscopic choledocholithotomy takes longer than straightforward laparoscopic cholecystectomy. Assuming that a surgeon's mean operative time for laparoscopic cholecystectomy is less than 1 hour, LCBDE may add approximately 1 hour or more to the procedure time. This period may be as little as 15 minutes when a transcystic basket is used, or several hours when the CBD disease is more complicated. Interestingly, this added time is not solely due to technical manipulations, but includes equipment set-up time and often the need to perform additional surgery. In addition, these patients often are older, with more chronic changes in the tissue of the porta hepatis, which makes dissection more difficult. Whereas the length of stay (LOS) for laparoscopic cholecystectomy is generally less than 24 hours, the LOS for patients undergoing LCBDE ranges from 1.3 to 7 days, depending on the severity of the disease, comorbid factors, access route, whether a T-tube was placed, and whether a biliary-enteric anastomosis was created. For transcystic LCBDE, the mean length of stay is 1.5 days in many large series. Length of stay for LCBDE via choledochotomy is generally longer than that for the transcystic approach.

Since 1990, surgeons throughout the world have developed a comprehensive laparoscopic solution to the problem of common bile duct stones. The success rate among accomplished laparoscopists approaches 90% or better. This compares favorably with treatment expectations in the prelaparoscopic era. Biliary tract surgeons practicing in this era should have the ability to treat all benign biliary tract disease laparoscopically in one setting, not requiring a series of costly, time-consuming, and potentially dangerous patient manipulations.

Suggested Reading

Decker G, Borie F, Millat B, et al: One hundred laparoscopic choledochotomies with primary closure of the common bile duct. Surg Endosc 2003;17:12–18.

Fletcher DR, Hobbs MS, Tan P, et al: Complications of cholecystectomy: Risk of the laparoscopic approach and protective effects of operative cholangiography: A population-based study. Ann Surg 1999;229:449–457.

Franklin ME, Pharand D: Laparoscopic common bile duct exploration. Surg Laparosc Endosc 1994;4(2):119–124.

Isla AM, Griniatsos J, Karvounis E, Arbuckle JD: Advantages of laparoscopic stented choledochorrhaphy over T-tube placement. Br J Surg 2004;91:862–866.

Lilly MC, Arregui ME: A balanced approach to choledocholithiasis. Surg Endosc 2001;15:467–472.

Nathanson LK, O'Rourke NA, Martin IJ, et al: Postoperative ERCP ± ES versus laparoscopic choledochotomy for clearance of selected bile duct calculi: A randomized trial. Ann Surg 2005;242:188–192.

National Institutes of Health State of the Science Statement on Endoscopic Retrograde Cholangiopancreatography (ERCP ± S) for Diagnosis and Therapy. Vol. 19(1), Jan. 16, 2002. Accessed at http://consensus.nih.gov/2002/2002ERCPsos020html.htm.

Perez G, Escalona A, Jarufe N, et al: Prospective randomised study of T-tube versus biliary stent for common bile duct decompression after open choledochotomy. World J Surg 2005;29:869–872.

Petelin J: Laparoscopic approach to common duct pathology. Am J Surg 1993;165:487–491.

Petelin JB: Laparoscopic common bile duct exploration: Lessons learned from >112 years experience. Surg Endosc 2003;17:1705–1715.

Rhodes M, Sussman L, Cohen L, Lewis MP: Randomised trial of laparoscopic exploration of common bile duct versus postoperative endoscopic retrograde cholangiography for common bile duct stones. Lancet 1998;351:159–161.

SALEH BAGHDADI AND
BASIL J. AMMORI

Laparoscopic Hepaticojejunostomy

The application of laparoscopy to biliary reconstruction began with the introduction of laparoscopic cholecystojejunostomy (LCJ) for palliation of malignant distal biliary obstruction in 1992. The technique was simplified by the introduction of endoscopic stapling devices, and benefited from the low demand for long-term patency due to the short life expectancy of these patients. Advanced biliary procedures were not approached laparoscopically until later. Laparoscopic choledochoduodenostomy is the simplest of advanced biliary reconstructive procedures, and a number of investigators have reported successful results. Laparoscopic hepaticojejunostomy (LHJ), however, is more complex because it requires an extensive dissection of the bile duct, the construction of a Roux-en-Y jejunal limb, and the fashioning of a more difficult high biliary-enteric anastomosis. Gagner and Pomp were the first to describe LHJ in 1994 as part of the reconstruction technique following pancreatoduodenectomy, and Rothlin and associates in 1999 described palliative LHJ with the construction of a Roux-en-Y jejunal loop and a sutured end-to-side anastomosis in patients with inoperable periampullary cancer. Subsequent reports of LHJ for benign and malignant diseases have been featured in the literature with good results.

OPERATIVE INDICATIONS

Laparoscopic biliary reconstructive procedures have been limited in part because of their complexity. Nevertheless, the advantages of the laparoscopic approach for other complex procedures, such as nephrectomy, adrenalectomy, and bariatric surgery, are well established and include reduced postoperative pain, hospital stay, and recuperation period. It is logical to think that such advantages also might be associated with a laparoscopic approach to biliary reconstruction; comparative studies with open surgery are needed, however, to examine this logic.

In selected patients, palliation of malignant distal biliary obstruction secondary to periampullary malignancy is one indication for LHJ. Some 80% or more of patients with periampullary malignancy have inoperable disease and commonly present with obstructive jaundice; their treatment merely is palliative. These patients' short life expectancy calls for minimally invasive palliative techniques with the intention to minimize intervention-related morbidity and fatality, shorten hospital stay, maximize quality of the patients' remaining life, and offer durable relief of obstructive jaundice.

Although endoscopic insertion of a metal biliary stent achieves good long-term biliary patency and should be considered the first choice in patients with longer expected survival, cannulation of the biliary tree is not always successful and may not be feasible in patients with proximal malignant duodenal obstruction. Failure of endoscopic palliation of distal biliary obstruction may be handled either by laparoscopic biliary bypass or by percutaneous transhepatic insertion of a metal biliary stent that may be followed, if necessary, by endoscopic insertion of an expandable metal duodenal stent. The choice between laparoscopic or radiologic approaches to relief of biliary obstruction is open to debate and depends on the local expertise available, the life expectancy of the patient, whether a LCJ or LHJ is required, and whether additional palliation of gastric outlet obstruction is indicated.

When considering laparoscopic biliary bypass, LCJ should remain the preferred option as it benefits from simpler technique, shorter operative time, and lower risk of morbidity. Although the gap in patency rate of the biliary-enteric anastomosis between LCJ and LHJ may be expected to widen after a year from surgery, this is a weak argument for routine application of biliary bypass to the bile duct, as the large majority of these patients do not survive beyond a year. LCJ requires, however, that the confluence of the cystic and common hepatic ducts be at least 1 cm proximal to the upper limit of the malignant biliary stricture in order to avoid occlusion of the cystic duct by disease progression before death. About one third of patients may be expected to satisfy this anatomic requirement at the time of presentation with obstructive jaundice. Fit patients who are expected to have better prognosis (e.g., locally advanced rather than metastatic disease; LCJ not possible or justified) may be offered LHJ. Surgical biliary bypass has the advantage of greater patency compared to biliary stents. The addition of a laparoscopic gastrojejunostomy, if necessary, is feasible and does not increase operative morbidity or fatality.

Another indication for LHJ is bypass of benign distal biliary obstruction, such as that caused by chronic pancreatitis not associated with pancreatic head mass, or by inflammatory stricture secondary to choledocholithiasis. The biliary bypass offers a definitive and long-term treatment option. In comparison, in such a patient there is little cause for repeated endoscopic biliary manipulation, and certainly there is no place for LCJ.

LHJ is part of the reconstruction technique after laparoscopic resection of the bile duct for benign (e.g., choledochal cyst) or malignant (e.g., pancreatoduodenectomy) disease. Cyst excision with Roux-en-Y hepaticojejunostomy is the standard treatment for type I and type IV choledochal cysts. Choledochal cysts, although most often seen and treated in childhood, occasionally are diagnosed in adults. Such cases are particularly well suited for a laparoscopic approach, given the relative patient size compared to that in the pediatric age group.

There are some further patient, disease, and anatomic requirements to consider when contemplating LHJ. The anticipated long operative time for LHJ calls for exclusion of patients with poor cardiopulmonary reserve and perhaps those with multiple risk factors for thromboembolism. Dilatation of the proximal bile duct certainly facilitates biliary reconstruction, and should be an important consideration for a laparoscopic approach, given the associated technical difficulty. Although some might prefer to avoid the laparoscopic approach in morbidly obese patients and patients with dense operative adhesions, these are not absolute contraindications to laparoscopic surgery, as the laparoscopic approach to bariatric surgery and to adhesiolysis is now well established.

PREOPERATIVE TESTING, EVALUATION, AND PREPARATION

Each patient should have an evaluation of cardiopulmonary reserve and fitness for prolonged surgery. The patients with periampullary malignancy should have performance status assessed. Nutritional status also should be assessed and addressed as needed; the consequences of anastomotic leak due to poor nutritional reserve, particularly in cancer patients, are quite serious. Although the role of preoperative biliary stenting in patients with periampullary malignancy undergoing pancreatoduodenectomy is controversial, it is advisable to address those with deep obstructive jaundice prior to LHJ by endoscopic or percutaneous biliary drainage. In addition, correction of coagulopathy and adequate hydration are achieved prior to surgery.

Each patient also should have an adequate study of the anatomy of the biliary tree to confirm the distal location of the biliary stricture, the extent of dilatation of the proximal biliary tree at the site of the intended biliary-enteric anastomosis, and a demonstration of the distance from the confluence of the cystic and common hepatic ducts to the upper limit of the malignant biliary stricture when bypass rather than resection is being considered. This information may be made available from endoscopic retrograde or percutaneous transhepatic antegrade biliary imaging (Fig. 22-1), from magnetic resonance cholangiography (Fig. 22-2), or from careful evaluation of reconstructed computed tomography images. Laparoscopic ultrasound is another alternative when the choice between LCJ and LHJ is being considered intraoperatively.

Confirmation of the underlying diagnosis and the appropriateness of operative intervention needs to be accomplished prior to surgery. Exclusion of malignancy in patients with distal biliary stricture secondary to chronic pancreatitis and a mass in the head of the pancreas, and in those with stone-associated stricture, may be challenging despite the availability of modern techniques, such as endoscopic ultrasound, fine-needle aspiration biopsy, endoscopic brush biopsy, and advanced cross-sectional imaging. In patients with choledochal cyst, the presence of anomalous

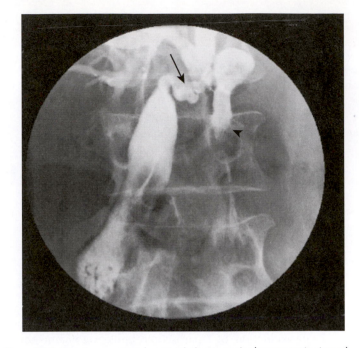

FIGURE 22-1 Percutaneous transhepatic cholangiography (postoperative image) showing insertion of the cystic duct (arrow) some 2 cm above the proximal end of the biliary stricture (arrowhead); this patient underwent a laparoscopic cholecystojejunostomy after a failed attempt at transhepatic insertion of a biliary stent, and contrast material could be seen entering the small bowel.

pancreatobiliary junction and the extent of intrahepatic ductal involvement, and the type of the disease according to the classification proposed by Todani, may be demonstrated by multimodality imaging. Patients with periampullary pancreatic or bile duct malignancy are offered pancreatoduodenectomy on the basis of careful evaluation of clinical and radiologic findings and without prior histologic confirmation.

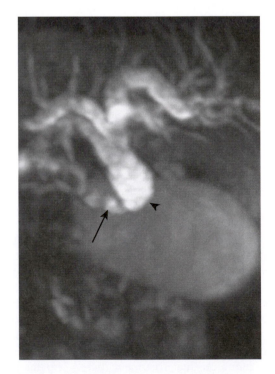

FIGURE 22-2 Preoperative magnetic resonance cholangiography in a jaundiced patient with unresectable pancreatic cancer showing insertion of the cystic duct (arrow) abutting the proximal end of the biliary stricture (arrowhead); this patient underwent a laparoscopic hepaticojejunostomy.

Finally, a periampullary malignancy should be evaluated for size and the reason for its inoperability. Large periampullary tumors, even if only locally advanced, may physically preclude a Roux loop from comfortably reaching the proximal bile duct, and undoubtedly will render the construction of a biliary-enteric anastomosis technically impossible. Patients with metastatic disease have short life expectancy (often less than 6 months) and should be offered biliary stenting rather than LHJ, unless the metastases are detected confidently and for the first time during a staging laparoscopy in a patient who remains jaundiced (i.e., without prior biliary stent) and in whom a concomitant LCJ is deemed appropriate. Patients who are found to have locally advanced nonmetastatic disease at staging laparoscopy and laparoscopic ultrasound may be considered for a concomitant LHJ if LCJ is not appropriate. Clearly, there is a consent issue here, and the prospect of laparoscopic biliary bypass should be discussed prior to staging laparoscopy.

PATIENT POSITIONING AND PLACEMENT OF TROCARS

Surgery is performed under general anesthesia with a single-lumen endotracheal tube and a 24-hour intravenous antibiotic cover. The patient is catheterized and urine output is monitored. The patient is placed either in a supine position with the operating surgeon and assistant standing on the patient's left side, or in modified "flat" Lloyd-Davis position with the surgeon standing between the patient's legs and the assistant on the patient's left. The operating table may be tilted 30 degrees head up to allow the colon to drop away from the infrahepatic space. An orogastric tube ensures that the stomach is deflated and could be removed at end of surgery.

The procedure may employ five to six ports (Fig. 22-3), 12 mm Hg of capnoperitoneum, and a 30-degree, 10-mm laparoscope. A triangular endoflex retractor (Mantis Surgical Limited, Newbury, Berkshire, U.K.) is introduced through the 5-mm port in the right anterior axillary line to retract the liver upward. Another triangular endoflex retractor may be introduced through the 5-mm port in the left anterior axillary line to retract the duodenum and colon downward, thus enhancing exposure of the bile duct.

OPERATIVE TECHNIQUE

Many of the important technical principles of laparoscopic biliary reconstructive surgery are the same as those in open biliary surgery. Surgeons performing these procedures should have extensive experience in both hepatobiliary surgery and advanced laparoscopic techniques. In particular, advanced intracorporeal suturing skills are necessary. Automatic suturing devices and knot-tying devices frequently do not allow for precise suture placement.

Preparation of the Biliary Tract

The anterior aspect of the supraduodenal common bile duct (CBD) and common hepatic duct (CHD) is displayed, and the overlying peritoneal sheath is incised transversely and longitudinally to expose the dilated bile duct. The aim will be to construct an end-to-side LHJ with concomitant cholecystectomy in patients with benign distal biliary stricture (see Figs. 22-4 to 22-7) or to apply the simpler side-to-side LHJ in patients undergoing palliative biliary bypass with preservation of the gallbladder (see Figs. 22-8 to 22-10). In the latter group of patients, a choledochotomy is deferred until a Roux-en-Y loop of jejunum has been prepared and brought up antecolically, and in the former group (Fig. 22-4), a cholecystectomy is performed at this stage and a cholangiogram is obtained, if necessary. Division of the cystic duct is delayed, however, as the cystic duct is a useful retraction tool that facilitates incision of the peritoneal sheath at the free margin of the foramen of Winslow, and it helps to expose the posterior aspect of the CBD in preparation for its circumferential dissection and division. Dissection of the CBD progresses from its left posterior border, taking care not to injure the right hepatic artery that often courses behind the duct or the portal vein. The CBD is held in a rubber sling with its ends secured by an endoclip, and the cystic duct then is clipped and divided (Fig. 22-5A). Traction

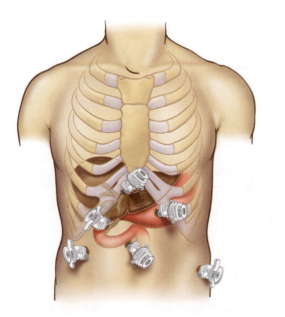

FIGURE 22-3 Diagram showing the sites of placement of the ports for a laparoscopic hepaticojejunostomy.

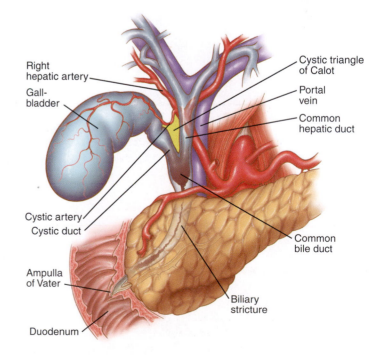

FIGURE 22-4 Anatomic drawing showing a distal smooth (benign) biliary stricture.

171

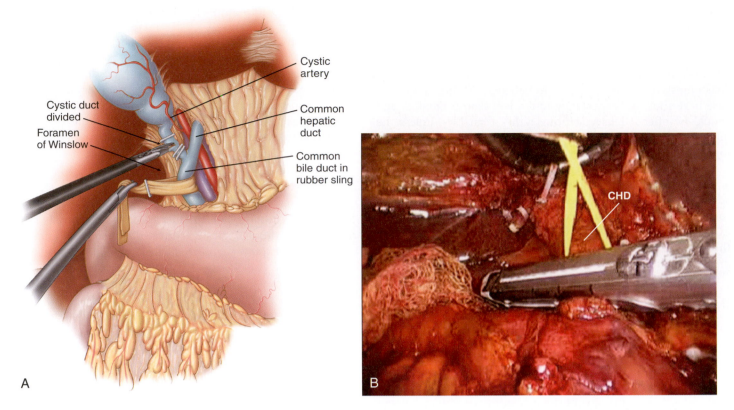

Cystic artery

Cystic duct divided

Foramen of Winslow

Common hepatic duct

Common bile duct in rubber sling

CHD

A

B

FIGURE 22-5 A laparoscopic cholecystectomy is being performed. The common hepatic and bile ducts have been mobilized and held up in a sling (diagram, **A**) in preparation for division of the common hepatic duct (CHD) using either a vascular stapler (operative picture, **B**) or an ultrasonic scalpel.

on the rubber sling tents the bile duct forward and enables dissection to progress safely in a proximal direction to expose the CHD. The CHD then is divided transversely above the insertion of the cystic duct using either a 35-mm vascular endostapler (Ethicon Endo-Surgery, Cincinnati, OH) (Figs. 22-5B and 22-6A and B) or an ultrasonically activated scalpel (UAS) (e.g., ACE, Ethicon Endo-Surgery). If divided with the UAS, the distal end will need to be sutured. The gallbladder is placed in a specimen retrieval bag, which then is tucked away in the left upper abdomen for removal at the end of the operation. The subhepatic space is packed with a gauze swab pending preparation of the Roux loop.

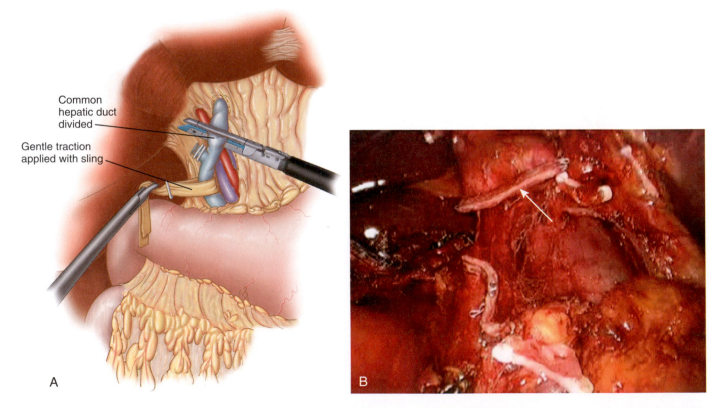

Common hepatic duct divided

Gentle traction applied with sling

A

B

FIGURE 22-6 The common hepatic duct has been divided using a vascular stapler (diagram, **A**; operative picture, **B**). *Arrow* indicates the staple line on liver side of the divided duct.

Construction of the Roux-en-Y Loop

For construction of the Roux-en-Y loop, the surgeon changes position and stands on the right side of the patient's head while the assistant stands on the left side facing a second monitor that is positioned above the patient's left thigh. The greater omentum is divided longitudinally with the UAS to expose the small intestine. The surgeon works through the two midclavicular ports and identifies a loop of jejunum 60 to 75 cm from the duodenojejunal flexure (longer if a concomitant side-to-side antecolic anterior gastrojejunostomy is intended). A window in the mesentery is opened with the UAS, the jejunum is transected with an endostapler, and the distal end is marked with a seromuscular 2-0 polyglactin suture for ease of identification. The mesentery is divided further with the UAS, dividing the first arcade of vessels. A 50-cm Roux loop is fashioned and a side-to-side stapled jejunojejunostomy is constructed (e.g., two firings of a 45-mm endostapler), and the common enterotomy is closed with a continuous 2-0 polyglactin suture. The mesenteric defect also is closed with a continuous 2-0 polyglactin suture.

The Hepaticojejunal Anastomosis

The surgeon and the assistant return to their original positions. In patients with benign disease, a window in the transverse mesocolon is made to the right of the middle colic vessels, and the suture-marked end of the Roux loop is delivered retrocolically to the subhepatic space. For patients with advanced malignancy undergoing palliative LHJ, the Roux loop is brought up antecolically to shorten operating time and to avoid passing the loop too close to the cancer.

In patients undergoing LHJ for benign disease, a sutured end-to-side biliary-enteric anastomosis is constructed. The first layer

of sutures is a continuous 3-0 polyglactin suture which takes seromuscular bites of the jejunum and through-and-through bites of the bile duct about 2 mm proximal to the staple line, thus incorporating the staple line (Fig. 22-7A). A transverse choledochotomy then is made with scissors, and a corresponding transverse enterotomy is made with the UAS. The posterior anastomotic line may be secured with a continuous 3-0 polyglactin suture that is tied extraluminally on either end of the anastomosis (Fig. 22-7B). The anterior anastomotic line is completed with interrupted 3-0 or 4-0 polyglactin suture (Fig. 22-7C), particularly if the duct diameter is not too wide; a continuous suture may be utilized if the duct is 15 mm or wider (Fig. 22-7D). The anastomosis is inspected circumferentially for integrity, a nonsuction 20-F tube drain is placed in the subhepatic space behind the anastomosis, and the gallbladder bag is retrieved from the abdomen.

For a palliative side-to-side LHJ, a transverse choledochotomy is made at least 1 cm above the stricture, and a transverse enterotomy is made 2 to 3 cm distal to the transected end of the Roux loop of jejunum (Fig. 22-8). A stapled side-to-side hepaticojejunostomy then may be created using a 35-mm vascular endostapler (Fig. 22-9) introduced through the 12-mm port above the umbilicus, with the laparoscope placed in the left midclavicular port. The common choledochotomy-enterotomy then is closed with interrupted 2-0 polyglactin suture (Fig. 22-10). No drain is employed in these patients in order to avoid drain-site tumor recurrence.

In 2000, Machado and associates reported a case with modification of the Roux loop technique that avoids the division of the mesenteric vessels. The technique involves side-to-side hepaticojejunostomy as a first step, followed by division of the jejunum proximal to the anastomosis. A side-to-side jejunojejunostomy then is performed to fashion a Roux loop. A continuous

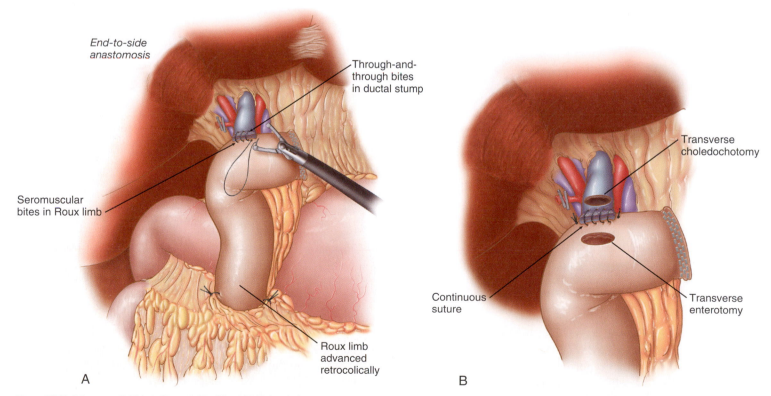

A   B

FIGURE 22-7 A Roux-en-Y 50- to 60-cm jejunal loop has been fashioned and brought out in a retrocolic manner. **A,** An end-to-side hepaticojejunal seromuscular continuous suture is placed, incorporating the staple line of the divided common hepatic duct. **B,** A transverse choledochotomy and enterotomy then are created.

Continued

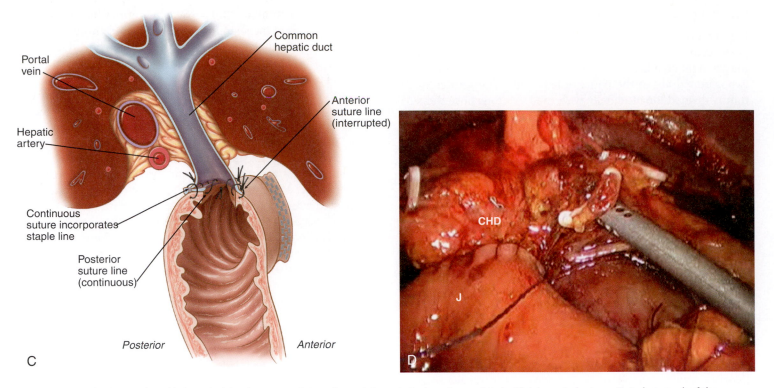

FIGURE 22-7 CONT'D **C**, An end-to-side hepaticojejunal anastomosis is performed; the anterior layer is completed with interrupted sutures. **D**, A photograph of the completed anastomosis. CHD, common hepatic duct; J, jejunum.

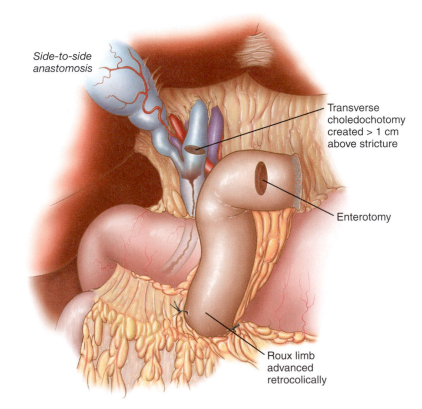

FIGURE 22-8 Drawing showing a cystic duct insertion within less than 1.0 cm from the upper end of a stricture of the common bile duct that shows shouldering indicative of malignancy; the common hepatic duct has been exposed and a transverse choledochotomy has been created. A Roux-en-Y antecolic 50-cm jejunal loop has been fashioned and a transverse enterotomy has been created.

intracorporeal suturing technique was used for the hepaticojejunostomy and a linear stapler was used for the jejunojejunostomy. Gentileschi and coworkers reported another modification of the technique in 2002 in which a laparoscopic gastrojejunostomy was constructed followed by lateral hepaticojejunostomy without using a Roux loop (i.e., using a simple loop).

Technical Issues

A bulky periampullary tumor may render access to the bile duct impossible. Careful preoperative evaluation of cross-sectional images is essential to avoid inappropriate patient selection. The retrocolic delivery of the Roux jejunal loop in patients with benign disease may be difficult. This is aided by taking down the hepatic

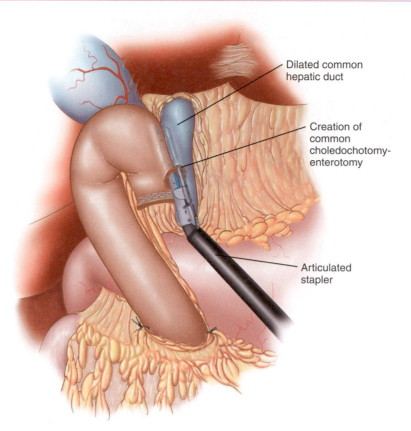

Dilated common
hepatic duct

Creation of
common
choledochotomy-
enterotomy

Articulated
stapler

FIGURE 22-9   A stapled side-to-side hepaticojejunostomy is created using a linear vascular 30-mm stapler. The narrow jaw of the stapler was introduced into the dilated common hepatic duct while the staple-harboring wider jaw was introduced into the jejunal limb.

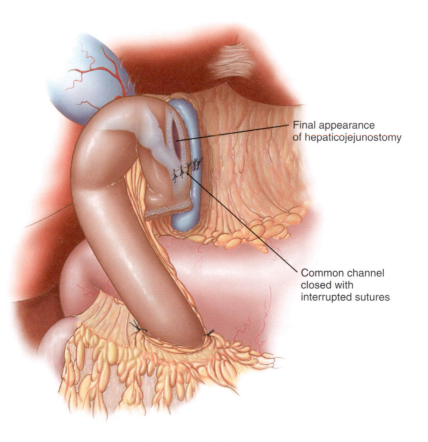

Final appearance
of hepaticojejunostomy

Common channel
closed with
interrupted sutures

FIGURE 22-10   The final appearance of a side-to-side stapled hepaticojejunostomy with the common choledochotomy-enterotomy closed with interrupted suture.

flexure of the colon, creating a window in the transverse mesocolon to the right of the middle colic vessels, and marking the proximal end of the loop with a suture for ease of identification.

There is no doubt that the construction of the biliary-enteric anastomosis is the most demanding part of the procedure. The magnification achieved by the laparoscope, however, may allow for better visualization of the operative field than in open surgery and facilitates reconstruction. It is essential to prepare the CHD circumferentially for this anastomosis. If the anterior aspect of the biliary-enteric anastomosis is being completed with interrupted sutures, then it would make suture placement easier if the last two or three sutures were left untied until they were placed. The temptation to transect the bile duct low in order to leave a long segment for ease of anastomosis should be resisted, as this may render the biliary end of the anastomosis ischemic. The surgeon should be adept at forehand and backhand intracorporeal suturing, and surgeons considering such procedures undoubtedly would benefit from acquiring contralateral-hand suturing skills to increase their maneuverability. The left midclavicular port is convenient for right-hand suturing and should be placed relatively high so that the needle holder approaches the biliary anastomosis almost in a transverse direction inline with the anastomosis. The technical challenges associated with intracorporeal suturing may be overcome by the use of recently developed robotic assistance devices, which use instruments with wrist-type end-effectors; the authors have no experience with these. Another option might be hand-assisted laparoscopic surgery. This procedure does not require the removal of a large specimen, however, so the added trauma and pain of a hand-assisted port is unnecessary in the authors' opinion and may prolong hospital stay.

POSTOPERATIVE CARE

The orogastric tube is removed before the patient is extubated; there typically is no indication for nasogastric tube drainage. Intravenous antibiotic cover is continued for 24 hours. Oral fluids may be introduced freely from the evening of surgery, and a liquid or soft diet may be allowed on the first postoperative day. The abdominal drain may be removed within 24 hours if there is no bile leak. The patient should be mobilized the first postoperative day; early mobility and chest physiotherapy decrease morbidity.

PROCEDURE-SPECIFIC COMPLICATIONS

Adherence to basic surgical principles is the mainstay of a safe outcome. Defining the biliary anatomy, dissecting out a suitable length of hepatic duct, creating an enteric loop of appropriate length to bring the bowel loop to the hepatic duct without tension, and creating a wide mucosa-to-mucosa biliary-enteric anastomosis are of paramount importance. Factors identified in association with morbidity and poor surgical outcome include history of recurrent cholangitis, proximal stricture, portal hypertension, cirrhosis, hepatic abscess, intra-abdominal abscess and bile collection, liver atrophy, advanced age, and surgical inexperience. Anastomotic leak or stricture requiring an open revision may occur. Some authors advocate placement of a percutaneous transjejunal biliary catheter for drainage and for postoperative radiologic assessment of the bilio-enteric anastomosis. Conversion to open surgery could result from severe adhesions, such as those from recurrent cholangitis or previous abdominal

surgery, or from high transection of choledochal cysts with subsequent retraction of the hepatic ducts into the liver substance.

RESULTS AND OUTCOME

LHJ for Distal Benign and Malignant Biliary Strictures

There is no doubt that, in expert hands, the laparoscopic approach to biliary bypass for palliation of malignancy offers clear benefits over open surgery in terms of operative morbidity and mortality rates, hospital stay, and quality of life. Open surgery for biliary bypass has been associated with high mortality and morbidity rates (8–33% and 20–60%, respectively). When compared to open surgery, laparoscopic palliation showed significantly lower postoperative morbidity rate (7%) and close to 0% mortality rate. In a case-controlled comparative study of laparoscopic versus open gastroenterostomy and hepaticojejunostomy, Rothlin and associates reported significantly lower operative morbidity and mortality rates and postoperative requirements of opiate analgesia, as well as reductions in postoperative hospital stay. The collective worldwide experience with this approach to early 2007 is summarized in Table 22-1.

It is well recognized that hepaticojejunostomy offers better long-term patency rate and lower risk of biliary reintervention compared with cholecystojejunostomy. Only a very small minority of cancer patients, however, might be expected to benefit from a universal policy of bypass to the bile duct, particularly when their short life expectancy is considered. A review of 1919 patients reported a reintervention rate for recurrent biliary obstruction of 7.5% with cholecystojejunostomy and 2.9% with hepaticojejunostomy. Moreover, the operating time for laparoscopic hepaticojejunostomy is considerably longer than that of cholecystojejunostomy. The authors have found that a cholecystojejunostomy is applicable in three quarters of patients with malignant obstructive jaundice requiring surgical bypass. If a patient has benign disease or a malignant obstruction within 1 cm of the cystic duct, then performance of LHJ should prevent the recurrence of jaundice.

LHJ after Excision of Choledochal Cyst

In 1998, the first case of laparoscopic excision of a type I choledochal cyst was reported. Since then, some 130 cases of laparoscopic or hand-assisted resections have been published, with 88% of the procedures performed in infants and children. More than two thirds of the resections in children were accomplished laparoscopically, with the remainder requiring a hand-assistance procedure or open conversion (overall conversion rate = 7%); one half of adult subjects underwent a hand-assisted approach. The feasibility of the purely laparoscopic approach, however, was demonstrated in the low rate of open conversion (<10%), low morbidity rate (<10%), and no deaths. Following laparoscopic excision, a prompt recovery has been reported with a purely laparoscopic approach; a typical mean hospital stay is 5 days. This compares favorably with the hospital stay of about 20 days in one series of laparoscopic hand-assisted resection of choledochal cyst with a Roux-en-Y hepaticojejunostomy. All patients with choledochal cyst require lifelong follow-up because of the increased risk of cholangiocarcinoma, even after complete excision of the cyst.

LHJ after Resection of Periampullary Malignancy

Although there have been only about 30 cases of laparoscopic and hand-assisted laparoscopic pancreatoduodenectomy reported

Table 22-1 Results of Laparoscopic Hepaticojejunostomy for Management of Distal Biliary Strictures

Authors	Diagnosis	Procedure	Operative Time (min)	Conversion	Morbidity	Mortality	Hospital Stay (days)	Follow-Up
Rothlin, et al., 1999	PC	LHJ and GJ (n = 3)	129 (30–330)*	0	Anastomotic leak (n = 1)	0	9.4*	NA
Machado, et al., 2000	PC	LHJ (n = 1)	NA	0	0	0	6	20 months
Gentileschi, et al., 2002	PC	LHJ (n = 1)	NA	NA	NA	NA	NA	NA
Ali and Ammori, 2003	PC	LHJ, GJ, BTS (n = 1)	NA	0	0	0	4	6 months
O'Rourke, et al., 2004	Choledocholithiasis, stricture	LHJ (n = 1)	272	0	0	0	3	15 months
Han and Yi, 2004	Recurrent CBD stones (n =5), benign biliary stricture (n = 2)	LHJ (n = 7)	358 (290–480)*	1	A self-limited episode of melena (n = 1)	0	NA	27.5* (5–60) months
Chowbey, et al., 2005	Iatrogenic biliary stricture	LHJ (n = 4)	285 (270–305)*	1	Open revision 18 months later for cholangitis (n = 1)	0	4*	3.1* years

*Data shown represent mean (range).
BTS, bilateral thoracoscopic splanchnicectomy; CBD, comman bile duct; GJ, gastrojejunostomy; LHJ, laparoscopic hepaticojejunostomy; NA, not available; PC, pancreatic cancer.

in the literature, there is no doubt that in selected patients this procedure can be performed safely, with three quarters of the patients achieving uneventful recovery, and with a mortality rate below 3%. The procedure is technically challenging and requires the expertise of a skilled laparoscopic pancreatic surgeon. The hand-assisted approach appears to shorten the operating time and to facilitate reconstruction after resection, including the hepaticojejunal anastomosis. Biliary complications following this procedure are uncommon according to the available literature, which attests to the safety of a laparoscopically constructed biliary-enteric anastomosis.

In conclusion, laparoscopic biliary reconstruction is safe and feasible, but it requires a long operative time, advanced laparoscopic skills, and significant experience in hepatobiliary surgery. Large studies will be needed to determine the long-term outcome and patency rates of laparoscopic biliary-enteric bypass and to compare the laparoscopic approach against endoscopic biliary stenting.

Suggested Reading

Ali AS, Ammori BJ: Concomitant laparoscopic gastric and biliary bypass and bilateral thoracoscopic splanchnotomy: The full package of minimally invasive palliation for pancreatic cancer. Surg Endosc 2003;17:2028–2031.

Ammori BJ, Baghdadi S: Minimally invasive pancreatic surgery: The new frontier? Curr Gastroenterol Rep 2006;8:132–142.

Chowbey PK, Soni V, Sharma A, et al: Laparoscopic hepaticojejunostomy for biliary strictures: The experience of 10 patients. Surg Endosc 2005;19:273–279.

Dulucq JL, Wintringer P, Mahajna A: Laparoscopic pancreaticoduodenectomy for benign and malignant diseases. Surg Endosc 2006;20:1045–1050.

Dulucq JL, Wintringer P, Stabilini C, et al: Are major laparoscopic pancreatic resections worthwhile? A prospective study of 32 patients in a single institution. Surg Endosc 2005;19:1028–1034.

Gagner M, Pomp A: Laparoscopic pylorus-preserving pancreaicoduodenectomy. Surg Endosc 1994;8:408–410.

Gentileschi P, Kini S, Gagner M: Palliative laparoscopic hepatico- and gastrojejunostomy for advanced pancreatic cancer. J Soc Laparoendosc Surg 2002;6:331–338.

Ghanem AM, Hamade AM, Sheen AJ, et al: Laparoscopic gastric and biliary bypass: A single-center cohort prospective study. J Laparoendosc Adv Surg Tech A 2006;16:21–26.

Han HS, Yi NJ: Laparoscopic Roux-en-Y choledochojejunostomy for benign biliary disease. Surg Laparosc Endosc Percutan Tech 2004;14:80–84.

Jeyapalan M, Almeida JA, Michaelson RL, Franklin ME, Jr: Laparoscopic choledocho-duodenostomy: Review of a 4-year experience with an uncommon problem. Surg Laparosc Endosc Percutan Tech 2002;12:148–153.

Machado MA, Rocha JR, Herman P, et al: Alternative technique of laparoscopic hepaticojejunostomy for advanced pancreatic head cancer. Surg Laparosc Endosc Percutan Tech 2000;10:174–177.

O'Rourke RW, Lee NN, Cheng J, et al: Laparoscopic biliary reconstruction. Am J Surg 2004;187:621–624.

Rothlin MA, Schob O, Weber M: Laparoscopic gastro- and hepaticojejunostomy for palliation of pancreatic cancer: A case controlled study. Surg Endosc 1999;13:1065–1069.

Shimi S, Banting S, Cuschieri A: Laparoscopy in the management of pancreatic cancer: Endoscopic cholecystojejunostomy for advanced disease. Br J Surg 1992;79:317–319.

Smith AC, Dowsett JF, Russell RC, et al: Randomised trial of endoscopic stenting versus surgical bypass in malignant low bile duct obstruction. Lancet 1994;344:1655–1660.

Urbach DR, Bell CM, Swanstrom LL, Hansen PD: Cohort study of surgical bypass to the gallbladder or bile duct for the palliation of jaundice due to pancreatic cancer. Ann Surg 2003;237:86–93.

Pancreas and Spleen

Malcolm M. Bilimoria, Constantine T. Frantzides,
Minh Luu, and Luis E. Laguna

Minimally Invasive Distal Pancreatectomy

23

The role of laparoscopy continues to evolve as part of the armamentarium of the modern day pancreatic surgeon. In the late 1980s and early 1990s, laparoscopy emerged as a tool to diagnose metastatic disease and assess tumor resectability in patients with pancreatic cancer. Laparoscopic evaluation of the abdomen prior to a major pancreatic resection can avoid a laparotomy in patients with metastatic disease not seen on a preoperative computed tomography (CT) scan. Today, with the improved sensitivity of CT scanning and magnetic resonance imaging, occult metastases uncovered by laparoscopy are becoming less common, and so many pancreatic surgeons have de-emphasized the staging laparoscopy. Some data suggest, however, that diagnostic laparoscopy can reveal small peritoneal metastasis in 5% to 15% of patients with a negative CT scan. The use of laparoscopic ultrasound for the determination of pancreatic tumor resectability has been partially replaced by high-resolution CT scanning and endoscopic ultrasound. Laparoscopic ultrasound still is useful, however, in the resection of pancreatic neuroendocrine tumors, because some of the tumors that are not found on preoperative imaging subsequently may be located with the ultrasound technology.

Since the mid-1990s, the use of laparoscopy for resection of pancreatic tumors has increased steadily. Resectional procedures range from the enucleation of neuroendocrine tumors to pancreaticoduodenectomy for periampullary carcinoma. In 2002, there were fewer than 70 reported cases of laparoscopic distal pancreatectomy; in 2006, however, there were more than 400 reported cases, and new series are being published at an increasing rate. This rapid growth of laparoscopic distal pancreatectomy has left many questions as to the benefit, complications, and overall indications for this technically difficult laparoscopic procedure. In this chapter we will present our perspective on this procedure and its related issues.

OPERATIVE INDICATIONS

There appears to be no consensus on whether any pancreatic disease should be excluded from a laparoscopic resection. One issue with laparoscopic resection for pancreatic cancer is port site metastasis. Currently, it is difficult to know whether a laparoscopic distal pancreatectomy for malignant disease, particularly adenocarcinoma, will produce a high rate of wound implants,

carcinomatosis, and a decreased overall survival. Recent data from the literature on colorectal cancer suggest that the incidence of port site metastasis after laparoscopic resection is not different from that of wound site implantation after open resection. Extrapolating the data from colon cancer to pancreatic cancer may be troublesome, so some authors continue to advocate laparoscopic distal pancreatectomy only for benign lesions. A multi-institutional prospective randomized study might determine the effectiveness of laparoscopic pancreatectomy for the treatment of adenocarcinoma, but whether such a trial is feasible is difficult to know. Precise preoperative indications and contraindications for laparoscopic pancreatic resection of a presumed malignancy have not been defined at this point in time.

PREOPERATIVE EVALUATION, TESTING, AND PREPARATION

Prior to embarking on a laparoscopic distal pancreatectomy the surgeon should try to obtain a tissue diagnosis. Endoscopic ultrasound (EUS) is useful for this purpose and is especially relevant if adenocarcinoma is suspected. When cases of intraductal papillary mucinous neoplasia are suspected, the EUS also can help determine the extent of disease. For suspected neuroendocrine tumors, an octreotide scan is important to rule out multifocal disease; in addition, preoperative serum biochemical markers should be drawn for the purpose of postoperative surveillance. If there is a reasonable probability that a splenectomy will need to be performed in conjunction with the distal pancreatectomy, then prophylactic vaccinations (pneumococcal, meningococcal, and *Haemophilus influenzae*) should be administered 2 weeks prior to operation.

PATIENT POSITIONING AND PLACEMENT OF TROCARS

The patient is placed supine on the operating table with the left side of the body rotated to no more than 45 degrees. Alternatively, the patient can be placed in the "French" position, which allows the surgeon to operate between the patient's legs. A Hasson cannula is placed infraumbilically, and a diagnostic laparoscopy is performed. Routine laparoscopic ultrasound of the liver may be performed for

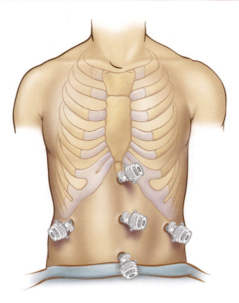

FIGURE 23-1 Positioning of trocars for laparoscopic pancreatectomy. The infraumbilical trocar is a Hasson cannula; the rest of the trocars are 5–12 mm.

sected (Fig. 23-3). The splenic flexure of the colon is mobilized next (Fig. 23-4), and then the transverse mesocolon is dissected away from the inferior border of the pancreas (Fig. 23-5). These maneuvers allow for complete visualization of the inferior portion of the spleen, the pancreatic tail, and the splenic artery (Fig. 23-6).

The laparoscopic ultrasound then is used to delineate the tumor and to determine the proximal extent of pancreatic resection. For an intraductal papillary mucinous neoplasia, the ultrasound specifically is used to assess any change in caliber of the main pancreatic duct. Once the proximal point of the pancreatic transection is noted, the anterior surface of the pancreas is marked with electrocautery to identify the level of the subsequent transection. If the spleen will be resected with the distal pancreas, then one method involves performing a lateral-to-medial dissection. The lateral attachments of the spleen are incised first; this begins the mobilization that will bring the spleen up to the anterior abdominal wall. The tail of the pancreas then is dissected with the splenic vessels away from the retroperitoneum, starting from the left side

disease staging. If any suspicious lesions are biopsied and sent for frozen section analysis, then the surgeon should wait for the results before proceeding with the operation. The positions of the additional trocars (five total) are shown in Figure 23-1; this particular configuration is better suited for the "French" position.

OPERATIVE TECHNIQUE

The resection starts by the surgeon grasping the anterior wall of the stomach and raising it toward the abdominal wall. Placing the patient in a reverse Trendelenburg position will facilitate this maneuver. An ultrasonic or bipolar scalpel then is used to enter the lesser sac through the gastrocolic ligament. The dissection is then carried cephalad along the greater curve of the stomach, and the short gastric vessels are divided (Fig. 23-2), which permits exposure of the anterior surface of the pancreas. If resection of the spleen is planned along with the distal pancreas, then all the short gastric vessels to the level of the esophageal hiatus should be tran-

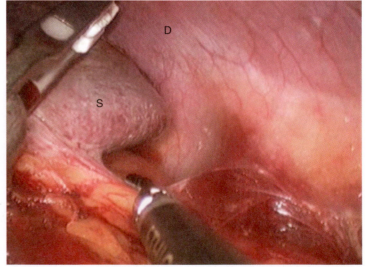

FIGURE 23-3 Division of the short gastric vessels to the esophageal hiatus. D, diaphragm; S, stomach; Sp, spleen.

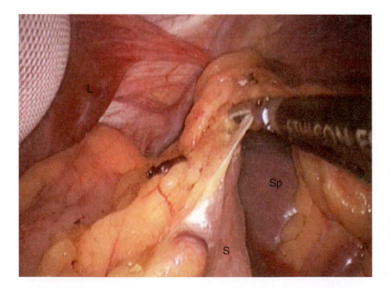

FIGURE 23-2 Division of the short gastric vessels and entry into the lesser sac. L, liver; S, stomach; Sp, spleen.

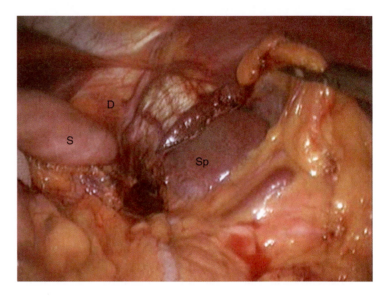

FIGURE 23-4 Division of the splenocolic ligament using the ultrasonic scalpel. D, diaphragm; S, spleen.

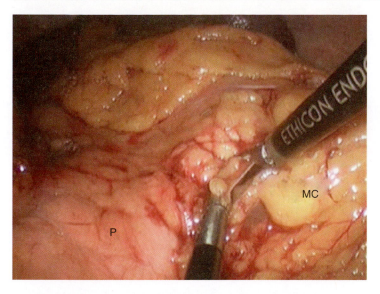

Figure 23-5 Mobilization of the inferior border of the pancreas (P). MC, mesocolon.

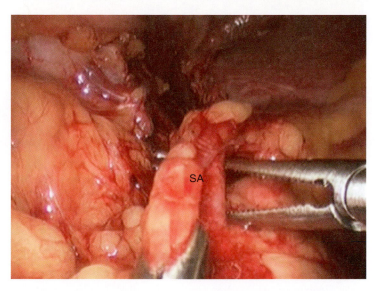

Figure 23-7 The splenic artery (SA) is dissected free of the superior edge of the pancreas with a right-angle dissecting forceps.

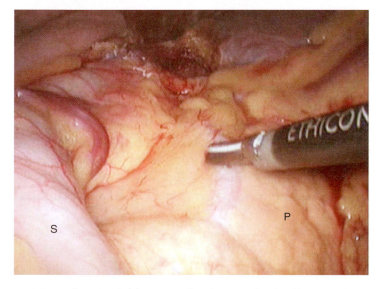

Figure 23-6 The stomach (S) is retracted to the patient's right, allowing visualization of the pancreas (P); the ultrasonic scalpel is indicating the position of the splenic artery along the superior border of the pancreatic tail.

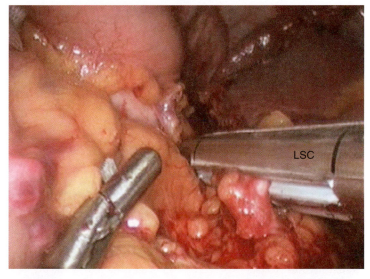

Figure 23-8 The splenic artery is divided with the linear stapler-cutter (LSC) loaded with a vascular cartridge (2-mm staples).

of the patient and moving medially. We prefer to perform this dissection with an ultrasonic scalpel, as opposed to individually clipping and dividing the vessels (the clips often interfere with the jaws of a stapler). After the pancreas has been mobilized to the point of transection, the pancreas, splenic artery, and splenic vein are divided with a linear stapler-cutter loaded with a vascular cartridge. If the pancreatic parenchyma is too thick, then a cartridge of 3.5- or 4.8-mm staples can be used.

Alternatively, in a medial-to-lateral dissection of the pancreas (as shown in the accompanying DVD), the pancreas and the splenic vessels are dissected circumferentially at the proposed transection site prior to splenic mobilization. In this instance, the splenic artery is mobilized at the selected transection level (Fig. 23-7) and then is divided with a 2-mm stapler cartridge (Fig. 23-8). The peritoneum on the inferior edge of the pancreas is incised with hook electrocautery, and dorsal dissection of the pancreas is performed in order to create a window for placement of the stapler. This can be accomplished easily with an esophageal retractor (Fig. 23-9). The pancreatic parenchyma (separately or

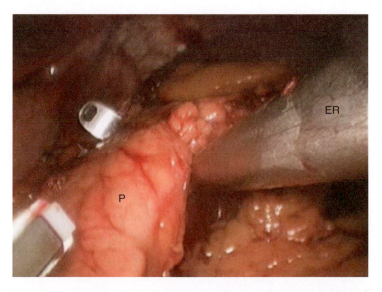

Figure 23-9 A window is created on the dorsal aspect of the pancreas (P) at the line of the planned transection with the use of the esophageal retractor (ER).

with the splenic vein) then is divided with the linear stapler-cutter, using 3.5- or 4.8-mm cartridges (Fig. 23-10), and the integrity of the staple line is confirmed (Fig. 23-11). After the pancreas has been divided, the pancreatic duct is secured with a 3-0 silk suture (Fig. 23-12). Individual ligation of the pancreatic duct with a nonabsorbable stitch has been associated with a fivefold relative risk reduction in the development of a pancreatic leak.

A different approach is utilized for the laparoscopic spleen-preserving distal pancreatectomy. The pancreas is exposed as described earlier; that is, the lesser sac is entered through the gastrocolic ligament, the short gastric vessels are divided, and the left colon is mobilized. After determining the level of pancreas transection, the dissection is begun at the leftmost lateral portion of the pancreas, away from the splenic vessels. It is important to establish dissection in the correct plane and maintain meticulous hemostasis for proper visualization. The peritoneum overlying the superior and inferior margin of the pancreas is incised with hook electrocautery or the ultrasonic scalpel. Careful blunt dissection of the dorsal aspect of the pancreas is performed. Small tributaries from the splenic artery and vein are divided with the ultrasonic scalpel. The dissection is continued medially to the

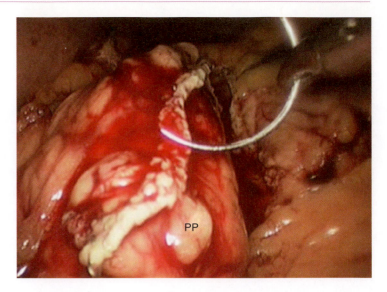

FIGURE 23-12 A figure-of-eight stitch is placed to secure the pancreatic duct. PP, proximal pancreas.

previously determined point of pancreas transection. The pancreatic parenchyma (not the splenic vessels) then is transected with the linear stapler-cutter as described previously.

Once the distal pancreas (with or without the spleen) has been freed, the specimen is placed in a plastic retrieval bag, and the umbilical port incision is extended to allow removal of the specimen (Figs. 23-13 and 23-14). This incision then is closed with suture, and the abdomen is re-insufflated. The abdomen is irrigated and hemostasis confirmed. If the spleen has been removed with the pancreas, the retroperitoneal bed high in the left upper quadrant should be inspected closely for hemostasis. Fibrin sealant (Tisseel, Baxter, Deerfield, IL) then is placed over the cut edge of the pancreas, and a closed-suction drain is left near the pancreatic stump. All port sites are closed with absorbable suture.

POSTOPERATIVE CARE

Following a laparoscopic distal pancreatectomy, a clear liquid diet is started on postoperative day 1 or 2, depending on the clinical course. Ambulation is encouraged at least by postoperative day 1.

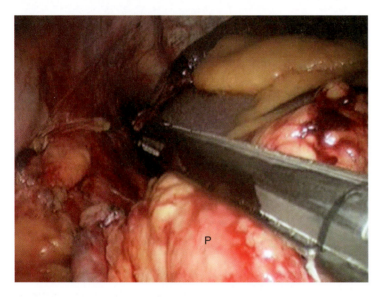

FIGURE 23-10 The pancreas (P) is transected with the linear stapler-cutter.

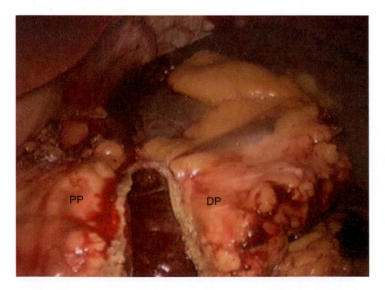

FIGURE 23-11 The pancreas has been divided, and the staple lines are intact on either side of the transection. DP, distal pancreas; PP, proximal pancreas.

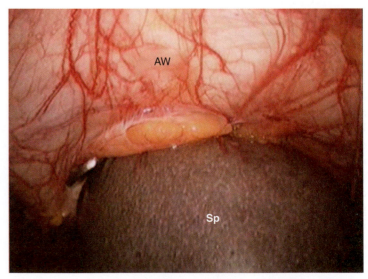

FIGURE 23-13 The specimen is shown in a specimen retrieval bag, which is being exteriorized through an infraumbilical curvilinear incision (i.e., an extension of the incision for the Hasson cannula). AW, anterior abdominal wall; Sp, spleen inside the bag.

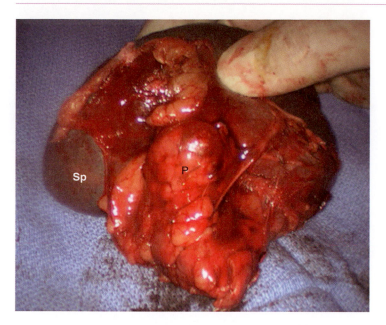

FIGURE 23-14 Specimen of a laparoscopic distal pancreatectomy (P) with splenectomy (Sp).

A low-fat diet usually is started on postoperative day 4 or 5. When the low-fat diet is initiated, the drain output is monitored closely. If an increased output is noted, then the fluid is assessed for amylase. If the patient is tolerating a low-fat diet without evidence of a pancreatic leak, then the drain may be discontinued.

PROCEDURE-SPECIFIC COMPLICATIONS

The most common procedure-specific complication after distal pancreatectomy (whether open or laparoscopic) is pancreatic leak. Reported leak rates are influenced by the number of patients in the study undergoing resection for chronic pancreatitis, because pancreatic resections in these patients have a lower risk of leak. Leak rates also vary based on the definition of a leak (i.e., symptomatic leak or elevated drain amylase). In a large series of open distal pancreatectomies (none for chronic pancreatitis), the symptomatic leak rate was noted to be 13% (17 of 126), and the biochemical leak rate (those patients with asymptomatic elevation of drain amylase three times greater than their serum amylase) was noted to be 6% (8 of 126). With the limited data available, it appears that the leak rates in open and laparoscopic distal pancresatectomy are comparable. Complicating this issue is the variable use of postoperative octreotide, which may or may not lower the rate of pancreatic leak after pancreatic resection. The use of fibrin glue on the pancreatic staple line may be associated with a lower risk of postoperative leak. If the patient has unexplained fever, elevated white blood cell count, or an inability to tolerate oral intake in the early postoperative period, then a CT scan of the abdomen with intravenous contrast agent should be obtained, with percutaneous drainage as needed. Fluid should be sent for chemistries and culture. The patient subsequently is supported with parenteral nutrition; most leaks will resolve with this type of management.

RESULTS AND OUTCOME

Small comparative studies have suggested that patients undergoing laparoscopic distal pancreatectomy have a shorter hospital stay and recovery period compared to those undergoing the open procedure; perioperative complication rates have appeared equivalent. The European Multicenter Laparoscopic Pancreas Study summarized the results from 25 European centers and described 127 minimally invasive procedures: 97 distal pancreatectomies (76%), 27 tumor enucleations, and 3 pancreaticoduodenectomies. The conversion rate was 14%. The rate of benign versus malignant disease was 87% and 13%, respectively. The median tumor size was 30 mm (range, 5–120 mm). Clinically evident pancreatic fistulas were noted in 17% of patients; the reoperation rate (6.3%) was somewhat higher than that in most smaller series. The median postoperative stay was 7 days (range, 3–67 days). At this point in time there are no controlled studies comparing open and laparoscopic distal pancreatectomy; because this is not a common procedure, such a study would be relatively difficult to accomplish. Similar to other more common procedures, it is likely that the general benefits of the minimally invasive approach would apply to distal pancreatectomy. Because this procedure is readily accomplished laparoscopically, the authors now carefully consider this approach with all distal pancreatectomies.

Suggested Reading

Ammori BJ, Baghdadi S: Minimally invasive pancreatic surgery: The new frontier? Curr Gastroenterol Rep 2006;8:132.

Ayav A, Bresler L, Brunaud L, et al: Laparoscopic approach for a solitary insulinoma: A multicentre study. Langenbecks Arch Surg 2005;390:134.

Bemelman WA, De Wit LT, Van Deleden OM, et al: Diagnostic laparoscopy combined with laparoscopic ultrasonography in staging of cancer of the pancreatic head region. Br J Surg 1995;82:820.

Bilimoria MM, Cormier JN, Mun Y, et al: Pancreatic leak after left pancreatectomy is reduced following main pancreatic duct ligation. Br J Surg 2003;90:190.

Dulucq JL, Wintringer P, Mahajna A: Laparoscopic pancreaticoduodenectomy for benign and malignant diseases. Surg Endosc 2006;20:1045.

Gagner M, Pomp A: Laparoscopic pancreatic resection: Is it worthwhile? J Gastrointest Surg 1997;1:20.

Gagner M, Pomp A, Herrera MF: Early experience with laparoscopic resections of islet cell tumors. Surgery 1996;120:1051.

Gouillat C, Gigot JF: Pancreatic surgical complications—The case for prophylaxis. Gut 2001;49:32.

Mabrut JY, Fernandez-Cruz L, Azagra JS, et al: Laparoscopic pancreatic resection: Results of a multicenter European study of 127 patients. Surgery 2005;137:597.

Palanivelu C, Shetty R, Sendhilkumar K, et al: Laparoscopic distal pancreatectomy: Results of a prospective nonrandomized study from a tertiary center. Surg Endosc 2006;16:45.

Pierce RA, Spitler JA, Hawkins WG, et al: Outcomes analysis of laparoscopic resection of pancreatic neoplasms. Surg Endosc 2006;19:660.

Root J, Nguyen N, Jones B, et al: Laparoscopic distal pancreatic resection. Am Surg 2005;71:744.

Velanovich V: Case-control comparison of laparoscopic versus open distal pancreatectomy. J Gastrointest Surg 2006;10:95.

Warshaw AL, Gu ZY, Wittenberg J, et al: Preoperative staging and assesment of respectability of pancreatic cancer. Arch Surg 1990;125:230.

ALBERT CHI, JOHN G. ZOGRAFAKIS, AND
MICHAEL J. DEMEURE

Minimally Invasive Splenectomy

24

Since the introduction of endoscopic and laparoscopic surgery in the 1990s, its application has expanded from cholecystectomy to operations involving virtually every organ system. As both the technology and surgical skills related to laparoscopy have advanced, minimally invasive surgery has become the standard treatment for many diseases. In the case of elective splenectomy, laparoscopic removal has proved to be safe and effective and is now the preferred method for splenectomy for most patients. Even in the case of a very large spleen, a hand-assisted laparoscopic approach provides many of the benefits associated with a minimally invasive approach. Laparoscopic splenectomy has been associated with a shorter hospital stay, less postoperative pain, an earlier return to daily activities, and better cosmetic results compared to open splenectomy.

OPERATIVE INDICATIONS

The indications for laparoscopic splenectomy are similar to those for open splenectomy and are summarized in Table 24-1. A splenectomy is indicated to control disease (e.g., idiopathic thrombocytopenic purpura) or alleviate symptoms of hypersplenism due to a number of hematologic disorders. Currently the two most common indications for splenectomy are trauma and hematologic disorders, and thrombocytopenia is the most common indication for splenectomy in the latter group. Immune thrombocytopenic purpura (ITP) is an acquired autoimmune phenomenon resulting in the destruction of platelets. The diagnosis is established by demonstrating normal or increased numbers of bone marrow megakaryocytes with peripheral thrombocytopenia in the absence of a systemic disease or the ingestion of drugs that are capable of inducing thrombocytopenia. In adults with ITP, a durable response to steroids, plasmapheresis, or immune globulin is uncommon. On the other hand, 75% to 85% of these patients respond to splenectomy with the platelet count rising above $100,000/mm^3$ within 7 days of operation. Refractory thrombocytopenia associated with systemic lupus erythematosus may respond to splenectomy. Splenomegaly in general can produce pancytopenia, thrombocytopenia, leukopenia, or anemia; 80% of patients with thrombocytopenia associated with splenomegaly (not secondary to portal hypertension) will have improved platelet counts after splenectomy. Splenectomy also is potentially therapeutic in pancytopenic patients with Hodgkin's disease, non-Hodgkin's lymphoma, chronic lymphocytic leukemia, and hairy cell leukemia. In addition, splenectomy is the treatment of choice for hereditary spherocytosis, a congenital disorder which produces spherical erythrocytes that undergo premature clearance by the spleen.

Partial splenectomy has been utilized in children with Gaucher's disease, congenital hemolytic anemias, or hereditary spherocytosis. The theoretical advantage of partial splenectomy is the resolution of the hypersplenism symptoms, while sparing the patient the increased risk of overwhelming postsplenectomy sepsis. Critics of partial splenectomy cite a greater operative blood loss due to hemostasis difficulties. Early case reports state that patients with benign splenic conditions, such as splenic cysts, are suitable for partial splenectomy without major blood loss. In children with hereditary spherocytosis, a partial splenectomy appears to control hemolysis while retaining splenic function. In congenital hemolytic anemias, partial splenectomy appears to control symptoms of hypersplenism and splenic sequestration. Partial splenectomy in the case of Gaucher's disease has been met with only limited success due to rapid splenic regrowth. In the hands of the experienced minimally invasive surgeon, laparoscopic partial splenectomy has been feasible in select cases. Relative contraindications to laparoscopic splenectomy include trauma, splenic artery aneurysms, splenic abscess, portal hypertension, and ascites. Massive splenomegaly (mass > 2000 g or length > 30 cm) and acute coagulopathy are stronger contraindications.

PREOPERATIVE EVALUATION, TESTING, AND PREPARATION

A preoperative ultrasound, computed tomography (CT), or magnetic resonance imaging (MRI) is done to evaluate splenic size and to look for accessory spleens. Failure to remove an accessory spleen is a common cause for persistent thrombocytopenia in patients with ITP. Using CT criteria for splenic length, there are three size categories: (1) normal (spleen < 11 cm long); (2) moderate splenomegaly (11–20 cm); and (3) severe/massive splenomegaly (>20 cm). Because spleens larger than 30 cm present special technical problems, spleens in this category have been referred to as "megaspleens." A megaspleen occupies excessive space within the abdominal cavity, making it difficult to place ports and to visualize the hilum, short gastrics vessels, and splenic attachments.

Table 24-1 Indications for Laparoscopic Splenectomy

Hematologic Disorders
Hemolytic anemias
  Hereditary spherocytosis
  Thalassemia major
  Sickle cell disease
  Hemoglobin SC disease
  Autoimmune hemolytic anemia
  Pyruvate kinase deficiency
Thrombocytopenias
  Idiopathic thrombocytopenic purpura (ITP)
  ITP related to HIV
  Thrombotic thrombocytopenic purpura
  Evan's syndrome
Myeloproliferative disorders
  Myelofibrosis
Neoplasia
  Hairy cell leukemia
  Hodgkin's lymphoma
  Non-Hodgkin's lymphoma
  Chronic lymphocytic leukemia

Miscellaneous disorders
Felty syndrome
Gaucher's disease
Sarcoidosis
Splenic cysts
Splenic tumors
Splenic vein thrombosis
Splenic artery aneurysm
Splenic abscesses
Trauma

In the patient with a hematologic malignancy, a coordinated effort must be made with the patient's hematologist in order to prepare the patient for the operation. The potential for blood product administration should be considered; due to previous transfusions some patients may have developed antibodies, which makes crossmatching difficult. Some authors suggest that patients with anemia or thrombocytopenia be transfused to a hemoglobin level of 10 g/dL and a platelet count above 50,000/mm^3; others recommend deferring transfusion until after the splenic artery has been ligated. Some patients with a hematologic malignancy may benefit from preoperative chemotherapy, which can reduce the size of the spleen by half. Generally it is recommended to wait 2 to 3 weeks after chemotherapy has been completed before proceeding with splenectomy. The patient on preoperative steroid maintenance may need additional perioperative steroid dosing. Another issue with splenectomy for hematologic disease is the increased risk of postoperative portal vein thrombosis. Some authors recommend an evaluation for a hypercoagulable state, including tests for antiphospholipid antibodies, lupus anticoagulant, and proteins S and C.

Overwhelming postsplenectomy sepsis is reported in approximately 3.2% of patients and is associated with a 1.4% mortality rate. The most common causative organism is *Streptococcus pneumoniae*, but other encapsulated pathogens such as *Neisseria meningitides* and *Haemophilus* have been associated with life-threatening infections. Sepsis due to gram-negative rods such as *Escherichia coli* and *Pseudomonas* species also have been associated with a high mortality rate in asplenic patients. As with elective open splenectomy, patients should receive a polyvalent pneumococcal, meningococcal, and *Haemophilus* flu vaccine 2 weeks prior to surgery. In the case of emergency splenectomy (e.g., for trauma), the vaccines

should be given just prior to discharge. Other immunizations to consider in asplenic patients include yearly influenza vaccinations and antimalarial prophylaxis (when traveling to or residing in endemic areas).

An early criticism of laparoscopic splenectomy was the inability of the surgeon to identify an accessory spleen(s), which could result in persistent hypersplenism. Accessory spleens are found in 10% to 20% of the general population, and an even greater percentage is found in patients with hematologic diseases. Most accessory spleens are found in the splenic hilum, near the tail of the pancreas in the retroperitoneum, in the greater omentum, in bowel mesentery, near the left broad ligament, near the pouch of Douglas (in females), or near the left testis (in males). Current methods of identifying accessory spleens include ^{99m}technetium or ^{111}indium scintiscans, CT, and ultrasonography. Most authors believe that the risk of a missed accessory spleen does not justify routine preoperative localizing studies prior to laparoscopic splenectomy. With knowledge of the common locations for accessory spleens, there does not appear to be an increased rate of missed accessory spleens in laparoscopic splenectomy when compared to open splenectomy.

An average spleen measures 11 cm in length and weighs 150 g. Special consideration should be given in the patient who has a massive or megaspleen (>30 cm or >2000 g) because exposure and bleeding issues are common. The most common complication associated with splenectomy is bleeding. Preoperative splenic artery embolization for the massive spleen may reduce intraoperative blood loss; some authors have suggested such embolization 2 hours prior to laparoscopic splenectomy in order to reduce the risk of hemorrhage. This practice is controversial; potential complications of splenic artery embolization include pain, pancreatitis, and acute gastric ulcers. Laparoscopic splenectomy may not be feasible for a spleen longer than 30 cm; however, a hand-assisted laparoscopic splenectomy may be a reasonable option in such a case.

PATIENT POSITIONING

Laparoscopic splenectomy may be performed using either an anterior or lateral approach. If an anterior approach is used, the patient is placed in a modified lithotomy ("French") position to allow the surgeon to operate from between the patient's legs; the assistants stand on either side of the patient. In the lateral position, the patient is placed in the full right lateral decubitus position; the table is "jack-knifed" or flexed in the middle in order to open up the space between the patient's left costal margin and the ipsilateral iliac crest.

OPERATIVE TECHNIQUE

Anterior Approach

For the anterior approach, a 12-mm bladeless optical trocar (left upper quadrant, subcostal position, midclavicular line) is used to initiate abdominal access and pneumoperitoneum (trocar 1; Fig. 24-1A). Four other trocars are placed: right subcostal in the midclavicular line (trocar 2), left subcostal in the anterior axillary line (trocar 3), subxiphoid (trocar 4), and midline between the xiphoid and the umbilicus (trocar 5). Trocar 1 should be a 12-mm port, for placement of the laparoscopic linear stapler-cutter. The 12-mm trocar allows the greatest flexibility for the introduction of retractors, clip appliers, and linear staplers. For better cosmetic results, some surgeons prefer 5-mm trocars at some of the port sites. For the lateral decubitus approach, trocars can be placed at different locations, as shown in Fig. 24-1B and C.

In the anterior approach, the surgeon operates from between the patient's legs, using trocars 1 and 2. A 30-degree laparoscope is placed through trocar 5 and is used to inspect the abdomen. The short gastric vessels are divided with the ultrasonic shears (Fig. 24-2). As the surgeon approaches the angle of His, care should be exercised in dividing the first short gastric pedicle, which often is closely adherent to the superior pole of the spleen (Fig. 24-3). An inflatable balloon retractor (Soft-Wand Balloon Retractor, Gyrus-ACMI, Southborough, MA) can be placed through trocar 4 in order to retract the left lobe of the liver or the greater curvature of the stomach.

Once the greater curvature of the stomach has been mobilized, the lesser sac, tail of the pancreas, and splenic artery are visible. Arterial supply to the spleen can be either distributive (multiple vessels branching in the splenic hilum from one common splenic artery trunk) or magistral (one common trunk of the splenic artery supplying the hilum of the spleen). This is relevant because the spleen often appears nodular with a distributive blood supply but tends to appear smooth with a magistral blood supply. This visual cue may allow the surgeon to anticipate multiple distal branches of the splenic artery.

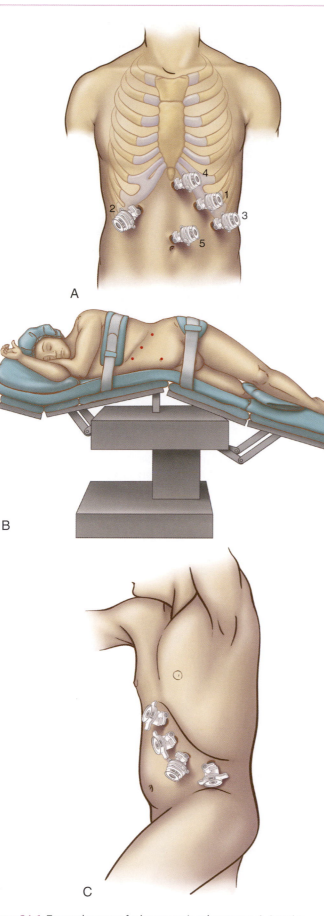

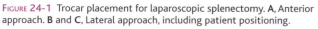

FIGURE 24-1 Trocar placement for laparoscopic splenectomy. **A**, Anterior approach. **B** and **C**, Lateral approach, including patient positioning.

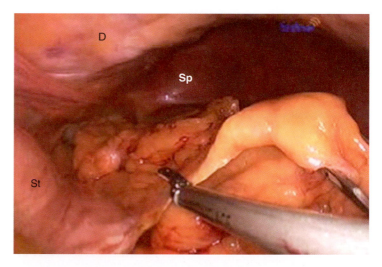

FIGURE 24-2 Division of the short gastric vessels using an ultrasonic scalpel. D, diaphragm; Sp, spleen; St, stomach.

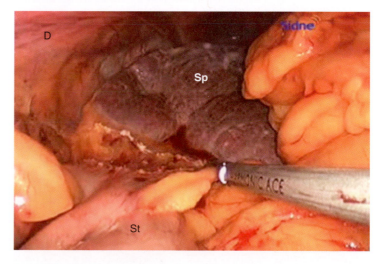

FIGURE 24-3 Division of attachments from the stomach to the spleen. D, diaphragm; Sp, spleen; St, stomach.

Using a curved dissector through trocar 1, the adipose tissue surrounding the splenic artery is dissected away to isolate the splenic artery for division. Advantages to dividing the splenic artery first include (1) better hemostasis during the subsequent dissection and (2) improved efficacy of platelet transfusion, if platelets are needed (e.g., for ITP). After circumferential isolation of the splenic artery close to the hilum, a laparoscopic linear stapler (45 mm × 2.5 mm [white load]) is used to transect the artery (Fig. 24-4). An alternative method of hemostasis utilizes SeamGuard, a bioabsorbable staple line reinforcement product (W.L. Gore & Associates, Flagstaff, AZ), which is loaded onto the stapler prior to firing. After dividing the splenic artery, the splenic vein should be found in an inferoposterior position; this vessel is divided in a similar manner. With the spleen devascularized, the splenic flexure of the colon is separated gently from the inferior pole of the spleen, carefully avoiding the tail of the pancreas. Slow dissection with ultrasonic shears is used to divide any remaining splenic attachments. Once free, the spleen can be placed in specimen retrieval device for morcellation and extraction (Fig. 24-5).

Lateral Approach

The lateral approach to the laparoscopic splenectomy offers several advantages over the anterior position, such as the fact that little force is necessary to retract the spleen in the lateral position; gravity will accomplish most of the retraction and exposure. The surgeon has easy access to the phrenocolic ligament in the lateral position and can leave a cuff here that can be used to retract the spleen. In addition, the tail of the pancreas generally is easier to identify in the lateral position. Furthermore, if hemorrhage occurs while operating in the lateral position, then the blood will tend to flow away from the operative field and not obscure the dissection.

For the lateral approach, four 12-mm trocars are placed along the left costal margin, which allows maximum flexibility for the camera, clip applier, linear stapler, and other instruments (see Fig. 24-1B and C). Three trocars are located anteriorly along the rib margin, and one is located in the left flank. Usually the most posterior trocar should not be inserted until after the splenic flexure has been mobilized. Enough distance between trocars (e.g., width of the palm) is required to preserve good working angles and easy triangulation. There is some advantage in placing the patient in slight reverse Trendelenburg position, which will move the spleen away from the diaphragm. With experience, some of the 12-mm trocars can be replaced with 5-mm trocars for improved cosmesis.

The abdomen is examined carefully for the presence of accessory spleens. The splenic flexure of the colon is mobilized using monopolar cautery (hook or scissors) or ultrasonic shears. The short gastric vessels are divided using ultrasonic shears, and then the splenophrenic ligaments are cut. The splenic artery is ligated with a proximal ligature and then may be divided with a stapler. The splenic vein also is divided with an endostapler. The investing fat aids in compression of the splenic vein and reduces bleeding at the staple line. Once freed, the spleen is placed into a specimen retrieval bag and removed via an enlarged umbilical incision or a small incision created by joining two left upper quadrant port sites. While in the bag, the spleen may be fractured with a ring forceps (morcellation) to facilitate removal; this technique still provides large tissue fragments for pathologic examination.

Hand-Assisted Laparoscopic Splenectomy

Hand-assisted laparoscopic surgery (HALS) refers to laparoscopic procedures performed with the aid of a hand port inserted in a 7.5- to 10-cm incision. Although a number of variations exist, a hand port consists of a sealed cuff that enables insertion and withdrawal of a hand in the abdomen without loss of pneumoperitoneum during the operation, thus allowing tactile abilities that are not possible with conventional laparoscopic surgery. For splenectomy, the HALS approach typically is done with the patient in the anterior position.

There is some debate over where to place the hand-port incision for a hand-assisted laparoscopic splenectomy. The decision depends on whether the surgeon is left- or right-handed. Incision placement has been described in the upper midline, the right upper quadrant, the left iliac fossa, and for a very large spleen, in a Pfannenstiel position. Most surgeons agree that the nondominant hand should be used in the hand-port. There are obvious advantages and drawbacks to this technique. The most apparent disadvantage is the longer abdominal incision. Moreover, this technique would seem to defeat the goal of developing surgical techniques that decrease surgical trauma even further. Nevertheless, comparative studies of laparoscopic splenectomy for large spleens (>700 g) seem to indicate outcomes similar to conventional laparoscopic techniques. Although the final role of the HALS splenectomy remains to be defined, it likely will have a

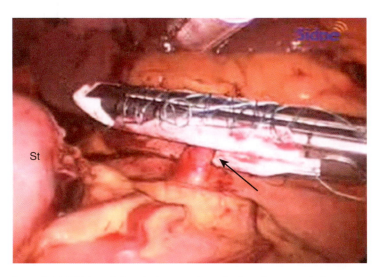

FIGURE 24-4 Division of the splenic artery (arrow) using a laparoscopic linear stapler. St, stomach.

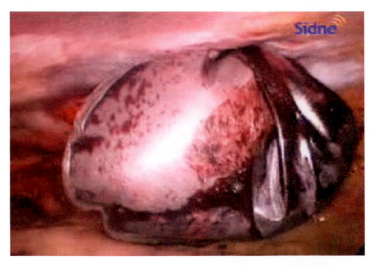

FIGURE 24-5 Extraction of the spleen in a specimen retrieval device.

place in the removal of large spleens and in the training of minimally invasive splenectomy. Of note, the HALS approach has curtailed the role of preoperative splenic artery embolization for the megaspleen.

Recommendations

In general, the authors prefer the lateral approach to laparoscopic splenectomy with the patient in the right decubitus position. An anterior approach is preferred when a concomitant procedure (such as cholecystectomy) is planned. The HALS approach may be beneficial in a patient with a massively enlarged spleen. Conventional laparoscopic management of a megaspleen also may be accomplished with preoperative splenic artery embolization or simply by open splenectomy. These recommendations are guidelines, however, and not strict rules.

POSTOPERATIVE CARE

In regard to postoperative antibiotic administration, there are two strategies in asplenic patients: daily antibiotics or empiric antibiotic therapy for fever. Although the risk of overwhelming postsplenectomy sepsis (OPSS) does not decrease with time after splenectomy, some guidelines recommend prophylactic antibiotics after splenectomy for children continue for 3 to 5 years or until adulthood. Daily antibiotic prophylaxis for children in several studies has resulted in decreased rates of infection. Daily penicillin given to children with sickle cell anemia and hyposplenism has yielded similar results. Critics of daily antibiotics suggest an increased risk of resistant strain selection with prophylactic use. Survivors of OPSS might be reasonable candidates for lifelong prophylaxis. All postsplenectomy patients should be advised to self-medicate with high doses of antibiotics and seek medical attention immediately if they experience a fever. Patients should be prescribed stand-by antibiotics. Appropriate antibiotic choices include Augmentin 875 mg, 1 g cefuroxime, or an extended spectrum fluoroquinolone (such antibiotics as 750 mg levofloxacin, 400 mg moxifloxacin, or 320 mg gemifloxacin) for beta-lactam–allergic patients. Medication should always be on hand and replaced when expired. Prophylaxis for dental procedures is not recommended.

PROCEDURE-SPECIFIC COMPLICATIONS

Leukocytosis is an important sign of potential sepsis or infectious process in the postsplenectomy patient, but leukocytosis (as well as thrombocytosis) can be a normal physiologic response to splenectomy. Patients should recover rapidly after a laparoscopic splenectomy. An atypical postoperative recovery or a persistently elevated white blood cell count should prompt close scrutiny. As documented in the literature, a white blood cell (WBC) count more than $15,000/mm^3$ or a platelet count/WBC ratio less than 20 after the fifth postoperative day should cause one to suspect an underlying infection in postsplenectomy patients. The patient suspected of developing postsplenectomy sepsis should be treated immediately with a high-dose penicillin or cephalosporin.

Postsplenectomy portal vein thrombosis (PVT) is a rare but potentially fatal complication that can produce intestinal ischemia and infarction. Risk factors for PVT include hypercoagulability, splenomegaly, myeloproliferative disorders, and thrombocytosis. Stasis of blood flow originating at the splenic vein may contribute to thrombus formation. There also may be a correlation between increased length of the splenic vein stump, vein diameter, and splenomegaly with postsplenectomy PVT. Patients with PVT have nonspecific symptoms, including abdominal pain, anorexia, fever, and diarrhea; the diagnosis may be difficult. Once the diagnosis of postsplenectomy PVT is made, however, prompt intervention is required. Multiple treatments may be implemented, including anticoagulation and regional/systemic thrombolytic therapy. In the asymptomatic patient at high risk for PVT, it may be prudent to screen with abdominal ultrasound at 3, 6, and 12 months postoperatively. Other less common complications of splenectomy include subphrenic abscess and pancreatic fistula, which generally can be treated with percutaneous measures.

RESULTS AND OUTCOME

Laparoscopic splenectomy was first described in 1992 and has now become the preferred technique for splenectomy for most elective indications. In general, laparoscopic splenectomy has resulted in fewer postoperative complications and shorter hospital stays than open splenectomy. The conversion rate of laparoscopic splenectomy for spleens less than 2000 g has been around 5%; for spleens greater than 2000 g, the conversion rate has been approximately 15%. Overall postoperative complication rates still can approach 50%, though, and the mortality rate is nearly 10% in some series. Increased morbidity and mortality rates are typical for splenectomy on organs greater than 2000 g or with blood loss greater than 1000 mL. If a patient is referred for laparoscopic splenectomy, then a careful evaluation should be performed for this potentially morbid procedure. Many patients undergoing splenectomy for hematologic diseases have been treated with steroids or other chemotherapy, which can impact wound healing. With shorter incisions, the laparoscopic approach is especially appealing in this scenario.

Suggested Reading

Brunt ML, Langer JC, Quasebarth MA: Comparative analysis of laparoscopic versus open splenectomy. Am J Surg 1996;172:596–601.

Carroll BJ, Phillips EH, Semel CJ, et al: Laparoscopic splenectomy. Surg Endosc 1992;6:183–185.

Delaitre B, Maignien B: Laparoscopic splenectomy: Technical aspects. Surg Endosc 1992;6:305–308.

Katkhouda N, Hurwitz MB, Rivera RT, et al: Laparoscopic splenectomy: outcome and efficacy in 103 consecutive patients. Ann Surg 1998;228:568–578.

Poulin EC, Mamazza J, Schlachta CM: Splenic artery embolization before laparoscopic splenectomy. Surg Endosc 1998;12:870–875.

Targarona EM, Balague C, Cerdan G, et al: Hand-assisted laparoscopic splenectomy (HALS) in cases of splenomegaly. Surg Endosc 2002;16:426–430.

Watson DI, Coventry BJ, Chin T, et al: Laparoscopic versus open splenectomy for immune thrombocytopenic purpura. Surgery 1997;121:18–22.

Kidneys and Adrenal Glands

MATTHEW D. DUNN AND JOSH HSU

Minimally Invasive Transperitoneal Nephrectomy

Prior to 1990, the standard for surgical removal of kidneys was through an open flank, abdominal, or thoracoabdominal incision. In 1991, Clayman and Kavoussi reported the first laparoscopic nephrectomy; this approach has changed the way renal extirpative surgery is performed. In fact, laparoscopy has become the standard for removal of most benign kidney disease and small renal tumors. Because the majority (90%) of small renal masses are picked up incidentally on imaging studies performed for unrelated reasons, laparoscopy provides the perfect minimally invasive treatment option for early-stage disease. The success of laparoscopy is based upon the demonstrated advantages of decreased blood loss, postoperative pain, and faster convalescence compared to open surgery, while maintaining the integrity of the operation. Laparoscopic removal of kidneys can be performed either purely laparoscopically (via a transperitoneal or retroperitoneal approach) or by a hand-assisted transperitoneal approach. The choice of method depends upon the patient's anatomy, suspected disease, prior surgical history, and the comfort level of the surgeon. In general, the most commonly used approach is the laparoscopic transperitoneal approach, which will be reviewed in this chapter. The techniques described herein can apply to the hand-assisted transperitoneal approach as well.

OPERATIVE INDICATIONS AND CONTRAINDICATIONS

The indications for laparoscopic transperitoneal nephrectomy are in evolution; currently accepted benign and malignant indications for this procedure include small renal tumors, nonfunctional hydronephrotic or chronically infected kidneys, donor nephrectomy for transplant, pretransplant native nephrectomy, and cytoreductive nephrectomy for limited metastatic renal cell carcinoma. At this point in time, clinical stage T1 (<7 cm) and certain early T2 tumors (7–10 cm) are considered candidates for laparoscopic removal; this size limit for laparoscopic removal of renal masses also appears to be evolving. Some experienced renal surgeons in high-volume practice have expanded the indications for laparoscopic nephrectomy, including tumors larger than 7 cm, the presence of a renal vein thrombus, limited adenopathy requiring an ipsilateral lymph node dissection, and morbidly obese patients.

Of note, the surgeon should not mistake transitional cell carcinoma (TCC) for renal cell carcinoma (RCC). TCC originates from the transitional urothelium, whereas RCC originates from tubular cells within the parenchyma. The patient suspected of having TCC may have multifocal lesions anywhere along the transitional epithelium, especially in the bladder. Such a patient needs a thorough evaluation of the entire collecting system. Management of upper urinary tract in a patient with TCC generally requires a nephroureterectomy with a removal of a cuff of bladder because of the high chance of local recurrence. Similarly, one should be careful of lymphoma, which can present as a large mass in the kidney similar to other malignancies. Lymphoma is not managed surgically but with chemotherapy. As such, a suspected renal lymphoma is one of the few indications for a biopsy.

Contraindications to laparoscopic nephrectomy include bulky adenopathy making hilar dissection difficult, excessively large tumors (>10 cm), severe perinephric scarring (e.g., by chronic infection or prior surgery), extension of tumor thrombus into the inferior vena cava, and chronic inflammatory (i.e., xanthogranulomatous pyelonephritis) or malignant conditions which infiltrate surrounding structures (e.g., liver, spleen, bowel, vena cava, aorta). The patient with a small renal tumor or the patient with renal insufficiency or a comorbid disease which puts him or her at risk for future renal insufficiency should be considered for nephron-sparing procedures (such as a partial nephrectomy or ablative therapy) instead of a total radical nephrectomy. There is growing evidence that for masses smaller than 4 cm, nephron-sparing surgery should be employed rather than total nephrectomy. Laparoscopic nephron-sparing surgery generally should be reserved for the high-volume institution that has familiarity with the procedure. Ablative therapy includes cryotherapy or radiofrequency ablation, which may or may not require laparoscopic exposure, depending on location of the tumor. Although still controversial in their applications, these ablative techniques are options for the patient who is not a good surgical candidate or who has minimal disease.

PREOPERATIVE EVALUATION, TESTING, AND PREPARATION

Radiographic imaging should include at least a computed tomography (CT) scan or magnetic resonance imaging (MRI) in order to (1) characterize the kidney in question, (2) evaluate the contralateral kidney, and (3) evaluate the vasculature for surgical planning. Any patient with a suspected malignancy should be thoroughly staged to rule out metastatic disease. For renal carcinoma (RCC), this should include a chest x-ray, with CT correlation for suspicious masses. Even in the face of limited metastatic disease in the chest, cytoreductive radical nephrectomy for RCC can be beneficial to patients before receiving immunotherapy.

The basic metabolic preoperative evaluation should include a comprehensive metabolic panel, complete blood count, coagulation parameters (prothrombin time, partial thromboplastin time), and urinalysis. Patients presenting with renal impairment or with comorbid medical conditions (typically hypertension or diabetes), which may increase the risk for subsequent dialysis, should be evaluated for nephron-sparing surgery. Patients with hematuria, either gross or microscopic (>3 red blood cells per high-power field on two out of three urinalyses), should be evaluated for transitional cell carcinoma or other uroepithelial causes of hematuria. If the patient has elevated liver transaminases or alkaline phosphatase or has complaints of bone pain, then he or she should be evaluated for metastatic spread to the liver and bone (the latter can be evaluated with a total body bone scan).

Preoperative preparation generally consists of a clear liquid diet the day before surgery, followed by a mechanical bowel preparation in order to decompress the intestines. This can be accomplished with one bottle of magnesium citrate, phosphosoda, or a small volume of Golytely the evening prior to surgery, followed by a second bottle as necessary. An antibiotic bowel preparation usually is not necessary, unless there is concern about mesenteric involvement from either an inflammatory or malignant process that may require a bowel resection. In that situation, one should proceed cautiously with the laparoscopic approach.

A patient should be typed and crossmatched for blood according to his or her condition (i.e., anemia) and per the surgeon's preference. As the surgeon develops a certain level of comfort with this procedure, the patient can receive a type and screen instead of a crossmatch. If the patient has a condition(s) that may make the operation difficult (e.g., obesity, adenopathy, multiple arteries, prior renal surgery), then having 2 to 4 units of crossmatched blood available may be prudent.

PATIENT POSITIONING IN THE OPERATING SUITE

Following anesthetic induction and endotracheal intubation, an orogastric tube and Foley catheter are placed. An arterial line is useful for blood pressure monitoring and, more important, serial blood gas monitoring to assess adequacy of ventilation. Placement of a central venous catheter may be deemed if the patient has serious comorbidities. The authors generally prefer a 30- to 45-degree modified flank position on a standard operating table (Fig. 25-1). This allows the bowel to fall medially out of the surgical field, while giving the surgeon proper access to the abdomen for trocar placement. The patient's downside should be well padded in order to provide stability and prevent a pressure-induced injury. An axillary roll should prevent injury to the axillary nerves and vessels. Flexing the table and utilizing the kidney rest are optional; these devices do not provide an advantage for the laparoscopic approach, but they are helpful in the event of an open conversion. The break should be placed above the iliac crest or at the level of the umbilicus so that the space between the iliac crest and costal margin can be widened.

Protection of the arms and legs and padding of all pressure points (ankle, knee, hip, elbow, axilla) is mandatory. Support for the suspended ipsilateral arm can be accomplished with an airplane arm holder for most patients; if the patient is small,

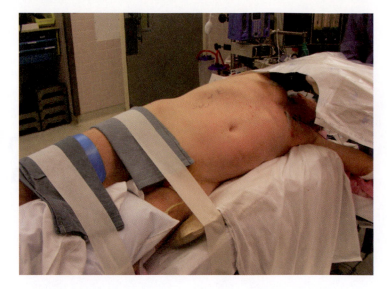

FIGURE 25-1 Modified flank position at about a 30- to 45-degree angle for a right nephrectomy. All pressure points are well padded, and the ipsilateral arm is well supported with an airplane arm holder. Patient is well secured to the table with 3-inch cloth tape.

however, then placing the arms in a "prayer" position between two pillows may be adequate. Other surgeons have used a Mayo stand to hold the ipsilateral arm but, in the authors' experience, this set-up is intrusive during dissection. The contralateral down arm is placed and secured on a regular armboard. The lower leg is bent at the knee and hip, and the upper leg is straight. Once in position, the patient is secured to the table with 3-inch cloth tape at the legs, hips, and shoulders so that the table can rotate during the procedure without the patient falling out of position.

POSITIONING AND PLACEMENT OF TROCARS

Creation of the pneumoperitoneum can be performed by either a Veress needle or with the Hasson approach, depending on the degree of comfort of the surgeon, as well as the potential for intra-abdominal adhesions. Suggested trocar arrangements for a right nephrectomy are shown in Figure 25-2A and B; port placement for a left nephrectomy would be the mirror image. In general, ports should be placed a handbreadth apart in order to minimize "crossing" of instruments. A relatively thin patient should have the camera port in the midline either at or above the umbilicus. In an obese patient, the midline will be too far away from the operative site, so the camera and other ports should be placed lateral to the rectus muscle in the midclavicular line. A trocar should not be placed into the belly of the rectus muscle because of risk of injury to the epigastric vessels. Retractors should be placed out of the way of working ports in order to prevent interference. For the left side, an additional 5-mm trocar at the anterior axillary line below the costal margin permits an instrument to either retract the kidney specimen laterally or to hold the spleen, pancreas, or colon out of the way. For the right side, a 5-mm subxiphoid port is ideal to hold the liver out of the way, and a 5-mm port subcostally in the anterior axillary line can be used for retraction of the renal specimen. Until the surgeon is comfortable with a routine, it is recommended to use 12-mm trocars for both working ports rather than 5-mm trocars. In an urgent situation, the 12-mm trocar allows more flexibility with instruments, such as using an Endo GIA (U.S. Surgical, Norwalk, CT) or a 10-mm clip applier to control bleeding.

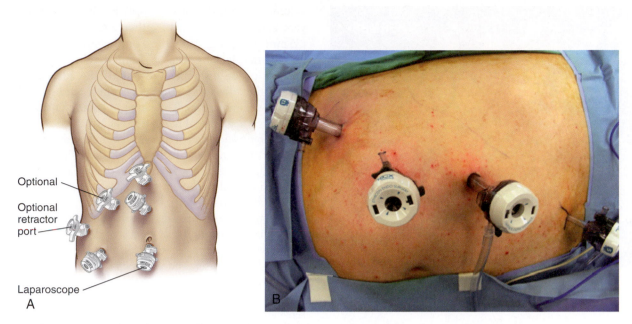

FIGURE 25-2 Trocar placement for a right nephrectomy. Placement of trocars for a left nephrectomy is the mirror image. **A,** Diagram. **B,** Intraoperative photograph; right of image is cephalad.

OPERATIVE TECHNIQUE

The key to success with a laparoscopic nephrectomy is to ensure adequate exposure, to avoid dissecting in a "hole" and to prevent injury to surrounding organs, such as the bowel, liver, and spleen. The kidneys are deep retroperitoneal organs that need to be dissected away from the surrounding structures. A radical nephrectomy for malignancy requires removal of the kidney with its surrounding fat and an intact Gerota's fascia. A simple nephrectomy for benign disease does not require keeping Gerota's fascia intact; when dealing with severe inflammation, however, it typically is easier to dissect outside Gerota's fascia. The technique for left and right nephrectomy will be described as separate procedures.

Left Nephrectomy

The dissection begins with the descending colon and spleen, which usually lie directly over the left kidney. The white line of Toldt is incised from the sigmoid colon up to and past the splenic flexure. This allows the left colon and spleen to be mobilized medially, exposing the anterior surface of Gerota's fascia (Fig. 25-3). The surgeon should not dissect posterolateral to Gerota's fascia, which may mobilize the kidney prematurely; the desired plane of dissection at this point is between the colonic mesentery and the anterior surface of Gerota's fascia. Excessive bleeding in this location may indicate that the surgeon has entered the colonic mesentery or that there may be parasitized blood vessels from a malignant renal tumor. Medial mobilization of the mesocolon will expose the renal hilum and the aorta. The medial dissection is complete after the aorta has been identified. The pancreas then is mobilized off the superomedial surface of Gerota's fascia in order to gain access to the upper renal pole and adrenal gland.

Inferiorly, the psoas muscle is exposed below the level of the kidney. The gonadal vein usually is the first vascular structure identified medial to the psoas muscle. In men, the gonadal vein crosses the psoas laterally toward the deep inguinal ring as part of the spermatic cord. In women, it will remain medial to the psoas to join the infundibulopelvic ligament. The ureter can be identified medial to the gonadal vein and within Gerota's fascia (Fig. 25-4). The ureter will be divided distally, just above where it crosses the

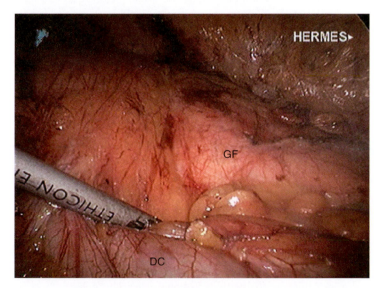

FIGURE 25-3 Medial mobilization of the descending colon (DC) and exposure of the anterior surface of Gerota's fascia (GF) during a left nephrectomy. Superior edge of photograph is lateral; left edge is cephalad.

common iliac artery; early ureteral transection of the ureter is not necessary, however, because it can provide a handle for retracting the kidney anteriorly during the hilar and posterior dissection. As the dissection progresses proximally toward the hilum, the ureter courses lateral to the gonadal vein. The gonadal vein then is followed cephalad up to its insertion into the left renal vein (Fig. 25-5). At this point the gonadal vein can be clipped and divided in order to facilitate exposure of an ascending posterior lumbar vein connecting to the posterior surface of the renal vein. Laceration of this tributary is a common cause of bleeding during this portion of the operation. Ligation and division of the posterior lumbar branch allow exposure of the renal artery posterior to the renal vein. The renal vein then is dissected circumferentially in order to identify the adrenal vein on the superomedial surface. If an adrenal-sparing nephrectomy is planned, then the adrenal vein should be left intact, with later division of the renal vein lateral to the insertion of the adrenal vein. Otherwise, the adrenal vein can be divided in

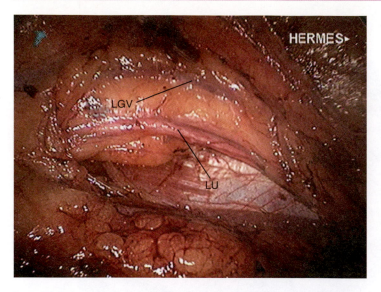

FIGURE 25-4 Exposure of the left ureter (LU) and left gonadal vein (LGV) during a left nephrectomy. Superior edge of photograph is lateral; left edge is cephalad.

order to increase the mobility of the renal vein. After the renal vein has been dissected with ligation of its various branches, it can be gently retracted to identify the renal artery posteriorly.

It is standard technique to take the artery before the vein during a nephrectomy. Taking the vein first would increase the vascular pressure in the kidney, which would predispose to troublesome backbleeding, renal rupture, or tumor rupture. The artery usually is identified inferior and posterior to the renal vein. An exception to this rule is in the minority of patients who have a retroaortic renal vein. In that situation the artery is situated anterior to the vein. This configuration can be identified on the preoperative CT scan or MRI. The artery may be wrapped in a plexus of lymphatic vessels, which can make it difficult to identify. After a circumferential dissection of the artery has been performed, it should be traced toward its origin from the aorta to obtain adequate length. The vessel can then be secured with co-polymer locking clips, a vascular Endo GIA stapler (35 mm), or multiple titanium clips. If clips are used, we recommend placing at least two co-polymer clips or three titanium clips on the aortic side. Following division of the artery, one should notice a partial collapse of the renal vein, consistent with ligation of the renal blood supply. If the vein retains a degree of turgor, then it would be prudent to dissect posteriorly in order to identify additional arterial branches.

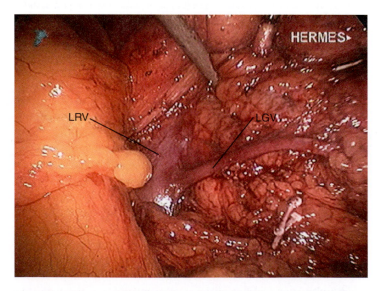

FIGURE 25-5 Insertion of left gonadal vein (LGV) into the left renal vein (LRV). Superior edge of photograph is lateral; left edge is cephalad.

Once the renal arterial supply has been controlled, the renal vein can be divided with either a vascular Endo GIA stapler (35 mm or 45 mm, depending on the size of the vein) or 10-mm co-polymer locking clips. Titanium clips should be avoided because of the dislodgement risk. If the adrenal gland is to be spared, then division of the renal vein should occur lateral to the adrenal vein insertion. The surgeon should ensure that no other structures (e.g., metal clips) are caught in the jaws of the Endo GIA stapler; such an occurrence could be catastrophic.

After the renal vein has been divided, the dissection proceeds to the superomedial aspect of the kidney. If the adrenal gland is to be taken (e.g., if there is a tumor in the upper pole or there is a suspected adrenal lesion), then dissection is performed medial to the adrenal gland, separating it from the lateral border of the aorta. There may be small arterial vessels in this area that are easily controlled with the harmonic scalpel. If a sizable branch is encountered, then it should be secured with clips. If the adrenal gland is to be spared, then the plane between the adrenal gland and upper pole of the kidney is developed and dissection continues up to the splenorenal attachments. The remaining attachments of Gerota's fascia to the posterior and lateral retroperitoneum then can be divided either with harmonic scalpel or electrocautery device. The ureter is ligated and transected next, which completes the dissection. The specimen is placed either on top of the spleen or in the pelvis so that the operative field can be evaluated for hemostasis at a low intra-abdominal pressure (e.g., 5 mm Hg). Specific areas to evaluate are the stumps of the renal hilar vessels, the adrenal bed, and the ureteral and gonadal vein stumps.

Right Nephrectomy

The liver poses more of a problem for a right nephrectomy than the spleen causes for a left nephrectomy. A retractor is necessary to keep the liver out of the way during the dissection on the right side. We prefer to employ a locking grasping forceps through a subxiphoid 5-mm port to lift the liver out of the way. This instrument can be fixed into position by grabbing the diaphragm on the right lateral wall or by attaching the instrument to a fixed-arm retractor holder.

The relationship of the colon to the right kidney is different than the left side in that the right colon usually lies over the renal hilum rather than overlying the whole kidney. Typically the prominence of the kidney is readily identifiable deep to the peritoneum. The exposure commences by incising the line of Toldt from the level of the cecum up to and slightly past the hepatic flexure to allow medial mobilization of the colon. The peritoneum lateral to the kidney fascia then is incised sharply; this incision is continued up toward the coronary ligament of the liver. This incision is joined to another perpendicular incision in the peritoneum directly under the liver edge, which is carried medially until the inferior vena cava is identified or the medial peritoneal incision is encountered. After the colon has been mobilized, the duodenum is exposed lying over the inferior vena cava. The duodenum is mobilized medially ("kocherized") with a combination of blunt and careful sharp dissections to expose the vena cava posteriorly. Once the vena cava has been identified, the renal vein should be visible branching laterally toward the kidney. In the authors' experience, identification of the renal vein at this point facilitates the subsequent steps.

The dissection then proceeds inferiorly, in a similar fashion as was described for the left nephrectomy. The psoas muscle is identified, followed by the gonadal vein and ureter in their medial position. The gonadal vein and ureter are traced cephalad; the gonadal vein inserts into the anterior surface of the vena cava near the level of the renal vein. In contrast to the left side, the right gonadal vein does not require routine ligation. It may be reflected medially and kept out of the way as the ureter is traced toward the hilum. The insertion of the gonadal vein into the cava should be identified, however, in order to prevent inadvertent tearing. The dissection proceeds by following the ureter up along the lateral surface of the inferior vena cava toward the renal vein. If the location of the renal vein is known ahead of time, then this step can proceed quickly. One has to be cautious of accessory renal vessels that insert into the lower pole of the kidney during this phase. After the renal vein has been identified and circumferentially dissected, it is retracted superiorly in order to identify the right renal artery posteriorly. In a similar fashion to the left nephrectomy, anterolateral retraction of the ureter exposes the posterior hilar elements, which facilitates the dissection of the renal artery. If the artery is difficult to identify or dissect from behind the renal vein, then the ureter can be transected early, which will allow the whole specimen to be mobilized superior and anterior, thus improving the exposure to the posterior hilum. The posterior-placed renal artery is divided as described for the left nephrectomy, followed by the renal vein. If the artery is superoposterior to the renal vein, then the adrenal vein coming off the posterior vena cava may need to be divided in order to improve exposure and prevent inadvertent vessel laceration.

If an adrenalectomy is planned, then the dissection proceeds along the lateral border of the inferior vena cava. Identification and ligation of the adrenal vein is crucial to complete the medial dissection. The hepatorenal attachments then are cut along the liver edge with the harmonic scalpel or similar hemostatic device. If the adrenal gland is to be spared, then the dissection proceeds between the adrenal gland and the upper pole of the kidney toward the liver edge. The adrenal vein is not taken in this situation. Superior and lateral attachments are divided sharply; at this point the kidney should be free from the surrounding tissue. The ureter is ligated and transected, which completes the dissection. The specimen is placed on the liver or in the pelvis, and the operative field is inspected for hemostasis at a low intra-abdominal pressure as described for the left nephrectomy.

Specimen Removal and Closure

The choice of specimen retrieval is based on the surgeon's decision to remove the specimen intact or to morcellate. For benign kidneys morcellation is perfectly acceptable and has the advantage of limiting the size of the incision required for extraction. For suspected malignant tumors, morcellation is somewhat controversial; general opinion is that these tumors should be removed intact to ensure accurate pathologic evaluation. For intact specimen removal, the simplest method is to make an incision and extract the specimen manually. It is preferable to place the specimen into a specimen retrieval bag, which allows the specimen to be milked out of a surprisingly small incision. Retrieval bags come in a variety of sizes. For an average-sized specimen, a 15-mm automatically deployed plastic bag should be large enough. Another option is the nylon-coated LapSac (Cook, Spencer, IN), which is more difficult to use because it does not automatically deploy itself. The surgeon must roll up the sack, feed it into the abdomen through a trocar, manipulate it open, and then work the specimen into the bag. The location of the specimen-extraction incision should be placed where a *muscle-splitting* rather than a *muscle-cutting* incision can be placed. This means either a lower quadrant incision (which can be an extension of a trocar incision) or a midline incision. Alternatively, the specimen can be removed through a modified Pfannenstiel incision. If specimen morcellation is chosen, then this can be accomplished with a commercially available device or simply with a Kelly clamp and ringed forceps. The advantage to morcellation is that it can be performed through one of the trocar incisions without an extension. Once the specimen has been removed, the open incision and trocar site is closed and infiltrated with a local anesthetic.

POSTOPERATIVE CARE

Postoperatively most patients are transferred to the medical/surgical ward after a brief stay in the recovery area. An intensive care unit or stepdown unit is not necessary, unless a patient has other comorbid medical issues that need close observation. A clear liquid diet may be started on the night of surgery as long as there are no issues with nausea or vomiting during recovery from anesthesia. The diet is quickly advanced to regular food as tolerated. Pain control can be accomplished with morphine, Demerol, or dilaudid on the first night. This is switched to oral pain medication as soon as a diet is tolerated. Sequential leg compression devices are the primary means of deep venous thrombosis prophylaxis until ambulation is started. For high-risk patients, subcutaneous heparin can be considered. Ambulation should be encouraged on the first postoperative day. The majority of patients are ready for discharge on postoperative day 2.

PROCEDURE-SPECIFIC COMPLICATIONS

In addition to massive hemorrhage during dissection of the renal hilum, potential complications of laparoscopic nephrectomy are related to the high retroperitoneal location of the kidney and include laceration of the spleen, liver, or diaphragm. In the former two situations, the pneumoperitoneum often can assist with tamponade of the viscera. This can be augmented with clotting aids, such as oxidized cellulose (Surgicel), or compression with local structures (allowing the kidney and Gerota's fascia to "sit" on top of the site). A laceration of the diaphragm should be repaired primarily to prevent formation of a diaphragmatic hernia.

RESULTS AND OUTCOME

In an early series on open nephrectomy, the overall 5-year survival rate for renal cell carcinoma was 52%, with a 66% 5-year survival rate for patients with localized disease. Owing to advances in imaging and earlier diagnosis, most contemporary series now report 5-year survival rates in the 75% to 95% range for organ-confined disease and in the 65% to 80% range if there is local extension. If laparoscopic nephrectomy is to be considered an equivalent oncologic operation to open radical nephrectomy, then long-term data (i.e., 5- and 10-year survival rates) need to be obtained. Multiple studies from various institutions have shown that the 5-year survival rate for laparoscopic nephrectomy in select patients (organ-confined disease, <7 cm in size) is in the 91% to 95% range. Some authors have reported a 10-year survival rate of 94%, with a 97% cancer-specific survival rate. The risk of local recurrence in laparoscopic radical nephrectomy has been documented to be 2.6%, which essentially is equivalent to the rate from open radical nephrectomy (2.2% to 2.8%). So far, the application of laparoscopy for renal extirpative surgery has been a success story. It is important to note, however, that the good outcomes described here for laparoscopic nephrectomy have been dependent on proper patient selection.

Suggested Reading

Bhayani SB, Clayman RV, Sundaram CP, et al: Surgical treatment of renal neoplasia: Evolving toward a laparoscopic standard of care. Urology 2003;62(5):821–826.

Fenn NJ, Gill IS: The expanding indications for laparoscopic radical nephrectomy. Br J Urol 2004;94:761–765.

Lam JS, Belldegrun AS: Long-term outcomes of the surgical management of renal cell carcinoma. World J Urol 2006;24:255–266.

Novick AC: Laparoscopic radical nephrectomy: Specimen extraction. Br J Urol 2005;95(suppl 2):32–33.

Ogan K, Cadeddu JA, Stifelman MD: Laparoscopic radical nephrectomy: Oncologic efficacy. Urol Clin North Am 2003;30:543–550.

Permpongkosol S, Chan DY, Link RE, et al: Laparoscopic radical nephrectomy: Long-term outcomes. J Endourol 2005;19(6):628–633.

Portis AJ, Elnady M, Clayman RV: Laparoscopic radical/total nephrectomy: A decade of progress. J Endourol 2001;15(4):345–354.

Saranchuk JW, Savage SJ: Laparoscopic radical nephrectomy: Current status. Br J Urol 2005;95(suppl 2):21–26.

EMERY L. CHEN AND RICHARD A. PRINZ

Minimally Invasive Adrenalectomy

26

Since Charles Mayo first excised a pheochromocytoma from Mother Mary Joachim in 1926, removal of the adrenal glands has been undertaken with a degree of trepidation. The paired adrenal glands are small, friable, and positioned deep within the retroperitoneum. They are seated between the level of vertebrae T11 and L1 and lie within a bed of adipose tissue. The right adrenal gland occupies a position superomedial to the kidney, close to the bare area of the liver, and slightly posterolateral to the inferior vena cava. The left adrenal gland lies in a similar superomedial position to its corresponding kidney, adjacent to the tail of the pancreas and splenic artery. Therefore, operating around the adrenal glands involves thorough anatomic knowledge of, and careful attention to, the surrounding vasculature and organs.

Due to the difficulty in gaining adequate exposure of the adrenal glands, a variety of surgical approaches have been described and used in the past. Traditionally, the three most common means of gaining access to the glands have included the anterior, posterior, and lateral approaches. The laparoscopic adrenalectomy was first described in 1992; since then, laparoscopic adrenalectomy has displaced all of the traditional methods to become the gold standard for the removal of most adrenal glands. Laparoscopic adrenalectomy not only provides superior visualization and exposure, but also reduces postoperative pain and length of hospitalization, without sacrificing safety and efficacy.

There are currently two main laparoscopic approaches to the adrenal glands. The most commonly performed laparoscopic technique is the lateral transperitoneal method. A useful alternate is the laparoscopic retroperitoneal approach, especially when patients have had previous abdominal surgery and intra-abdominal adhesions are anticipated. In addition, there are now a few endocrine units experienced with robot-assisted adrenalectomy as well as "augmented reality"–assisted adrenalectomy. However, these are essentially variations and enhancements of laparoscopic adrenalectomy. The next paradigm shift may lie with natural orifice transluminal endoscopic surgery (NOTES); although still experimental, NOTES has been useful for appendectomy, cholecystectomy, and splenectomy. It remains uncertain whether NOTES will have any benefit over our current laparoscopic technique for adrenalectomy.

OPERATIVE INDICATIONS

Adrenal lesions are very common. Up to 4% of all abdominal computed tomography (CT) scans done for any reason reveal an adrenal mass or abnormality. Indications for laparoscopic adrenalectomy should necessarily be clear and well defined. Otherwise, many unnecessary operations will be performed. The indications fall into three main categories: (1) biochemically active adenomas; (2) nonfunctioning adenomas with characteristics that suggest an increased risk of malignancy; and (3) nonfunctioning tumors that are symptomatic from local mass effect (Table 26-1). The first category includes (a) Cushing's syndrome due to a benign cortisol-producing adenoma; (b) Cushing's disease (cortisol-secreting pituitary adenoma) that has not improved with other forms of therapy; (c) Conn's syndrome (hyperaldosteronism) due to a unilateral adenoma; and (d) benign-appearing pheochromocytomas. The second category includes adenomas or incidentalomas between 4 and 6 cm in size or those that increase in size during observation. An example of the final category is a symptomatic angiomyolipoma. We caution against laparoscopic adrenalectomy for primary or metastatic malignant tumors larger than 6 cm. because of the risk of tumor implantation. Although some surgeons have reported laparoscopic removal of extra-adrenal pheochromocytomas (paragangliomas) and malignant pheochromocytomas, we would again caution against this because of variations in vascular anatomy in the former and the possibility of inadequate curative resection in the latter.

PREOPERATIVE EVALUATION, TESTING, AND PREPARATION

Preoperative imaging is crucial, not only to demonstrate the size and location of the abnormality, but also to show its relationship to surrounding structures. For example, a large right lobe of the liver that extends down toward the pelvis may make access to the right adrenal gland difficult, if not impossible, with standard approaches. Likewise, the variable location of the left adrenal gland can be better anticipated by preoperative imaging. Rare vascular anomalies (e.g., left-sided inferior vena cava) can make imaging invaluable for preoperative planning and intraoperative

Table 26-1 Indications for Laparoscopic Adrenalectomy	
Category	**Examples**
Biochemically active adenomas	Aldosteronoma Pheochromocytoma Cushing's syndrome Cushing's disease that has failed treatment Virilizing tumors

Nonfunctioning adenomas with
  characteristics that suggest an
  increased risk of malignancy
	Lesions 4–6 cm in largest dimension
	Enlarging in size during observation

Nonfunctioning tumors that are symptomatic from local mass effect	Myelolipomas Ganglioneuromas

identification of the adrenal vein. Our preferred method of obtaining this information is spiral CT with intravenous contrast. Although others may favor magnetic resonance imaging, we have not found that it adds any appreciable information. With hormone-producing lesions, the diagnosis should be secure, fluid and electrolyte deficits corrected, and the state of the hormone excess reversed or blocked, if possible, prior to undertaking adrenalectomy.

PATIENT POSITIONING AND PLACEMENT OF TROCARS

Patient positioning is very important with the lateral transperitoneal approach. The patient is placed in the lateral decubitus position (Fig. 26-1). This allows the viscera to fall away by gravity from the area of dissection. To maximize the region between the lower ribs and the iliac crest, the operating table should be flexed to stretch this area by lowering the head and legs. The table should also have a kidney rest, and the patient's contralateral flank between the twelfth rib and the iliac crest should be positioned on it. The kidney rest should then be elevated to magnify the flexion

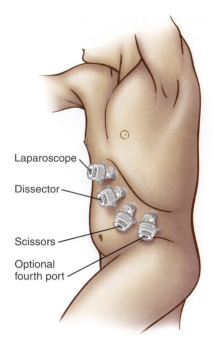

FIGURE 26-2 Port placement for laparoscopic left adrenalectomy.

and push the adrenal gland and kidney on the side of the operation up and away from the other retroperitoneal structures. An axillary roll is placed, and careful padding of all pressure points is done to prevent any nerve or skin injury. Once the patient and the table are positioned, a safety belt or strap and wide adhesive tape are used to secure the patient on the operating table. This is important because the table will be rotated from side to side, and from the Trendelenburg position to the reverse Trendelenburg position, to utilize gravity and position for optimal retraction and exposure. The surgical drapes leave exposed the entire area between the spine laterally, the costal margin superiorly, just beyond the midline medially, and the iliac crest inferiorly.

Four ports are usually employed for right adrenalectomy. They are placed at least 1 to 2 cm below the costal margin along the subxiphoid, midclavicular, anterior, and midaxillary lines. Three ports are generally used on the left: along the midclavicular, anterior, and midaxillary lines (Fig. 26-2). If the ports are placed too close to the costal margin, pressure on the lower ribs can cause postoperative pain. These ports should be spaced at least 5 cm apart to allow adequate freedom of movement. A fourth port is mandatory for retraction of the liver on the right, whereas a fourth port is usually not necessary on the left, as gravity is employed to medially retract the spleen and pancreas. However, if more retraction is needed, an additional port should be placed without hesitation on either side.

OPERATIVE TECHNIQUE

Right Laparoscopic Adrenalectomy

The patient is placed in the left lateral decubitus position (left side down). The surgeon and the cameraperson stand on the left side of the table, facing the patient's abdomen, and the assistant stands on the right side, facing the patient's back. The table is rotated slightly away from the surgeon to bring the midclavicular line into a superior position. Along this line a Veress needle is introduced into the peritoneal cavity 1 to 2 cm below the costal margin, passing through three layers of fascia. Care must be taken to avoid injury

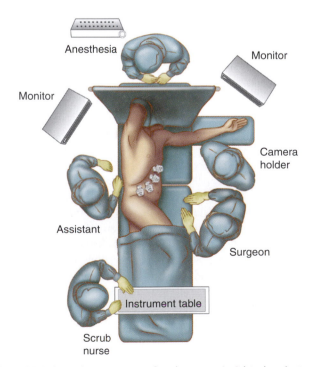

FIGURE 26-1 Operating room set-up for a laparoscopic right adrenalectomy.

to the liver. Once the position of the Veress needle is confirmed to be intraperitoneal, carbon dioxide pneumoperitoneum is established to a pressure of 15 mm Hg. If there is difficulty placing the Veress needle or uncertainty about its position or if the patient has undergone prior abdominal surgery, an open approach (i.e., Hasson cut-down) using a blunt cannula should be used, usually in the periumbilical region.

Once the abdomen is insufflated, the Veress needle is withdrawn and replaced by a 10-mm trocar. The laparoscope is then introduced through this port and the peritoneal cavity is inspected. Under direct vision through the laparoscope, two 10-mm ports are placed along the anterior axillary line and midaxillary line 2 cm below the costal margin. A 5- or 10-mm port is then placed beneath the xiphoid process just to the right of midline.

The dissection is begun by sharply dividing the right triangular ligament. This allows the right lobe of the liver to be reflected medially and superiorly with a fan retractor placed through the subxiphoid port. In displacing the right lobe of the liver, the superior pole of the right adrenal gland and the retrohepatic portion of the inferior vena cava (IVC) will be brought into view. It should be stressed that mobilization of the right lobe of the liver is a critical initial step to allow adequate exposure of the IVC without the need to mobilize the colon or duodenum. Extreme caution is advised when approaching this portion of the IVC, as bleeding in this area is difficult to control. The IVC should be identified early in the course of the dissection, and the surgeon should always be aware of its location throughout the procedure.

The peritoneum overlying the medial border of the adrenal gland and the lateral border of the IVC is then dissected, and the retroperitoneal tissue is entered. The adrenal gland is displaced laterally and the plane between it and the IVC is gently dissected while maintaining gentle superomedial retraction on the liver. Dissection of the space between the adrenal gland and the IVC then proceeds from a superior to inferior direction. The main adrenal vein should be identified at its origin from the IVC, about 1 to 2 cm caudal to the IVC's entry into the liver. The vein is relatively constant in its location at the superomedial aspect of the gland. Although the right adrenal vein is short, it is usually long enough to safely apply a sufficient number of clips (one or two clips on the gland side and three on the side of the IVC). If the vein is too large, a vascular stapling device may be used to divide the vein from the IVC. The dissection proceeds inferiorly once the adrenal vein is divided. The posterior limit of dissection is obtained when muscle fibers of the diaphragm are seen. The gland and perigland tissues can then be mobilized from a medial to lateral direction. Arterial branches arising from the inferior phrenic artery and aorta are usually quite small and can often be transected with cautery. Larger vessels may need to be dissected, clipped, and divided carefully. Use of a coagulator-sealer device (e.g., LigaSure, Valleylab, Boulder, CO) or a harmonic scalpel can help facilitate this portion of dissection. When dissecting the inferior aspect of the right adrenal gland, care must be taken to avoid injury to the right renal artery, which can course obliquely down from the aorta and lie very close to the medial inferior border of the gland.

The adrenal gland should not be grabbed or retracted directly. It is best to dissect in the periadrenal fat to be sure that the entire gland is removed and that the capsule is not entered. Once the gland has been completely mobilized and dissected from the surrounding structures, it is removed by placing it into a sterile bag that is withdrawn through the 10-mm port site. The importance of handling the gland gently throughout the entire operation cannot

Table 26-2   Keys to Right Adrenalectomy
Division of the triangular ligament and medial-superior retraction of the liver
Bloodless dissection of the lateral border of the inferior vena cava
Early identification and control of the short adrenal vein

be overstated. Every effort should be made not to grasp the gland directly. Indirect retraction using the periglandular tissues and fat is recommended. Rupturing of the gland may result in recurrence of disease (e.g., in a patient with Cushing's disease) or precipitation of a life-threatening alteration in blood pressure (as with pheochromocytomas). Similarly, this principle must be adhered to when removing the gland from the abdominal cavity through a port site. Rupture of the bag (especially if the gland is disrupted) can have detrimental consequences. To avoid such an occurrence, the surgeon should make a sufficient opening to allow ease of delivery of the specimen and should use a stronger plastic bag. We do not favor morcellization of the gland as advocated by some groups to facilitate removal without having to enlarge the incision.

The operative field must be thoroughly inspected for adequate hemostasis. Irrigation is usually used to remove clots and any tissue debris before completing the operation. A drain is not necessary. All trocar sites greater than 5 mm should be closed at the level of the fascia with absorbable sutures. Skin closure is done according to surgeon preference. A long-acting local anesthetic is infiltrated around each trocar site, and a sterile dressing is applied to each of the wounds (Table 26-2).

Left Laparoscopic Adrenalectomy

The patient is in the left lateral decubitus position (right side down). The surgeon and the cameraperson stand on the right side of the table, facing the patient's abdomen. The assistant stands opposite the surgeon on the left side. An assistant may not be needed unless a fourth port is placed for retraction. The table is then rotated slightly away from the surgeon to place the midclavicular line in a superior position. A Veress needle is placed along this line into the peritoneal cavity approximately 1 to 2 cm below the costal margin. The three layers of the anterior abdominal wall have to be penetrated. Standard methods of confirming the intraperitoneal position of the needle are performed before beginning insufflation. As with the right side, if there are difficulties encountered with placement of the needle, if the position of the needle is uncertain, or if the patient has had prior upper abdominal surgery, the recommended means of establishing pneumoperitoneum is through an open approach in the periumbilical region.

Carbon dioxide pneumoperitoneum to a pressure of 15 mm Hg is then established. A 10-mm trocar is then placed in the midclavicular line through the incision made for the Veress needle. The laparoscope is passed through this trocar into the peritoneal cavity. A 0- or 30-degree scope can be used, depending on the operator's preference. The peritoneal cavity is inspected through this initial port. Under direct vision, two 5-mm trocars are placed in the anterior and midaxillary lines, just below the costal margin. The incisions for the trocars should be aligned, if possible, so they can be connected as a single incision should conversion to an open operation become necessary. Although three trocars generally provide an adequate number of camera and operating ports, the surgeon should not hesitate to place additional ports if the need arises.

Using endoscopic scissors, blunt dissection, and judicious use of electrocautery, the spleen is mobilized medially with division of

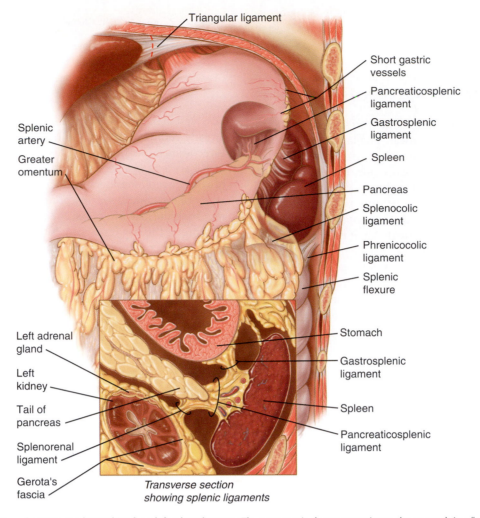

FIGURE 26-3 Relevant ligaments and anatomic relationships for a left adrenalectomy. The pancreas is shown posterior to the stomach in a "phantom" view. Main (upper) figure orientation: anterior (coronal). Inset orientation is cross section (transverse, as seen with a CT scan).

its attachment to the diaphragm and lateral peritoneum (Fig. 26-3). Similarly, the transverse colon at the splenic flexure is mobilized in a caudal direction with division of the splenocolic ligament and the white line of Toldt. This maneuver gains access to the retroperitoneum, often likened to opening the covers of a book. The tail of the pancreas is exposed and visualized as the spleen is medially rotated. It can, however, be mistaken for the left adrenal gland if the surgeon is not familiar with the anatomy and characteristic brownish orange color of the adrenal gland. The pancreas can be gently retracted medially with the use of a laparoscopic "cotton peanut" or other nontraumatic instruments (e.g., an inflatable balloon retractor). The dissection should focus on the continued medial mobilization of the spleen and pancreas. The lateral and diaphragmatic attachments of the spleen should be divided up to the point where the greater curvature of the stomach can be seen and the spleen is able to freely fall medially (Fig. 26-4). The mobilization of the pancreatic tail off the retroperitoneum should proceed in the avascular plane with care not to disrupt the thin pancreatic capsule or its vascular parenchyma. Medial superior traction on the spleen and pancreas and medial inferior countertraction on the splenic flexure of the colon will help delineate the proper planes. The left kidney should be palpable by instruments after the splenic flexure of the colon has been mobilized inferomedially. The adrenal gland will then become visible superomedial to the upper pole of the kidney.

Dissection of the adrenal gland should begin along its medial-inferior margin, with the goal of early identification of the adrenal

vein. Gentle blunt dissection and careful use of hook electrocautery on a low setting is helpful. Once the adrenal vein is identified, it should be followed to its confluence with the left renal vein. The surgeon must be careful not to injure the renal artery or vein. The adrenal vein should be skeletonized, securely clipped (one or two clips on the gland side and three on the renal vein side), and divided (Fig. 26-5). Dissection of the superior pole of the gland can then proceed, moving in an inferior to superior direction. An effort should be made to look for or anticipate an accessory adrenal vein coming from the inferior phrenic vein, which is a variation of normal anatomy. The inferior phrenic arterial branches supplying the superior pole are usually small enough to allow them to be safely transected with cautery. If they are larger, they can be clipped and divided. The use of a harmonic scalpel or LigaSure device for this portion of the dissection may be helpful, but is not always necessary. The small arteriole branches that may be encountered are similarly divided with cautery. Again, the gland should be delicately handled and carefully removed from the retroperitoneum with the aid of a sterile bag as described for the left side. Similar attention is paid to hemostasis, irrigation, and wound closure (Table 26-3).

POSTOPERATIVE CARE

Postoperatively, close monitoring of vital signs and urine output is mandatory. Appropriate attention should be paid to analgesia. Infiltration of long-acting local anesthetic, after closure of the

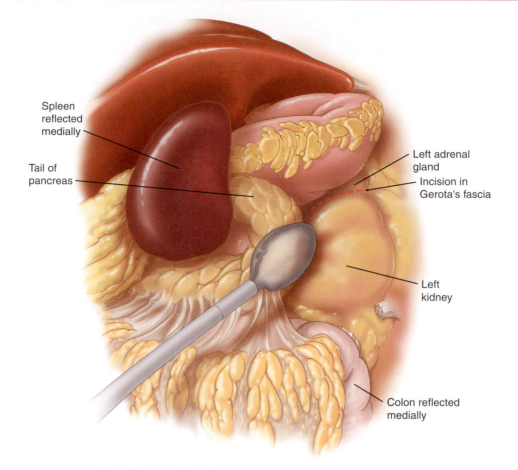

Spleen reflected medially

Tail of pancreas

Left adrenal gland

Incision in Gerota's fascia

Left kidney

Colon reflected medially

FIGURE 26-4 Medial mobilization of the spleen and pancreatic tail during a laparoscopic left adrenalectomy.

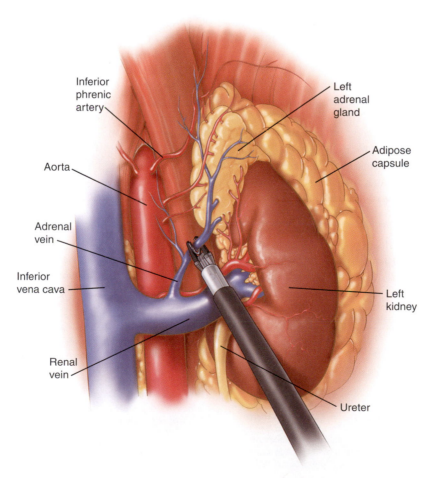

Inferior phrenic artery

Left adrenal gland

Aorta

Adipose capsule

Adrenal vein

Inferior vena cava

Left kidney

Renal vein

Ureter

FIGURE 26-5 Clipping of the left adrenal vein.

Table 26-3   Keys to Left Adrenalectomy
Division of the splenoparietal and splenocolic ligaments as well as the white line of Toldt to allow generous retraction of the spleen and colon at the splenic flexure
Identification and medial rotation of the tail of the pancreas
Control and ligate the adrenal vein and anticipate an accessory adrenal vein

wounds, makes pain much more tolerable. Oral analgesia is generally sufficient, but intravenous boluses of narcotics for breakthrough pain are occasionally necessary. Patient-controlled analgesia is rarely needed. Beyond routine early mobilization and resumption of oral intake, there are a few specific postoperative issues to look out for, depending on the adrenal disease being treated (Table 26-4).

For patients with Conn's syndrome, spironolactone should be stopped and serum potassium monitored in the first week after adrenalectomy. If spironolactone and potassium replacement are continued, the patients can develop hyperkalemia. Patients with Cushing's syndrome or those who have undergone bilateral adrenalectomy should be given stress steroids and discharged home with a maintenance dose. The dose will be higher for patients with Cushing's syndrome because they will require replacement until they can be slowly weaned off for unilateral disease or down to a maintenance dose if they have Cushing's disease. Finally, patients with pheochromocytoma should have their blood sugar closely monitored for the first 24 hours because of the risk of hypoglycemia from relative hyperinsulinemia.

PROCEDURE-SPECIFIC COMPLICATIONS

The most dangerous complication is uncontrolled hemorrhage. The location of the adrenal glands, deeply seated in the upper abdominal retroperitoneum in close proximity to great vessels, makes vascular control difficult. Careful hemostasis must be maintained throughout the entire procedure, as an apparently minor amount of bleeding may impair the view of the operative field, creating a potentially hazardous situation. When bleeding becomes more pronounced, control may be temporarily achieved using direct pressure from forceps or "laparoscopic peanuts" or inflatable balloon retractors. If this lessens or halts the bleeding, the field can be irrigated and inspected for definitive control with vascular clips, bipolar cautery, or intracorporeal suturing. With massive and uncontrolled hemorrhage, the operation should be immediately converted to an open procedure to obtain vascular control and avoid further injury.

Other potential complications to be wary of include injuries to the adjacent viscera. This can occur during placement of the Veress needle and ports or during retraction and dissection. On the right side, the organs at increased risk of injury include the liver, duodenum, hepatic flexure of the colon, and the right kidney. On the left side, structures at risk include the spleen, splenic flexure of the colon, tail of the pancreas, stomach, and left kidney. Injury to solid organs, typically a small puncture or laceration incurred during retraction and dissection, can often be managed with local pressure, electrocautery, or suture. With injury to the pancreas, drains should be placed and not removed until the patient is eating and there is no evidence of pancreatic fluid leakage. If the injury is extensive and hemorrhage becomes a problem, conversion to an open procedure is warranted and should be done without delay.

Injury to the diaphragm can occur with dissection of the adrenal glands high in the abdomen. This can happen when mobilizing the spleen and, especially, when mobilizing the liver in thin patients. The intra-abdominal pressure of the pneumoperitoneum can be transmitted into the chest, and tension pneumothorax may result from such an injury. It is very rare that this would require conversion to open surgery. If the patient is hemodynamically stable, the surgeon should reduce the intra-abdominal pneumoperitoneal pressure. The anesthesiologist should be instructed to increase the respiratory frequency, and a laparoscopic repair of the diaphragmatic injury should be carried out, with interrupted nonabsorbable stitches (see Chapter 32).

RESULTS AND OUTCOME

Pheochromocytoma and hyperaldosteronism are the two most common indications for laparoscopic adrenalectomy. A review of our experience revealed that pheochromocytomas are more challenging to operate on than aldosteronomas, based on the length of operating time. This may be due to the fact that pheochromocytomas tend to be bigger and up to 73% occur on the right side. Conversely, aldosteronomas are left-sided 85% of the time and smaller when compared to pheochromocytomas in our series. Our conversion rate from laparoscopic to open adrenalectomy is approximately 4%, but it can range from 0% to 13% as reported in the literature for most large series. The complication rate in our series is 15%, with significantly more occurring in patients with pheochromocytomas. Death from laparoscopic adrenalectomy is extremely rare. In our series and others like it, the mortality rate was well below 1%.

Suggested Reading

Assalia A, Gagner M: Laparoscopic adrenalectomy. Br J Surg 2004;91(10):1259–1274.

Baron TH: Natural orifice transluminal endoscopic surgery. Br J Surg 2007;94(1):1–2.

Barresi RV, Prinz RA: Laparoscopic adrenalectomy. Arch Surg 1999;134(2):212–217.

Brunt LM: Minimal access adrenal surgery. Surg Endosc 2006;20(3):351–361.

Carlson MA, Frantzides CT: Control of vena cava hemorrage during laparoscopic adrenalectomy. J Laparoendosc Surg 1996;6:349–351.

Gagner M, Lacroix A, Bolte E: Laparoscopic adrenalectomy in Cushing's syndrome and pheochromocytoma [letter]. N Engl J Med 1992;327:1033.

Gagner M, Lacroix A, Prinz RA, et al: Early experience with laparoscopic approach for adrenalectomy. Surgery 1993;114:1120–1125.

Lal G, Duh QY: Laparoscopic adrenalectomy—Indications and technique. Surg Oncol 2003;12(2):105–123.

Morino M, Beninca G, Girando G, et al: Robot assisted vs. laparoscopic adrenalectomy: A prospective randomized controlled trial. Surg Endosc 2004;18(12):1742–1746.

Prinz RA, Rao R: Minimally invasive endocrine surgery. In Frantzides CT (ed): Laparoscopic and Thoracoscopic Surgery. St Louis, Mosby-Year Book, 1995.

Table 26-4 Postoperative Care after Adrenalectomy		
Operative Indication	**Complication**	**Prevention of Complication**
Aldosteronoma (Conn's syndrome)	Hyperkalemia	Discontinue spironolactone and potassium supplements
Pheochromocytoma	Hypoglycemia	Close glucose monitoring for 24 hours after surgery
Hypercortisolism (Cushing's syndrome due to an adenoma, and Cushing's disease)	Adrenal insufficiency (Addison's disease)	Steroid replacement therapy with a slow wean for unilateral adrenalectomy and maintenance steroids for bilateral adrenalectomy

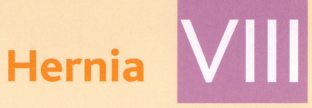

GEORGE S. FERZLI AND
ERIC D. EDWARDS

Laparoscopic Preperitoneal Inguinal Hernia Repair

27

The existence of the preperitoneal space has been known for over 150 years, but the importance of it to surgeons interested in herniorrhaphy was largely unappreciated until the late 1950s. In 1823, Bogros first detailed the lateral preperitoneal space when describing an approach to repair aneurysms of the iliac arteries. This was followed in 1858 by Retzius's description of the prevesicular portion of the preperitoneal space. After these initial descriptions, Eduardo Bassini in 1884 published a description of his hernia repair technique that relied on dissection in the preperitoneal space as one of its components. The work of Nyhus, followed by Stoppa and Wantz's description of giant prosthetic reinforcement of the visceral sac, firmly established the use of the preperitoneal space in the repair of groin hernias. The introduction of the tension-free "plug and patch" mesh repairs ushered in a new era of herniorrhaphy that was based less on anatomic principles and more on mechanics. Recurrence rates with this approach declined dramatically, but some of the anatomic concepts of hernia repair were lost. With the advent of laparoscopy, interest in applying the principles of hernia pioneers of Stoppa and Wantz was reborn. The importance of the myopectineal orifice of Fruchaud has again become a subject of great interest. Herein we present a simple stepwise approach to the laparoscopic preperitoneal hernia repair. The technical aspects of this operation are not difficult. Rather, it is a thorough knowledge of the anatomy that allows one to be successful with this operation.

OPERATIVE INDICATIONS

Initial reports of laparoscopic preperitoneal hernia repair were limited to repair of small, previously untreated groin hernias. Today, this approach has been applied with success to bilateral hernias, large scrotal hernias, recurrent hernias after open repairs, and recurrent hernias after prior laparoscopic repairs. It is recommended that one should become facile with repair of smaller, primary hernias before moving on to more complex cases. Some have argued that this technique has no role in the treatment of unilateral primary inguinal hernias. We disagree with that argument, because a significant number of patients are found to have occult contralateral hernias on laparoscopic exploration. Our practice is to explore both sides and repair these occult hernias, if found. Recently, it has been argued that not all groin hernias need to be repaired. The watchful waiting approach does seem prudent in high-risk, asymptomatic patients. Whether or not this approach should be applied to all who present with an asymptomatic hernia remains to be proved.

PREOPERATIVE PREPARATION

Patients should undergo an appropriate medical evaluation if necessary to determine their fitness for general anesthesia. Spinal anesthesia is an alternative for patients at high risk of pulmonary complications. This operation can also be performed with local anesthesia supplemented with intravenous sedation. Airway control can be supplemented with a laryngeal mask airway in these instances. No bowel preparation is necessary. A single dose of a first-generation cephalosporin is administered prior to incision.

PATIENT POSITIONING AND TROCAR PLACEMENT

The patient is placed supine on the operating table with both arms tucked at the sides. Care is taken to ensure adequate padding of all pressure points. The operating table is placed in a slight Trendelenburg position. Sequential compression devices are placed on the lower extremities. Patients void prior to entering the operating room, so urinary catheters are not needed. A single monitor is placed at the foot of the operating table. The operating surgeon stands on the side of the table opposite the affected side. A total of three trocars, one 10 mm and two 5 mm, are placed in the midline for this procedure (Fig. 27-1A and B). This operation is unique when compared to intraperitoneal procedures, in that placement of the initial trocar is intimately tied to the operative dissection. Furthermore, placement of additional trocars cannot easily remedy poor initial trocar placement. Specific details regarding port placement will be discussed below.

OPERATIVE TECHNIQUE

Relevant Anatomy

There are two preperitoneal spaces that are of particular interest in the laparoscopic repair of inguinal hernias (Fig. 27-2). The first is the space of Retzius, which is familiar to urologists as the prevesicular or retropubic space. The space of Bogros is a lateral extension of the space of Retzius that extends to the level of the anterior superior iliac spine. The opening of these spaces by blunt dissection is critical to successful completion of the repair. The myopectineal orifice of Fruchaud is the area from which all inguinal hernias arise (anterior

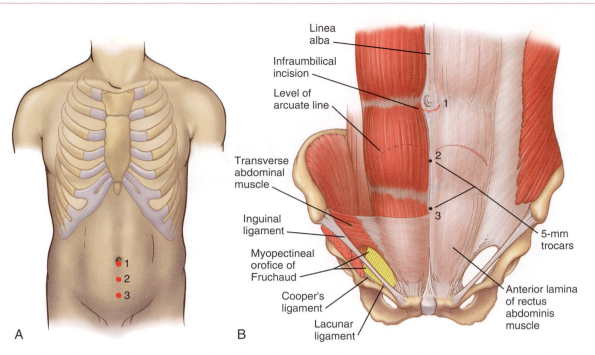

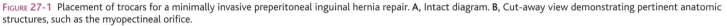

FIGURE 27-1 Placement of trocars for a minimally invasive preperitoneal inguinal hernia repair. **A,** Intact diagram. **B,** Cut-away view demonstrating pertinent anatomic structures, such as the myopectineal orifice.

view in Fig. 27-1B; posterior view in Fig. 27-3). This space is bound superiorly by the aponeurotic arch of the internal oblique and the transversus abdominis muscle, inferiorly by Cooper's ligament, medially by the lateral border of the rectus muscle, and laterally by the iliopsoas muscle. The inguinal ligament and iliopubic tract pass obliquely through this area. Complete mesh coverage of the myopectineal orifice is the ultimate objective of the operation.

Placement of Trocars

Placement of the initial trocar is critical to the success of the procedure, and mistakes in the initial placement cannot be easily rectified. A curvilinear infraumbilical incision large enough to accommodate a Hasson trocar is first made (see Fig. 27-1A and B). Sharp dissection is carried down to the level of the rectus sheath. The anterior rectus sheath is sharply incised transversely, not

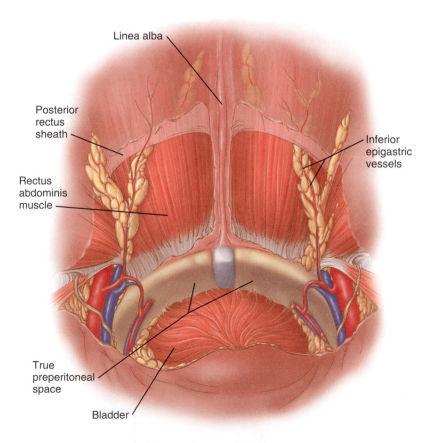

FIGURE 27-2 Relevant anatomic spaces that are developed during a minimally invasive preperitoneal inguinal hernia repair. The space of Retzius is anterior to the bladder; the space of Bogros extends laterally on both sides of the anterior superior iliac spines.

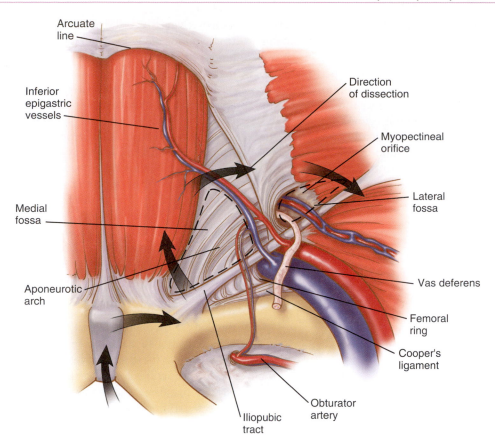

FIGURE 27-3 Anatomy of the inguinal region (posterior view, as seen through the laparoscope). The boundaries of the myopectineal orifice of Fruchaud are the arch of the internal oblique and transversus abdominis muscles superiorly, the rectus abdominis muscle medially, Cooper's ligament inferiorly, and the ileopsoas muscle laterally (not shown).

in the midline, but to one side or the other. The rectus muscle then is retracted laterally. An index finger is inserted into the preperitoneal space and, once below the line of Douglas, is swept side to side (Fig. 27-4). Occasionally a patient will have a linea alba that extends beyond the line of Douglas (variably known as the linea semicircularis, semicircular line, or the arcuate line of the abdomen). In this instance, it is necessary to open the rec-

tus sheath bilaterally and use finger dissection to bluntly dissect the linea alba. At this point the linea alba can be sharply incised, which opens up the preperitoneal space so that the trocars may be placed. This dissection also can be done with a commercially available balloon dissector, but this adds considerably to the cost of the procedure as well as to the operative time, so this dissector is not necessary. Care should be taken during finger dissection to

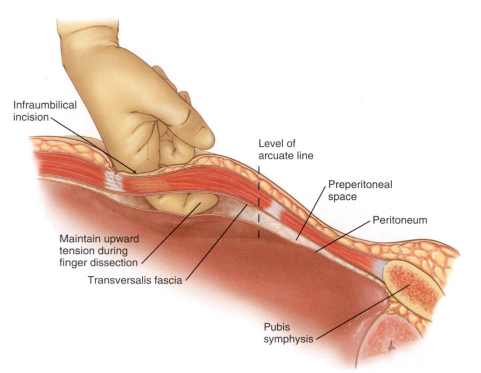

FIGURE 27-4 Finger dissection of preperitoneal space.

apply upward tension while sweeping from side to side, in order to avoid making a rent in the peritoneum. A Hasson cannula then is placed into the preperitoneal space and secured with two interrupted 2-0 Vicryl sutures in the skin. Pneumoperitoneum to a pressure of 10 mm Hg then is achieved. A 10-mm, 30-degree laparoscope then is advanced into the preperitoneal space. The scope is directed blindly toward the pubis symphysis. Once this structure is encountered, the scope can be gently swept from side to side, dividing loose areolar tissue found in the preperitoneal plane. At this point two additional 5-mm trocars can be placed under direct vision in the midline, as shown in Figure 27-1A.

Dissection of the Hernia Spaces

Four potential sites of hernia formation are associated with the myopectineal orifice: the indirect space, the direct space, the femoral canal, and the obdurate canal (the last site actually lies outside the traditional boundaries of the myopectineal orifice). The first step is to bluntly clear off Cooper's ligament in a medial to lateral direction (see Fig. 27-3). This maneuver allows visualization of the femoral space and the obdurate space. The next step is to identify the direct space located medial to the epigastric vessels. The epigastric vessels are identified and are elevated superiorly so that they stay with the rectus muscle. Dissection above the epigastric vessels inevitably leads to bleeding. Blunt dissection just lateral to the epigastric vessels will allow the Bogros space to be opened. This maneuver is critical to allow placement of an appropriately sized mesh. The indirect space is identified by finding the cord structures as they pass through the internal ring (see Fig. 27-3).

Reduction of Hernia Sac

Direct hernias usually are identified medial to the epigastric vessels. The direct hernia sac will obscure the view of Cooper's ligament. The sac can be bluntly peeled from the attenuated transversalis fascia without much difficulty. The key to reducing a direct hernia is gentle traction and countertraction (Fig. 27-5). Sharp dissection rarely is required. In a male with an indirect hernia, the sac can be

seen overlying the cord structures, obscuring the vas deferens. Prior to attempting reduction of an indirect sac, the cord structures must bluntly be separated from the sac. This is more easily accomplished if all lipomas of the cord are reduced first, as one would do in an open herniorrhaphy. Failure to reduce lipomas of the cord has been associated with a high recurrence rate. Reduction of the indirect sac is accomplished by first sweeping the cord structures posteromedially while holding the sac superolaterally. The hernia sac then is pivoted medially and posteriorly while sweeping the cord structures posterolaterally. Alternating between these two maneuvers results in separation of the cord structures from the hernia sac (Fig. 27-6). In female patients, the round ligament should be treated like the vas deferens. In male patients, once the vas deferens and testicular vessels are separated from the sac, it can be reduced with constant tension by passing it hand over hand.

If a femoral hernia is present, great care should be taken to avoid injury to the femoral nerve or the associated blood vessels during reduction of the sac. Incarcerated obturator hernias also can be repaired using this technique. Occasionally it is helpful to divide the floor of the inguinal canal (transversalis fascia and muscle) to allow reduction of the hernia sac. This can be done with electrocautery medial to the epigastric vessels for direct hernias, and lateral to the cord structures for indirect hernias. Any concern about bowel viability mandates that the peritoneum be opened and the bowel inspected. If the bowel is found to be viable, then the peritoneum can be closed and a mesh repair performed.

Large scrotal hernias present a particular challenge to the laparoscopic surgeon. One may need to divide the epigastric vessels in order to reduce the hernia. An additional 5-mm trocar placed in the anterior axillary line at the level of the anterior superior iliac spine will allow an additional instrument to aid with retraction. Once the contents of the hernia sac are reduced, it may be necessary to amputate the sac, leaving the distal end in the scrotum.

Whether done accidentally during dissection or intentionally to inspect bowel viability, a rent in the peritoneum can be problematic. If this occurs, one does not necessarily need to decompress the peritoneal cavity with a Veress needle, as

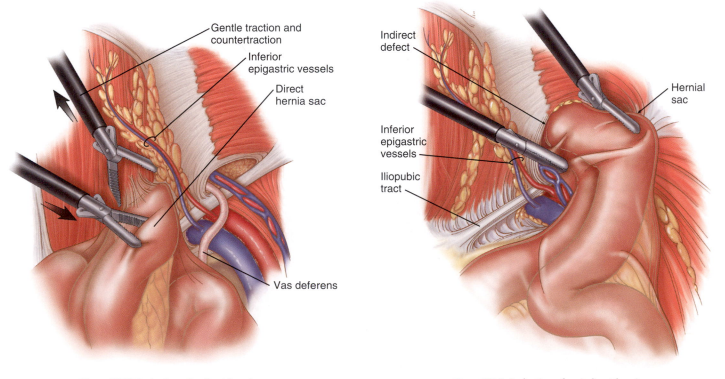

FIGURE 27-5 Reduction of a direct hernia.

FIGURE 27-6 Reduction of an indirect hernia.

suggested by some authors. We believe that such decompression is of questionable help and may be dangerous. If a small tear is away from the site of mesh placement, then the tear may be left alone. Large tears, or those adjacent to the myopectineal orifice, should be closed with a Vicryl Endo-loop (Ethicon, Somerville, NJ). A hole in the peritoneum can make the operation more difficult, but a good dissection of the Retzius and Bogros spaces usually preserves an excellent working space.

Mesh Placement

Various types of mesh are available for the laparoscopic repair of groin hernias, and a full discussion of their individual merits and shortcomings is beyond the scope of this chapter. We use a 15 × 15 cm polypropylene mesh that is introduced through the 10-mm trocar. The mesh is unfolded in a medial to lateral direction. The mesh should cover the entire myopectineal orifice, from the symphysis pubis to the anterior superior iliac spine (see Figs. 27-1B, 27-2, and 27-3). Bilateral hernias require two pieces of mesh that are overlapped in the midline. Fixation of the mesh with a surgical tacker is not necessary. The inherent adhesiveness of the polypropylene when in contact with body fluid, in conjunction with intra-abdominal pressure, serves to keep the mesh in place. If one chooses to use a tacker, then tack placement should be done with great care, as injury to large blood vessel and sensory nerves can occur (please refer to Chapter 28 for a description of mesh fixation).

Conclusion of Procedure

After mesh placement is complete, the two 5-mm trocars are removed and the pneumoperitoneum is released under direct vision. The 10-mm trocar then is removed and the defect in the anterior layer of the rectus sheath is closed with an absorbable suture. The skin is then closed with a subcuticular stitch or skin staples.

POSTOPERATIVE CARE

Patients typically are discharged home on the same day of surgery. Incisional pain can be controlled with oral narcotics or nonsteroidal anti-inflammatory drugs. Male patients may develop ecchymosis of the scrotum. Patients should be made aware that they will likely still have their hernia "bulge" postoperatively. This usually represents a self-limiting seroma and not an early recurrence. Specific restrictions on physical activity are not given.

PROCEDURE-SPECIFIC COMPLICATIONS

The most common intraoperative problem is making an inadvertent rent in the peritoneum, which is discussed earlier. Bleeding is particularly problematic in laparoscopic surgery. Even small amounts of blood can obscure the field, both directly and by absorbing light from the laparoscope. If the trocars are not placed in the midline, then branches of the epigastric vessels can be injured. Bleeding from such injuries may not manifest until well after the operation. If bleeding is encountered from the epigastric vessels or one of their branches, then a 5-mm clip applier can be used for hemostasis. Bleeding from small preperitoneal vessels can be controlled with judicious use of cautery, although they usually stop bleeding spontaneously. Injury to the femoral vessels mandates a conversion to an open procedure.

Nerve injury can be particularly problematic because often there is not a good solution that remedies the situation. During repair one must avoid the "triangle of pain," so named because of the many nerves coursing through it. This triangle is a theoretical space bounded by the gonadal vessels medially, the reflected peritoneum laterally, and the iliopubic tract superiorly. In this region one will find the femoral nerve (L2–L4), the genitofemoral nerve (L1, L2), the anterior femoral cutaneous nerve (L2–L4), and the lateral femoral cutaneous nerve (L2–L3) (Fig. 27-7).

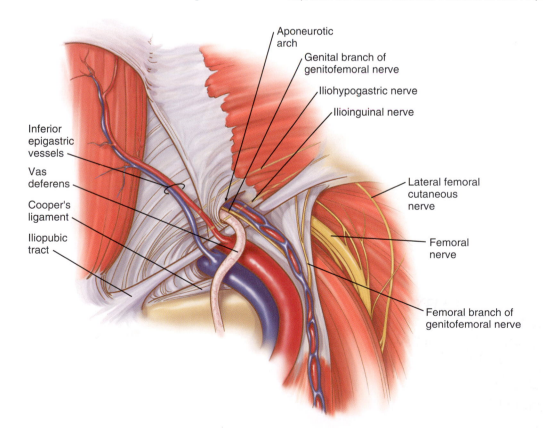

Inferior epigastric vessels

Vas deferens

Cooper's ligament

Iliopubic tract

Aponeurotic arch

Genital branch of genitofemoral nerve

Iliohypogastric nerve

Ilioinguinal nerve

Lateral femoral cutaneous nerve

Femoral nerve

Femoral branch of genitofemoral nerve

FIGURE 27-7 Relevant nerves encountered during a minimally invasive preperitoneal inguinal hernia repair. If staples or tacks are to be used for mesh fixation, then the surgeon should avoid placement of them in the region lateral to the iliac vessels and inferior to the iliopubic tract.

The ilioinguinal and iliohypogastric nerves are located anterior to the transversus abdominis and superior to the inguinal ligament, so these nerves usually are not visualized during a laparoscopic hernia repair. Vigorous application of the hernia tacker during mesh fixation, however, can cause entrapment of these nerves.

Hernia recurrence probably is the most common complication and a main reason why this operation has not been as widely embraced as it might have been. There are two main reasons why patients develop recurrences after a laparoscopic herniorrhaphy: failure to expose the entire myopectineal orifice and improper utilization of the mesh. Failure to completely expose the myopectineal orifice often results in missing hernias or lipomas. All four potential sites of herniation (direct, indirect, femoral, and obdurate) must be examined prior to placement of the mesh. Further, the cord structures or the round ligament must be completely parietalized. Common mistakes involving the mesh include selecting a mesh size that is too small to adequately cover the myopectineal orifice and putting a keyhole or slit in the mesh to accommodate the cord structures. We believe that the mesh must be at least $10 \times 15\,cm$ to adequately cover all potential sites of hernia formation. We also feel that any defects in the mesh can serve as a doorway for hernia recurrence, and thus, we do not advocate slitting the mesh.

RESULTS AND OUTCOME

Recurrence rates after laparoscopic inguinal herniorrhaphy has been a subject of intense debate in recent years. Recent studies comparing laparoscopic to open techniques appear to have serious flaws, so the conclusions drawn from these studies may be questionable. The concept of this operation is sound from an anatomic perspective, and its validity has been demonstrated in open preperitoneal repairs for several decades. In over 1500 cases of laparoscopic inguinal herniorrhaphy spanning 14 years, the senior author (GSF) has a recurrence rate of 0.5%, with most recurrences occurring within 3 months after the repair. This recurrence rate is similar if not better than that seen with open tension-free mesh repairs. The key to this low recurrence rate is having a thorough knowledge of the anatomy. We believe that this is best accomplished by collaborating with a skilled mentor for the first 10 to 15 cases.

Suggested Reading

Bowne WB, Morgenthal CB, Castro AE, et al: The role of endoscopic extraperitoneal herniorrhaphy: Where do we stand in 2005? Surg Endosc 2007;21:707–712.

Brick WG, Colborn GL, Gadacz TR, Skandalakais JE: Crucial anatomic lessons for laparoscopic herniorrhaphy. Am Surg 1995;61(2):172–177.

Ferzli GS, Khoury GE: Treating recurrence after a totally extraperitoneal approach. Hernia 2006;10(4):341–346.

Ferzli GS, Kiel T: The role of the endoscopic extraperitoneal approach in large inguinal scrotal hernias. Surg Endosc 1997;11(3):299–302.

CONSTANTINE T. FRANTZIDES, JOHN G. ZOGRAFAKIS, AND
MARK A. CARLSON

Laparoscopic Transabdominal Preperitoneal Inguinal Hernia Repair

28

A substantial advantage may be gained by using the preperitoneal space during the repair of inguinal hernia. The tissue planes often are relatively clean, the relevant anatomy is easy to appreciate, and the mesh may be applied posterior to the defect, which has a theoretical mechanical advantage over anterior placement. The laparoscopic approach to groin hernia repair is able to utilize these advantages. To date, laparoscopic transabdominal preperitoneal (TAPP) and total extraperitoneal (TEP) inguinal hernia repair both have been demonstrated to be acceptable methods to treat groin hernia. Some controversy remains regarding the superiority of one technique over the other, whether laparoscopic repair is better than open repair, in which patient a particular procedure is indicated, and so on. Because the data on these issues currently are not conclusive, this chapter will not focus on these debates, but instead provide an overview for the technique of the laparoscopic TAPP repair.

OPERATIVE INDICATIONS

Traditionally the mere presence of an inguinal hernia was an indication for repair in the patient who could tolerate the procedure, regardless of whether the patient had symptoms or not. An inguinal hernia can lead to life-threatening complications; the rate at which this occurs, however, is controversial, and whether this risk justifies routine inguinal hernia repair in an asymptomatic patient has been the topic of debate. Certainly a patient who has a symptomatic inguinal hernia should undergo an elective repair. In actuality, there is a continuous spectrum of symptomatology in these patients, from very little to severe. Most general surgeons do not actually see "asymptomatic" groin hernias, because they do not do primary care. The typical decision the surgeon needs to make is whether the degree of symptoms that a particular patient has from a groin hernia will justify repair of that hernia. Because most of these patients have been referred to the surgeon for repair of their groin hernia, a decision in favor of repair typically is made. The practice of the authors is to carefully question each patient to determine how much of a problem is caused by the groin hernia and then to make an individualized decision.

If a groin hernia repair is chosen, then a further decision the surgeon typically needs to make is the operative approach: open or laparoscopic, TAPP or TEP, and so forth. Currently, the indications for each procedure are relative, and the deciding factors will derive from patient and surgeon preference. In addition to the advantages of the laparoscopic approach described earlier, the specific advantages of the TAPP procedure include the ability to instantly scout for an inguinal hernia on both sides. If bilateral hernias are found, then both may be repaired. In addition, the working space with TAPP is much larger than it is with TEP, and the surgeon also may perform a diagnostic laparoscopy if other questions of intra-abdominal disease exist. TAPP also may be easier to perform than TEP in the patient who has had a previous violation of the preperitoneal space (e.g., secondary to a retropubic extraperitoneal prostatectomy). The contraindications to a TAPP repair include the inability to tolerate a general anesthetic, the presence of infection, and moderate coagulopathy.

PREOPERATIVE EVALUATION, PREPARATION, AND POSITIONING

The preoperative TAPP patient should undergo the necessary evaluation in preparation for a general anesthetic. In Western societies, each patient over age 50 should have screening for colorectal cancer prior to the hernia repair, as recommended by the American Cancer Society. Aspirin and other nonsteroidal anti-inflammatory drugs should be discontinued for 1 week prior to surgery. Shaving of the operative field, if done at all, should only be performed immediately prior to the procedure (i.e., not the evening before). All patients should receive a dose of a first-generation cephalosporin (or equivalent antibiotic to cover skin organisms) 30 minutes prior to skin incision.

The patient is placed supine on the operating room table, and general anesthetic is administered. We prefer to use an alcohol-based surgical scrub for skin preparation. Both upper extremities are tucked, taking care to pad appropriately the elbows and any other exposed bony prominences. The patient should be secured to the table using a lower body and upper body padded strap. If the patient voids prior to the procedure, then Foley catheterization is not routinely necessary. If the surgeon anticipates that the procedure may be prolonged, then Foley placement would be helpful to keep the bladder decompressed and out of the operative field. A video monitor is placed at the foot of the operating room table. The surgeon may stand on the same side of the hernia or the contralateral side (depending on the surgeon's preference or dominant hand), and the camera operator stands opposite the surgeon.

Trocar Placement

We prefer to initiate the pneumoperitoneum by placement of a Hasson cannula through a curvilinear infraumbilical incision. At least one 10-mm trocar will need to be placed in order to introduce the mesh into the abdominal cavity; we employ the umbilical site for this purpose. A pneumoperitoneum of 15 mm Hg is established; this pressure typically is decreased at a later phase of the procedure. An initial abdominal diagnostic laparoscopy then is performed with a 10-mm, 30-degree laparoscope with the patient in slight Trendelenburg position. Two additional trocars then are placed, either 5 or 10 mm, depending on surgeon's preference. The trocars are both placed at the same level as the initial infraumbilical trocar, but lateral to the rectus abdominis muscle on both sides (Fig. 28-1).

Operative Technique

The inguinal hernia is identified by diagnostic laparoscopy (Fig. 28-2). If the hernia sac is occupied with intra-abdominal contents, then these usually can be reduced with gentle traction. If an intra-abdominal structure is incarcerated into the sac, then removal may need to wait until after the peritoneal flap has been developed. Prior to developing the flap, however, it is helpful to elevate the peritoneum from the anterior abdominal wall. A grasper is inserted into the inguinal defect, and the hernia sac is evaginated into the abdominal cavity with steady, backward traction. As this maneuver is performed, the hernia sac and surrounding peritoneum are lifted away from the anterior abdominal wall. This separation of peritoneum from underlying musculoaponeurotic structures will create the space in which the surgeon will work after the peritoneal flap is developed. This maneuver is analogous to the insufflation of the balloon dissector during a TEP repair. The surgeon should take care not to tear the peritoneum during this step; while a tear will not hamper the procedure as it would in a TEP approach, it generally is better to have an intact peritoneal flap when the mesh needs to be covered at the procedure's completion.

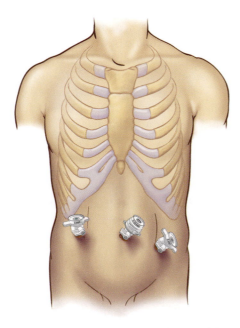

FIGURE 28-1 Trocar placement for a laparoscopic right transabdominal preperitoneal (TAPP) inguinal hernia repair. Umbilical trocar typically is a 10-mm port; trocars 2 and 3 may be 5 or 10 mm.

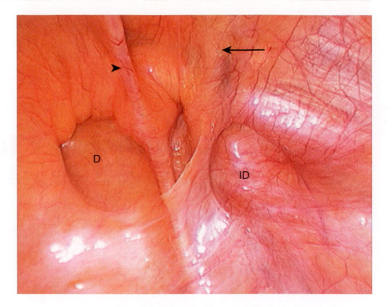

FIGURE 28-2 Laparoscopic view of a combined direct (D) and indirect (ID) right inguinal hernia (i.e., pantaloon hernia). *Arrow* indicates epigastric vessels in the lateral umbilical fold; *arrowhead* points to medial umbilical fold. Top of image is anterior.

After the peritoneum has been elevated from the anterior abdominal wall, the peritoneum is incised in the transverse direction with the hook electrocautery about 2 cm above the hernia defect, from the median umbilical ligament to a point about 10 cm laterally. The inferior epigastric vessels are identified and preserved as they come up from the internal inguinal ring and run along the anterior abdominal wall. Dissection of the preperitoneal space then is accomplished in the avascular plane between the peritoneum and the underlying musculoaponeurosis. Traction on the peritoneal flap is maintained with a grasper while blunt dissection is performed with a palpation probe or similar device. Preperitoneal adipose tissue in the medial portion of the field is dissected until Cooper's ligament is exposed overlying the superior pubic ramus. Not infrequently there is a small blood vessel overlying Cooper's ligament that originates from the obturator artery. The surgeon should be cautious not to injure this vessel when tacking the mesh to Cooper's ligament. The medial portion of Cooper's ligament is cleaned off, which allows the surgeon to view the inguinal floor medial to the epigastric vessels. The pubic tubercle is identified as the medial extent of the dissection (Fig. 28-3A and B).

A traditional classification of inguinal hernia is direct or indirect hernia. The former is a weakness or defect in the inguinal floor medial to the epigastric vessels, and the latter represents a protrusion through an enlarged internal inguinal ring. In addition, there are combined direct/indirect hernias and hernias with protrusion of retroperitoneal structures. Regardless of the hernia type, the approach and treatment are the same: reduction of the hernia sac and contents and coverage of the hernia defect with prosthetic mesh. If the hernia sac was not completely reduced earlier, then the surgeon may now dissect it from the surrounding cord structures (in the male) under direct vision. This part of the procedure can be difficult and time-consuming and should be done carefully with sharp dissection in order to avoid damaging the cord structures. Often there is mass of preperitoneal fat ("cord lipoma") adherent to the sac and cord; this fat should also be dissected away from the cord and reduced into the abdominal cavity. It is important to completely reduce the hernia sac in order to reduce the chance of hernia recurrence.

We prefer to develop the space underneath the cord structures in anticipation of passing the mesh around the cord so that

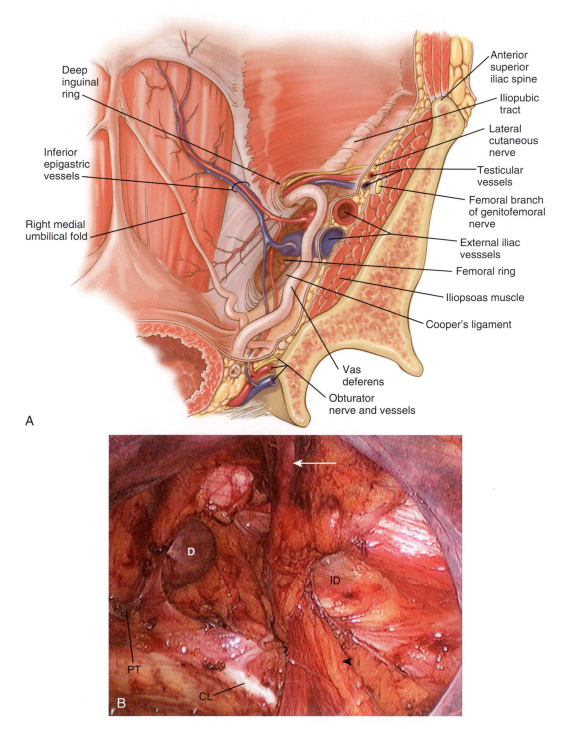

FIGURE 28-3 View of right inguinal anatomy after dissection: **A,** Drawing. **B,** Laparoscopic appearance. *Arrow* indicates epigastric vessels; *arrowhead* shows spermatic cord. CL, Cooper's ligament; D, direct hernia; ID, indirect hernia; PT, pubic tubercle.

the latter lies within the mesh's "keyhole" (see later discussion). Caution should be exercised when dissecting underneath the cord structures in this location, however, because of the proximity of the external iliac vessels. These vessels typically are covered with a layer of adipose tissue and do not need to be disturbed unless there is evidence of a femoral hernia. If a femoral hernia is present, then careful dissection in this area should be performed in anticipation of covering this area with the mesh. Once the sac and preperitoneal fat have been completely reduced, the spermatic cord (i.e., vas deferens with spermatic vessels) should be easy to identify. A "window" underneath the cord should be developed with blunt dissection, which will allow later passage of the mesh.

After the hernia sac and spermatic cord have been delineated, the lateral portion of the field should carefully be dissected. When developing this lateral preperitoneal space, most of the adipose tissue should be left on the muscle layer; this will minimize the risk of injury to crossing nerves in this region. At this point the surgeon should have a clear view of all the pertinent structures, including the pubic tubercle, Cooper's ligament, the internal ring, all hernia defects, the spermatic cord, the inferior epigastric vessels, and the arch of the transversalis aponeurosis. If these structures are clearly visible, then the surgeon is ready to perform the mesh repair.

Although there are a number of prefabricated mesh products available, we prefer to use a simple sheet of polypropylene mesh which has a beginning dimension of 8 × 15 cm. Some surgeons prefer to lay this sheet of mesh intact over the myopectineal orifice and cord together; we prefer to cut a "keyhole" into the mesh, and bring the spermatic cord through this slot. In most patients the 15-cm width of the mesh is excessive, so the width of the operative field should be measured laparoscopically using an instrument with a known dimension (e.g., the open jaws of a grasper), and the mesh is trimmed as needed prior to insertion into the abdomen. A slot then is cut into the lateral one third of the mesh along its long axis; this cut creates a superior and inferior wing of the keyhole. The superior edge of the mesh is inked with an indelible surgical marker, and a stitch of 0 polyglactin (with 2-cm tails) is placed into the upper outer corner of the inferior wing; these maneuvers will help the surgeon orientate and position the mesh after it has been inserted into the abdomen. The mesh then is rolled around a 5-mm instrument and pushed into the abdomen through a 10-mm trocar.

After the mesh has been inserted and unfurled, it is positioned around the spermatic cord by passing a grasper underneath the cord and dragging the marking suture on the inferior wing through the window. The surgeon should take care that the inferior wing does not become twisted or folded as it is brought underneath the cord. The mesh then is flattened out against the myopectineal orifice. The surgeon should ensure that the inguinal floor, femoral triangle, and internal ring are all well covered by the mesh prior to its fixation. If there is difficulty in obtaining this coverage, then the dissection probably was not taken to completion.

Fixation of mesh during laparoscopic inguinal hernia repair is controversial. Mesh fixation would seem to make empiric sense in order to prevent slippage or migration of the mesh with subsequent recurrence. Firing of tacks or staples from a posterior approach into the anterior abdominal wall has been suspected, however, of causing chronic abdominal wall pain, presumably from nerve entrapment. Some surgeons have demonstrated salutary results with mesh inguinal herniorrhaphy without conventional fixation (Stoppa's original technique of open retroperitoneal groin herniorrhaphy employed minimal mesh fixation). We have taken a somewhat intermediate approach in our practice with the judicious use of fixation staples fired only in select areas.

The mesh can be fixed with any of a variety of staplers or tackers; we prefer to use a multifire straight hernia stapler. Although this instrument requires a 10-mm trocar, the ability to partially fire the staple and thereby grab, hook, and reposition structures is important to us. In addition, we feel that the force that the surgeon needs to exert on the stapler for an adequate purchase of tissue is less than that required with the use of a helical tacker. In any event, the surgeon should consider closing the keyhole first with the tacker or stapler prior to actually anchoring the mesh in place, so that a proper fit around the cord can be obtained without interference from an anchoring staple. If the multifire straight hernia stapler is utilized, then the superior wing can be approximated to the inferior wing by partially firing a staple, hooking into the superior wing, dragging it slightly over the inferior wing, and then completing the staple firing. The mesh should be closed around the cord such that a 5-mm instrument can be slid easily alongside the cord.

After the keyhole has been closed, staples are fired into the pubic tubercle and the medial portion of Cooper's ligament. If these structures have been exposed properly, then only slight pressure on the stapler is required to anchor the mesh. Several staples then can be placed along the superior edge of the mesh into the arch of the transversalis aponeurosis, medial to the inferior epigastric vessels. One or two staples then can be placed just lateral to these vessels, and the fixation is completed (Fig. 28-4A and B). Specifically, a staple should not be fired inferior to the iliopubic tract or more than 3 cm lateral to the internal inguinal ring. Many surgeons describe a "two-handed" stapling technique, in which the dominant hand manipulates the stapler/tacker and the nondominant hand provides counterforce on the abdominal wall against the head of the stapler/tacker. This certainly will ensure a deep bite of tissue by the staple or tack, but the surgeon needs to balance this against the risk of injuring a vessel or nerve in the abdominal wall. If the anchoring structures have been well dissected, then relatively little force is required to push the staple through the pores of the polypropylene mesh and into the underlying fibrous tissue.

Upon completion of the mesh anchorage, the field is inspected for hemostasis, and then the peritoneal flap is used to cover the mesh. Staples are fired with gentle pressure to secure the flap over the mesh (Fig. 28-5). Decreasing the pneumoperitoneum pressure prior to closing the flap will facilitate this step. No portion of the polypropylene should be visible after the flap has been repositioned. The pneumoperitoneum then is evacuated, and all 10-mm ports are closed with 0 polyglactin. After the drapes have been removed, the surgeon should ensure that both testicles are present in the scrotum; occasionally a testicle will have been pulled into the inguinal canal during the reduction of the hernia. If the patient has incurred a massive pneumoscrotum, then this can be rapidly decompressed at this time with an 18-gauge angiocatheter.

POSTOPERATIVE CARE

One dose of intravenous ketorolac can be administered in the operating room for analgesia; additional doses of ketorolac may be given later that day. Typically the patient is discharged home on the day of surgery on a regular diet and with a prescription for oral analgesics. Physical activity should be restricted for at least 4 weeks (no lifting greater than 10–15 pounds). The patient should be seen 1 week after surgery in order to evaluate the incisions. Most patients can return to work (light activity) within 10 days of surgery; earlier return to light activity is reasonable if the patient is motivated. The surgeon should not compromise on the period of lifting restriction, though.

PROCEDURE-SPECIFIC COMPLICATIONS

Complications specific for the TAPP procedure include bladder injury, epigastric vessel laceration, spermatic cord injury or constriction, hematoma, and chronic groin pain. The risk of bladder injury may be minimized by maintaining bladder decompression. If the bladder is injured, then suture repair with decompression is indicated. If possible, insertion of permanent mesh should be avoided in this scenario. Epigastric vessel laceration typically is caused by trocar insertion; this can be avoided by transilluminating the abdominal wall with the laparoscope prior to placing the lateral trocars (see Fig. 28-1). If the patient is not excessively obese, then abdominal wall transillumination should reveal the location of the inferior epigastrics. A bleeding inferior epigastric vessel can be ligated using a suture and a laparoscopic needle passer. Injury to spermatic cord can be avoided by using

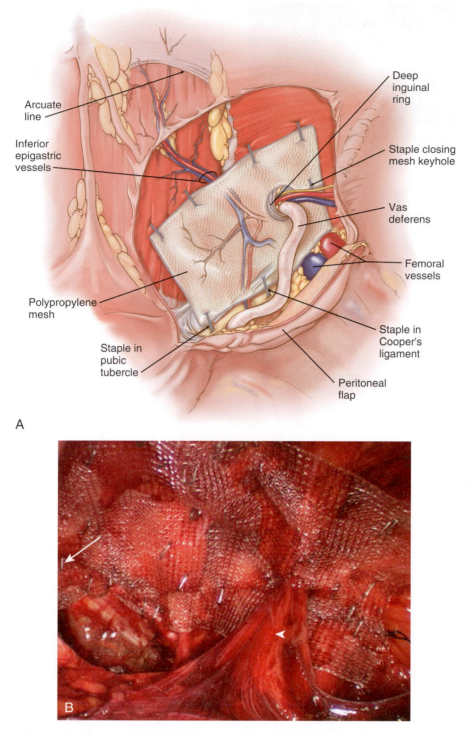

FIGURE 28-4 Placement of polypropylene mesh with a cut keyhole for a laparoscopic right transabdominal preperitoneal (TAPP) inguinal hernia repair. **A,** Drawing. **B,** Laparoscopic appearance. *Arrow* shows pubic tubercle; *arrowhead* shows spermatic cord.

careful sharp dissection in the vicinity of the cord and by ensuring that the mesh keyhole has not been closed too tightly around the cord. If the spermatic artery is interrupted, then it is likely the testicle will undergo acute necrosis or atrophy. A hematoma often is the result of excessive blunt dissection or an underlying coagulopathy. If incurred, a hematoma usually will be amenable to nonoperative management of rest, scrotal elevation, and ice as needed. The risk of chronic groin pain can be minimized by judicious mesh fixation, as described earlier. Chronic groin pain arguably is a greater problem after mesh herniorrhaphy (either open or laparoscopic) than recurrence. The treatment of postherniorrhaphy pain has variable success, but is beyond the scope of this chapter.

RESULTS AND OUTCOME

Documented recurrence rates after laparoscopic repair of inguinal hernia in the hands of specialists have been only 1% to 2%. Interestingly, a recent randomized trial comparing open to laparoscopic repair documented a 10% recurrence rate in the laparoscopic group, which was significantly greater than the rate in the open group. There was a slight advantage in the laparoscopic group with respect to pain and return to activity. Not surprisingly, this study came under heavy criticism from proponents of the laparoscopic approach. The contrast in results between retrospective series from "expert centers" and a randomized trial (performed in the abovementioned case within

is critical and that individual results may vary depending on subtle technique differences that may or may not be obvious to us or any other group of authors. Our individual results (unpublished) do not reflect a 10% recurrence rate; we are confident that the TAPP procedure is effective, safe, and durable, and so we will continue to utilize this operation for the repair of inguinal hernia.

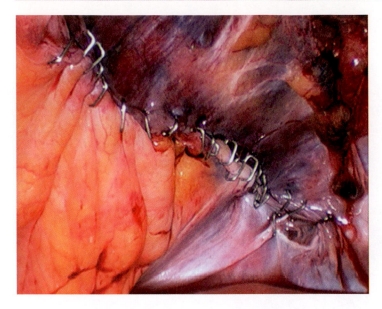

FIGURE 28-5 Coverage of the mesh with the peritoneal flap.

the Veterans Administration setting) has been seen before with other procedures, not just with inguinal hernia repair. This discrepancy suggests that the actual technique of the herniorrhaphy

Suggested Reading

Fitzgibbons RJ, Jr, Giobbie-Hurder A, Gibbs JO, et al: Watchful waiting vs. repair of inguinal hernia in minimally symptomatic men: A randomized clinical trial. JAMA 2006;295:285–292.

Kapiris SA, Brough WA, Royston CM, et al: Laparoscopic transabdominal preperitoneal (TAPP) hernia repair: A 7-year two-center experience in 3017 patients. Surg Endosc 2001;15:972–975.

Leibl BJ, Schmedt CG, Kraft K, et al: Recurrence after endoscopic transperitoneal hernia repair (TAPP): Causes, reparative techniques, and results of the reoperation. J Am Coll Surg 2000;190:651–655.

Lovisetto F, Zonta S, Rota E, et al: Laparoscopic transabdominal preperitoneal (TAPP) hernia repair: Surgical phases and complications. Surg Endosc 2007;21:646–652.

Neumayer L, Giobbie-Hurder A, Jonasson O, et al: Open mesh versus laparoscopic mesh repair of inguinal hernia. N Engl J Med 2004;350:1819–1827.

Stoppa R, Petit J, Henry X: Unsutured Dacron prosthesis in groin hernias. Int Surg 1975;60:411–412.

Wara P, Bay-Nielsen M, Juul P, et al: Prospective nationwide analysis of laparoscopic versus Lichtenstein repair of inguinal hernia. Br J Surg 2005;92:1277–1281.

CONSTANTINE T. FRANTZIDES, MARK A. CARLSON, AND
JOHN G. ZOGRAFAKIS

Laparoscopic Ventral Hernia Repair

Similar to cholecystectomy, ventral hernia repair is one of the most common procedures performed by general surgeons. Perhaps the abundance of ventral herniorrhaphy is a sad reflection on our ability to obtain secure and durable closure of the long abdominal incision (and, incidentally, also could be a strong pitch for minimally invasive surgery). The literature on ventral hernia repair contains a large number of technical descriptions on how to fix the abdominal wall defect. There also is a large number of publications describing the experience of a single surgeon/institution in which the recurrence rate (the primary outcome measure of ventral herniorrhaphy) is astoundingly low, in the range of 0% to 1%. Yet it has been documented that the recurrence rate after ventral herniorrhaphy for all operators is much higher, in the range of 10% to 30% (and that is with the use of mesh). This suggests that, perhaps as much or more than any other common general surgical procedure, the long-term outcome of ventral hernia repair is dependent on operative technique.

One technical aspect of ventral hernia repair that has received increasing emphasis is the importance of utilizing mesh. Ventral herniorrhaphy with mesh has been shown in both controlled and uncontrolled settings to have a lower recurrence rate than repair without mesh. This statement, however, is hopelessly broad; it makes no mention of important technical details, such as what type of mesh to use, where the mesh should be placed in relation to musculoaponeurotic layers, how large the mesh should be in relation to the defect, how the mesh should be secured, and so on. We believe that within these technical details resides the source of the abovementioned variability in recurrence.

Currently there is a smoldering controversy about the superiority of laparoscopic versus open ventral hernia repair. Without the benefit of an adequate clinical trial, this issue is difficult to resolve. Not surprisingly, we believe in the laparoscopic approach, and feel somewhat justified in taking this position by the volume of uncontrolled data that support this approach. It would be irresponsible, however, to imply that open hernia repair is inferior or below the fabled "standard of care."

In using the term "ventral hernia," we refer to all defects of the anterior abdominal wall, whether they involve a previous surgical incision, a primary umbilical defect, a recurrent ventral hernia of any type, and so forth. In line with our other contributions to this atlas, we will make no claim of possessing the "best" or "purest" technique, because very little of what we will advocate has been tested in a controlled trial. We simply will describe in detail what has worked well for us; moreover, as there is more than one author of this chapter, it will become apparent that this chapter contains more than one technique of ventral herniorrhaphy.

OPERATIVE INDICATIONS

The primary indication to repair a ventral abdominal hernia is the presence of symptoms, which include pain, pressure, cosmesis, partial or complete obstruction, and strangulation. An asymptomatic ventral hernia typically does not need to be repaired, especially in an older, frailer patient. A common predicament that arises in a symptomatic patient, however, is the presence of comorbidities that can be a relative contraindication to repair. For example, should a 48-year-old man with a body mass index (BMI) of 51 and a mildly symptomatic incisional hernia from a previous colon resection undergo a minimally invasive ventral herniorrhaphy? Or would such a patient be better suited to have medical/surgical treatment of his morbid obesity? This comorbidity likely was the main predisposing factor for his incisional hernia and, left untreated, would put him at an elevated risk for perioperative complication and recurrence after a hernia repair. If such a patient were experiencing disabling symptoms or developed a severe complication (e.g., strangulation), then certainly early/immediate operative intervention would be indicated. Nevertheless, it is our preference in the mildly symptomatic patient to first address a comorbidity, such as morbid obesity, prior to proceeding with a minimally invasive ventral hernia repair. In addition, there was some initial concern about utilizing the laparoscopic approach for a "giant" incisional hernia (Fig. 29-1); however, many authors have demonstrated that laparoscopic technique for this indication is feasible (and even preferable).

PREOPERATIVE EVALUATION

The goals of the preoperative evaluation for minimally invasive ventral hernia repair may be organized as follows: (1) to assess by physical examination the presence, location, size, and extent of the ventral hernia; (2) to determine whether the patient's symptoms are severe enough with respect to associated comorbidities such that a herniorrhaphy is justified; (3) to identify and characterize any previous abdominal operations; and (4) to make an operative plan. Routine testing should include blood chemistries, blood count,

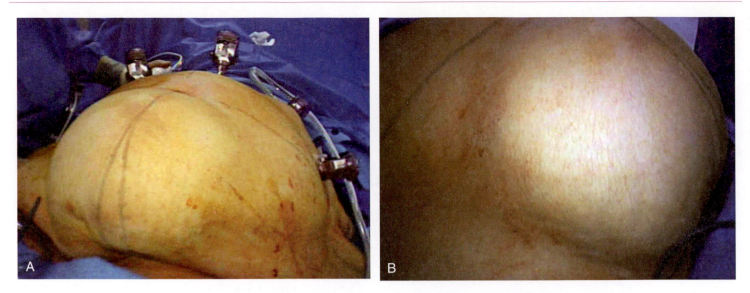

FIGURE 29-1 External views of "giant" incisional hernias. **A,** Inferior view. **B,** Lateral view.

and if indicated by the history and physical exam, a cardiopulmonary evaluation. If the diagnosis of ventral hernia in a symptomatic patient is questionable (e.g., because of a thick abdominal wall), then an abdominal computed tomography (CT) scan may be performed.

A giant ventral hernia is not a contraindication to a laparoscopic approach. Nevertheless, the surgeon should take into consideration the possible intraoperative or postoperative derangements in pulmonary function that may occur in a patient whose large hernia has been repaired. Such a patient may be helped with pulmonary consultation and optimization prior to surgery. Some authors have advocated the use of preoperative treatments of pneumoperitoneum for several weeks prior to repair of a giant ventral hernia; however, we do not have experience with this technique. On the day prior to surgery, the patient may undergo a bowel preparation consisting of polyethylene glycol lavage and oral antibiotics.

PATIENT POSITIONING AND PLACEMENT OF TROCARS

For a minimally invasive ventral hernia repair, the patient is placed supine on the table, with both arms tucked. Belts or straps are placed around the upper chest and upper thighs so that extreme table movements can be performed safely. The surgeon may stand on either side of the patient and faces the monitor on the contralateral side. The surgeon may decide to cover the patient's skin with an adhesive iodine-impregnated drape (or similar shield) as an additional protective measure against mesh contamination.

Establishment of pneumoperitoneum for a ventral hernia repair can be complicated because many of the patients have had a previous abdominal procedure. Avoidance of visceral injury during this step is paramount. We prefer to use the optical bladeless trocar at a position well away from the hernia site. Alternatively, a Hasson cannula (i.e., open technique) may be utilized. The Veress needle also is a possibility, but we are reluctant to recommend the use of this device in a previously operated abdomen. We generally place three trocars on one side of the abdomen, typically one or two 12-mm ports (one for the camera, another for the 10-mm hernia stapler, if used) and one or two 5-mm ports. Additional trocars may be placed on the contralateral side as needed to complete the dissection of the hernia and the subsequent fixation of the mesh.

Similar to many other laparoscopic procedures, there are no absolute rules to trocar positioning for minimally invasive ventral herniorrhaphy, yet poorly positioned trocars can be this operation's undoing. If the trocars are placed too close to the hernia defect, then it is difficult to visualize the operative field, and the mesh may end up covering the trocar. If the trocars are placed too far away (i.e., too lateral) from the hernia defect, then there is risk of perforation of the colon along the left flank. In addition, standard-length instruments may not reach all of the hernia if the ports are placed too lateral. The optimal trocar position is intermediate between these two extremes.

OPERATIVE TECHNIQUE

The first objective of the procedure is to expose the entirety of the anterior abdominal wall. Many, if not most, patients with a ventral hernia will have some degree of obesity, and a large omentum often is the main or sole tissue occupying the hernia defect (Fig. 29-2). Usually this can be reduced relatively quickly using

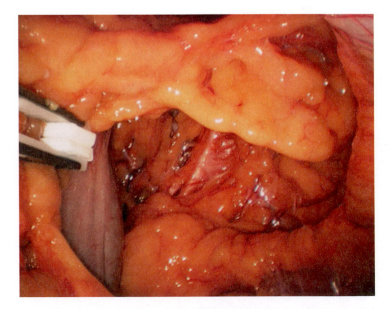

FIGURE 29-2 Laparoscopic view of a large incisional hernia containing omentum and small intestine.

a combination of tension on the omentum and sharp dissection where the omentum has formed adhesions to the hernia sac. If loops of bowel are incarcerated in the hernia sac, then the surgeon should apply gentle traction on these with an atraumatic grasper and cut the adhesions with scissors but without cautery. The extra time spent performing a careful, meticulous dissection on an incarcerated bowel in order to avoid a full-thickness injury is preferable to the uncomfortable scenario of having to deal with a bowel injury after a hasty dissection. In some cases, proper mobilization of an incarcerated bowel can extend the duration of the procedure substantially, so the surgeon should be prepared for this.

The entire anterior abdominal wall requires exposure so that the surgeon can be certain that all hernia defects are visualized (Fig. 29-3). In the common case of a long midline incision, the anterior wall from the xiphoid to pubis should be dissected clean. After this has been done, the surgeon can decide which area of the abdominal wall needs to be repaired. Typically this is obvious secondary to a large fascial hole with an associated sac. In some patients with attenuation of their musculoaponeurotic layers, however, the decision of what to fix may not be obvious after the hernial adhesions have been lysed. The surgeon should rely on his or her knowledge of the precise location of the patient's pain/symptoms along with careful intra-abdominal inspection of the previous incision (if present), using transillumination with the laparoscope to highlight any weak spots. It may be helpful for the surgeon to mark out the defects requiring repair with a sterile marking pen on the patient's skin during the procedure.

After the hernia defect or defects have been identified, the surgeon chooses the mesh type and size for the repair. Mesh repair for minimally invasive ventral herniorrhaphy essentially is standard, as virtually every hernia in over 6000 published cases (which we reviewed recently) utilized mesh. The choice of mesh type is somewhat surgeon-dependent; we have preferred to use a double-sided polytetrafluoroethylene (PTFE) mesh (DualMesh, W.L. Gore & Associates, Flagstaff, AZ), which has a corduroy-style surface for tissue incorporation (to face the abdominal wall) and a smooth side for minimal tissue reaction (to face the viscera). Probably more important than the type of mesh is how large the mesh should be in relation to the abdominal wall defect; in general, the mesh should overlap the hernia defect by 3 to 5 cm on all sides. In other words, a defect 6 cm in diameter should be covered with a piece of mesh that is at least 12 cm in diameter. The diameter of the hernia defect(s) can be measured with an umbilical tape or with an open grasper that has a known inter-jaw distance.

Multiple techniques of mesh fixation that utilize sutures, tacks, staples, or a combination thereof have been described; none has been proved superior in a controlled trial. Most surgeons would agree that mesh fixation in minimally invasive ventral herniorrhaphy is critically important in order to prevent mesh slippage and hernia recurrence, yet it is difficult to arrive at a consensus of just exactly how the mesh fixation should be accomplished. The authors of this chapter use different techniques, which will be described here.

The first technique involves fixation with staples only. Prior to insertion of the mesh into the abdomen, four cardinal sutures of 2-0 polypropylene with long tails are placed into the mesh margin at the 3, 6, 9, and 12 o'clock positions (corresponding to left lateral, inferior, right lateral, and superior on the patient). The mesh then is rolled up, like a "cigar," and inserted through a 12-mm port into the abdomen. If the mesh is too large to fit through a 12-mm port, then this can be upsized (e.g., to 15–18 mm). Alternatively, the rolled-up mesh can be inserted into a polyethylene bag, and

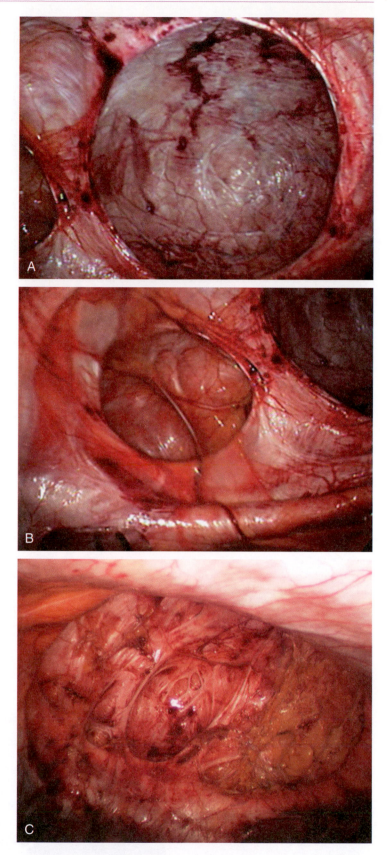

FIGURE 29-3 A to C, Laparoscopic views of anterior abdominal wall after large incisional hernias have been reduced. Empty hernia sacs are visible in each image.

this bag can be fed through the 12-mm trocar incision with the port removed. We feel that it is important to avoid mesh contact with the skin, so we would discourage stuffing the mesh without a protective cover through a skin incision. In addition, we like to change our gloves immediately prior to handling the mesh.

The mesh is unfurled once it has been placed into the abdomen; if a double-sided PTFE mesh is being utilized, then the corduroy surface faces the anterior abdominal wall. Each of the four cardinal sutures is brought through the abdominal wall using a laparoscopic suture-passer (Carter-Thomason CloseSure System, Inlet Medical, Trumbull, CT), at the 3, 6, 9, and 12 o'clock positions on the abdominal wall (Fig. 29-4). These sutures are meant for temporary suspension of the mesh so that it can be stapled to the anterior abdominal wall; the sutures will be removed at the end of the procedure. The periphery of the mesh then is fixed using a 10-mm hernia stapler (Endopath EMS, Ethicon Endo-Surgery, Albuquerque, NM). Each staple is positioned radially at the mesh margin, so that the inner arm of each staple hooks into the mesh, and the outer arm bites into tissue (Fig. 29-5). A "two-handed technique" is preferred, in which one hand of the surgeon operates the stapler, while the other hand compresses the abdominal wall into the head of stapler. This technique ensures a deep tissue bite for each staple. Staples are place at 1-cm intervals around the mesh periphery. The surgeon should not allow redundancy or folds to form in the mesh, but rather the mesh should be kept taut and stretched out. Completed hernia repairs with PTFE and polyester mesh are shown in Figure 29-6. Once the abdomen is desufflated, any fold or redundancy in the mesh will become exaggerated, so it is best to avoid introducing these features.

A second and possibly a third inner row of staples is placed after the mesh periphery has been secured. A radial distance of 2 cm should separate the rows. The staples of the inner row(s) also are fired with a two-handed technique, but obviously both arms of each staple now have to traverse the mesh. After the stapling has been completed, the cardinal sutures are cut from within the abdomen with laparoscopic scissors. Hemostasis is checked, the abdomen is irrigated as needed, the pneumoperitoneum is evacuated, and the fascia of all ports greater than 5 mm is closed.

An alternative method used by one of the authors of this chapter is to secure the mesh with a combination of permanent sutures and tacks. For this technique, the exposed skin of the surgical field should be covered with an iodine-impregnated adhesive drape. The mesh to be used is set upon the abdomen, centered over the defect, and a trace of the mesh is drawn on the adhesive drape with an indelible surgical marking pen. For a 15 × 19 cm oval sheet of double-sided PTFE, we will place 8 transabdominal fixation sutures (2-0 polypropylene) evenly spaced around the mesh margin; for a 26 × 34 cm oval sheet of PTFE, 16 such sutures are used. Each suture takes a 3- to 4-mm bite of mesh; the suture is tied down onto the mesh, and each suture tail is cut to a length of 15 to 20 cm. The tails are tightly coiled and

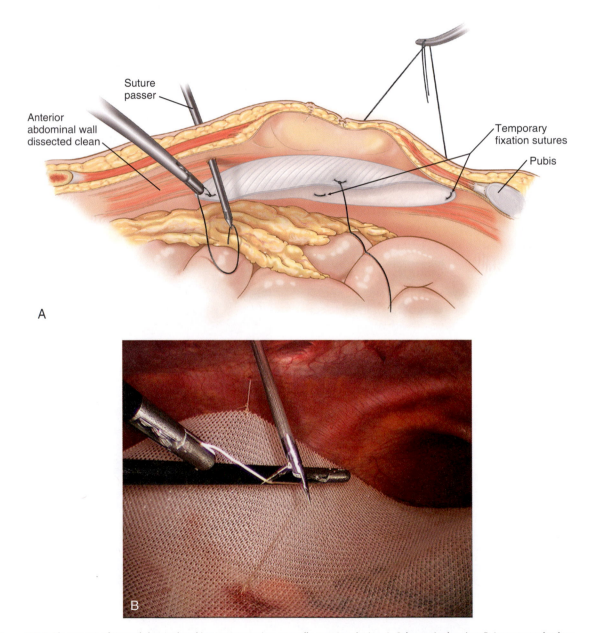

FIGURE 29-4 Placement of transabdominal tacking sutures using a needle-passing device. **A,** Schematic drawing. **B,** Laparoscopic view.

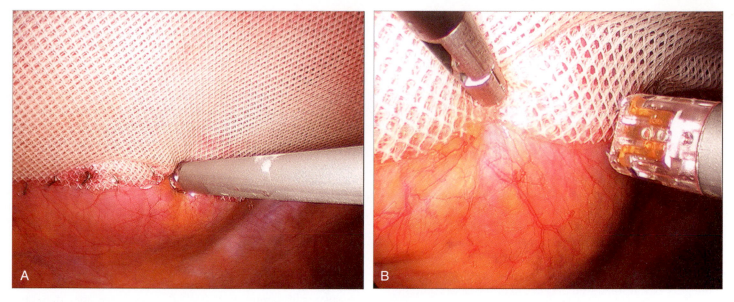

FIGURE 29-5 Technique of mesh stapling. Each staple is fired in a radial orientation at the edge of the mesh, such that the inner arm of the staple hooks into the mesh and the outer arm of the staple bites into the abdominal wall. **A**, Wide view. **B**, Close-up view.

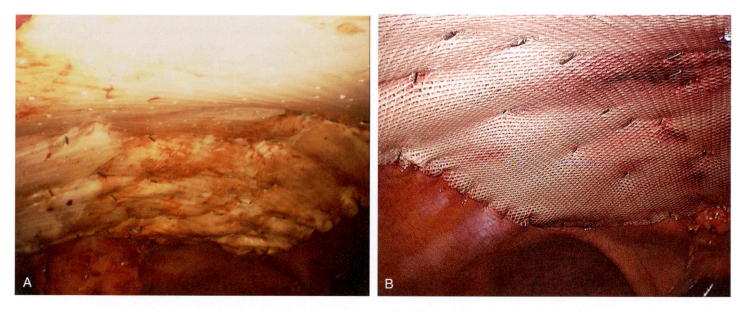

FIGURE 29-6 Laparoscopic view of completed minimally invasive ventral hernia repairs. **A**, PTFE herniorrhaphy. **B**, Parietex herniorrhaphy.

taped down to the mesh with an adhesive strip; one end of each adhesive strip is bent back upon itself and marked with indelible ink for subsequent ease of removal. The sutures are consecutively numbered with indelible ink on the corduroy side of the mesh adjacent to each suture and also on each adhesive strip. In addition, a large arrow pointing in the superior direction is marked on the corduroy surface for subsequent ease of orientation. The mesh then is tightly wound and inserted into the abdomen, as described previously.

Once inside the abdomen, the mesh is unfurled and oriented with the arrow pointing superiorly. The future exit site of each suture is marked with a number on the outside of the abdomen, directly on the iodine-impregnated adhesive drape. In general, each exit site should be marked about 3 cm outside of the previously traced outline of the mesh. This lateral location will help keep the mesh on stretch when the transabdominal sutures are tied. Beginning with a suture site on the side contralateral to the laparoscope, a stab incision (~5 mm) is made with a No. 11 scalpel. Inside the abdomen, the adhesive strip of the suture number corresponding to the outside site is pulled off the mesh with a

5-mm grasper. A laparoscopic suture-passer then is passed from the outside to the inside, through the stab incision and perpendicular to the abdominal wall; one of the suture tails then is grabbed and pulled back through the incision. The process is repeated with the other tail, but making sure that the suture-passer does not follow the same pathway through the abdominal wall. Each entry of the suture passer into the abdomen is monitored with the laparoscope to ensure that there will be some tissue caught between the suture tails when they are tied.

This process is repeated for each transabdominal fixation suture, moving from the most distal to the most proximal to the laparoscope. If visualization of this process becomes awkward or impossible on the side ipsilateral to the laparoscope, then the surgeon may need to place trocars on the contralateral side in order to complete the procedure. After all sutures have been brought through the appropriate stab incisions, the pneumoperitoneum pressure is reduced to 10 mm Hg (exposure permitting) or less, the sutures are tied (carefully, avoiding string breakage), and the tails are trimmed. Upon tying the sutures, the mesh should be drawn up to a taut position against the anterior abdominal wall.

The anchorage of the mesh then is completed by placing one row of helical fasteners (e.g., Autosuture and Protack, U.S. Surgical, Norwalk, CT) or similar tacks around the periphery of the mesh at 1-cm intervals. A second row may be placed if the mesh appears lax in some areas. Hemostasis is checked, the abdomen is irrigated as needed, the pneumoperitoneum is evacuated, and the fascia of all ports greater than 5 mm is closed.

POSTOPERATIVE CARE

An abdominal binder is placed in the operating room before transfer to the recovery room. The binder should remain on at all times possible during the day, especially after repair of a large defect. The binder may be removed during sleep. If the patient has a relatively small hernia, then same-day discharge is possible. A patient with a large defect or prolonged procedure typically is hospitalized for 1 to 2 days. If the surgeon has a concern regarding the integrity of intestinal wall because of an extensive adhesiolysis, then a longer period of in-hospital observation may be warranted. Clear liquids may be given in the evening after surgery; a regular diet may be given on postoperative day 1. Ambulation and incentive spirometry are strongly encouraged right after surgery. The patient should have clear instructions to avoid lifting anything greater than 15 pounds (7 kg) and strenuous activity for a minimum of 3 months. Walking is encouraged and expected. The patient also should receive instructions on how to recognize symptoms of a delayed intestinal perforation (e.g., fever, malaise, abdominal pain, incisional drainage).

PROCEDURE-SPECIFIC COMPLICATIONS

Enterotomy is the most problematic intraoperative complication and can occur even with the most experienced surgeon. An enterotomy creates a dilemma of whether to use permanent mesh or not. If the bowel has undergone mechanical and antibiotic preparation, then an enterotomy with no spillage should not necessarily preclude the use of mesh. On the other hand, if there is gross spillage of enteric contents, then it may be more prudent to defer mesh placement for a later operation. Usually an interval of several days (with the patient receiving some intravenous antibiotics) is sufficient before a redo herniorrhaphy may be safely attempted. A more difficult decision arises in the patient who has had an enterotomy with a "little bit" of spillage. It is difficult to provide a strong recommendation in this situation, so this will fall into the judgment of the operating surgeon.

Delayed perforation/leak is the most problematic postoperative complication of minimally invasive ventral hernia repair. The surgeon should have a high index of suspicion for this complication, because often the patient can have minimal symptoms. If a perforation is suspected, then the first diagnostic procedure should be a contrast CT scan. If this indicates a leak, then a mesh explantation should be performed. Whether or not this can be performed laparoscopically depends on the status of the patient's abdomen. Distention of the bowel with florid peritonitis probably should be managed with a laparotomy.

Small bowel obstruction after minimally invasive herniorrhaphy may occur secondary to herniation of the bowel over the mesh, which may be a result of poor mesh anchorage or inadequate mesh overlap. In order to avoid this scenario, mesh overlap and anchorage should be performed as described earlier. Alternatively, the patient may have a simple adhesive obstruction. A suspected bowel obstruction after this procedure should be managed like any other postoperative bowel obstruction.

Seroma occurs in virtually all patients. The utilization of a binder may minimize formation of a seroma. An asymptomatic seroma may be managed expectantly, as these will resolve spontaneously. In this situation there is no need to aspirate or drain the fluid collection; doing so may cause an infection. If the patient has signs or symptoms of infection within the seroma, however, then a diagnostic tap would be indicated, followed by appropriate operative management.

RESULTS AND OUTCOME

A few small, randomized trials have demonstrated the superiority of minimally invasive ventral hernia repair over the open approach with respect to perioperative results (e.g., length of hospital stay, pain, recovery time, infection rate). In addition, multiple retrospective analyses support the notion that the incidence of recurrence is lower with the laparoscopic approach. In a review of over 6000 minimally invasive ventral hernia repairs performed by experienced surgeons, the overall recurrence rate was 3%. The issue of recurrence in laparoscopic versus open ventral herniorrhaphy ultimately will need to be settled with randomized trials that have large numbers of patients observed for more than 5 years. Admittedly, minimally invasive herniorrhaphy can be challenging and tedious, especially in the patient with a massive hernia and extensive adhesions. The authors of this chapter abandoned open hernia repair in the early 1990s. Similar to cholecystectomy, the advantages of the laparoscopic approach in the repair of ventral hernia seemed to be quite obvious.

Suggested Reading

Carlson MA, Frantzides CT, Shostrom VK, Laguna LE: Minimally invasive ventral herniorrhaphy: An analysis of 6266 published cases. Hernia 2008;12:9–22.

Condon RE: Incisional hernia. In Nyhus LM, Condon RE (eds): Hernia. Philadelphia, Lippincott, 1995, pp 319–328.

Frantzides CT, Carlson MA: Technical factors predisposing to recurrence after minimally invasive incisional herniorrhaphy. In Schumpelick V, Fitzgibbons RJ (eds): Recurrent Herniation. New York, Springer Verlag, 2007, pp 170–178.

Frantzides CT, Carlson MA, Zografakis JG, et al: Minimally invasive incisional herniorrhaphy: A review of 208 cases. Surg Endosc 2004;18:1488–1491.

Heniford BT, Park A, Ramshaw BJ, Voeller G: Laparoscopic repair of ventral hernias: Nine years' experience with 850 consecutive hernias. Ann Surg 2003;238:391–399; discussion 399–400.

LeBlanc KA: Incisional hernia repair: Laparoscopic techniques. World J Surg 2005;29:1073–1079.

Rudmik LR, Schieman C, Dixon E, Debru E: Laparoscopic incisional hernia repair: A review of the literature. Hernia 2006;10:110–119.

Stoppa RE: The treatment of complicated groin and incisional hernias. World J Surg 1989;13:545–554.

Wantz GE: Atlas of Hernia Surgery. New York, Raven Press, 1991.

CONSTANTINE T. FRANTZIDES, ATUL K. MADAN, AND
MARK A. CARLSON

Laparoscopic Repair of Diaphragmatic Hernia Not Involving the Hiatus

The most common diaphragmatic hernia in the adult involves the esophageal hiatus. Unless otherwise specified, diaphragmatic hernia in this chapter will refer to a hernia not involving this hiatus. Diaphragmatic hernia in adults can be congenital or acquired (e.g., from trauma). Traumatic diaphragmatic hernia can be acute or chronic. Acute traumatic diaphragmatic hernia traditionally was approached via a laparotomy, and chronic traumatic diaphragmatic hernia was approached via thoracotomy. It now is feasible to approach both acute and chronic traumatic diaphragm hernias through the laparoscope. Congenital diaphragmatic hernias, though uncommon in adults, typically occur from incomplete fusion of the posterolateral foramina of the diaphragm (Bochdalek hernia) or at anterior midline through the sternocostal region of diaphragm (Morgagni hernia) (Fig. 30-1). The Bochdalek hernia is the more common of the two, and it occurs on the left side in 90% of the cases. Operative management of diaphragmatic hernia is not altered by the specific cause of the hernia. The benefits of laparoscopic repair of diaphragmatic hernia include improved operative visualization, less postoperative pain and narcotic requirement, shorter hospital stay, and quicker recovery.

OPERATIVE INDICATIONS

The presence of a diaphragmatic hernia typically is indication for repair in the patient who can tolerate a general anesthetic, because these hernias have a high risk of developing a complication. The timing of operation usually is dictated by the patient's symptoms. For patients who have obstructive symptoms such as nausea, vomiting, or pain, urgent repair is necessary. For those patients in whom the hernia is found incidentally, an elective repair can be performed. Any patient with a diaphragmatic hernia who will be observed should be followed carefully, with immediate repair undertaken if signs or symptoms of strangulation or obstruction occur.

PREOPERATIVE EVALUATION, TESTING, AND PREPARATION

A symptomatic hernia presents with nausea, vomiting, pain, or difficulty breathing. In patients who have traumatic diaphragmatic hernias, a history of trauma may or may not be obvious. There may be a vague history of trauma years before the diagnosis of the diaphragmatic hernia. The asymptomatic hernia typically is incidentally found on a radiologic examination performed for some other indication. The first diagnostic test should be an upright chest x-ray. Air-fluid levels above the diaphragm may be apparent. If the chest x-ray is nondiagnostic, then a computed tomography (CT) scan can be obtained. In addition, upper or lower gastrointestinal radiologic studies may diagnose a diaphragmatic hernia. A contrast study should be performed with water-soluble medium if a diaphragmatic hernia is suspected. After diagnosis, typical preoperative testing will depend on the patient's overall medical condition. A bowel preparation may be performed if there is a concern of colon involvement. If there is evidence of a subacute colonic obstruction secondary to the hernia, then standard bowel preparation may be risky secondary to the risk of colonic perforation.

PATIENT POSITIONING AND TROCAR PLACEMENT

The patient is placed in the low lithotomy position with the addition of reverse Trendelenburg positioning. A bean bag and straps are helpful in securing the patient to the operating room table. The surgeon stands between the patient's legs, while the camera operator stands on the patient's right and the first assistant stands on the patient's left. In addition to the laparoscopic equipment and instrumentation, a thoracostomy tube or thoracic decompression needle should be available in case a tension pneumothorax develops. The patient's abdomen and thorax are sterilely prepared and draped from the neck to the groin in case a thoracostomy tube is required.

The placement of the trocars resembles that for a Nissen fundoplication (Fig. 30-2; see also Chapter 3). All trocar incisions are made after infiltration of local anesthetic at the port site. The camera is placed in the more caudad midline trocar (trocar 5). The liver retractor (if needed) is placed in the subxiphoid trocar (trocar 4). The surgeon utilizes the right upper quadrant trocar (trocar 2) for the left hand and the more medial left upper quadrant trocar (trocar 1) for the right hand. The assistant utilizes the most lateral left upper quadrant trocar (trocar 3). Either the assistant or camera operator can retract the liver.

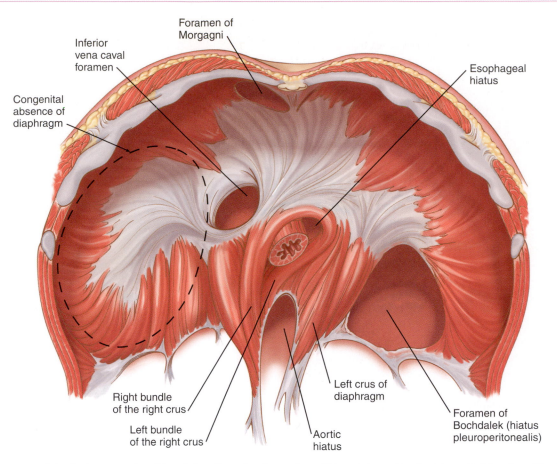

FIGURE 30-1 Typical anatomy of the diaphragm, as viewed from below. Note that the esophageal hiatus is formed by the right and left bundles of the right diaphragmatic crus; typically, the left crus is not involved.

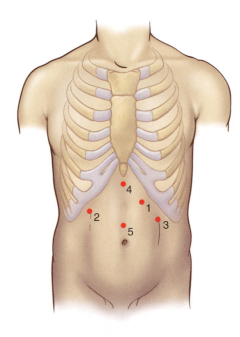

FIGURE 30-2 Port placement for a laparoscopic diaphragmatic hernia repair (same placement as performed for a laparoscopic Nissen fundoplication; see Chapter 3).

OPERATIVE TECHNIQUE

Exposure

The amount and type of the hernia contents can determine the difficulty of the procedure (Fig. 30-3). The key instruments required for this repair are atraumatic graspers, a stapler, and a suturing device. After the trocars have been placed, the area of the diaphragm involved with the hernia should be exposed. If necessary, the left lobe of the liver can be mobilized by dividing the left triangular ligament. If the defect is on the right side, a balloon retractor can be utilized to push the liver caudad. On the left side, the left lobe of the liver and the spleen may need to be retracted to expose the hernia and its incarcerated contents. All these manipulations should be done with atraumatic instruments and retractors.

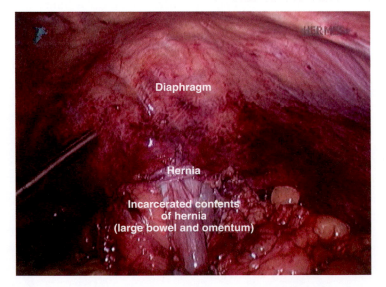

FIGURE 30-3 Intraoperative view of a diaphragmatic hernia, demonstrating incarceration of the omentum and colon.

Dissection

The dissection of the diaphragmatic hernia requires reduction of the hernia contents and the sac. The reduction of the hernia contents often is the most challenging task of this procedure. The reduction of the hernia contents and sac might be accomplished with some traction from atraumatic graspers (Atraugrip, Specialty Surgical Instrumentation, Nashville, TN) (Fig. 30-4). More commonly, however, the reduction can be tedious and difficult. The best method is to employ sharp dissection along the edge of the defect and the hernia contents. Care should be taken not to injure the herniating viscera. Sometimes the reduction can be facilitated by incising the diaphragm and enlargening the hernia defect. After reduction of the hernia contents, a thorough inspection of the reduced viscera should be done to ensure that there is no injury or areas of ischemia.

Communication with the anesthesiologist is important during the hernia reduction, because a tension pneumothorax can develop. Often the chest cavity can be seen after the reduction (Fig. 30-5), so the surgical team should be aware of this risk. The pneumothorax can decrease the lung volume and increase the peak inspiratory pressures. If the patient is stable, then the elevated pressures can be compensated by increasing the patient's respiratory rate in order to maintain the same minute ventilation (see "Procedure-Specific Complications").

Defect Closure

After reduction of the hernia contents and the sac, closure of the defect sometimes can be accomplished with sutures. The Endo Stitch device (U.S. Surgical, Norwalk, CT) is useful in performing a diaphragmatic herniorrhaphy because the rigidity of its arms facilitates suturing at awkward angles. Extracorporeal or intracorporeal suturing can be utilized. We prefer extracorporeal tying, because it is easier to control the amount of tension on the suture. Sutures alone may be sufficient with an acute traumatic diaphragmatic hernia. Prior to tying the last suture, the anesthesiologist should give the patient a sustained, large tidal volume while the intra-abdominal pressure is lowered. This step will expand the lung and evacuate the air from the thorax into the peritoneal cavity.

For chronic hernias, mesh usually is needed for the repair. If the defect is closed under tension, an onlay patch should be placed over the suture line. Suture repair of a traumatic diaphragmatic hernia is shown in Figure 30-6; because this suture line appeared to be under tension, an onlay patch subsequently was placed. Occasionally the diaphragmatic defect is so large that mesh is required to bridge the diaphragmatic gap. Mesh reinforcement may be considered for almost all diaphragmatic hernias (either as an onlay or as a bridge). The exception is the small acute traumatic diaphragmatic hernia that can be closed without tension.

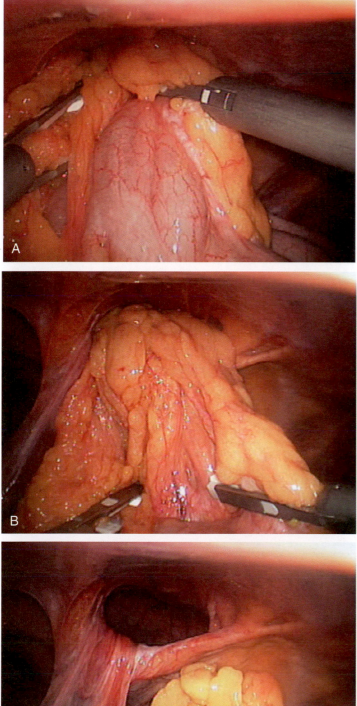

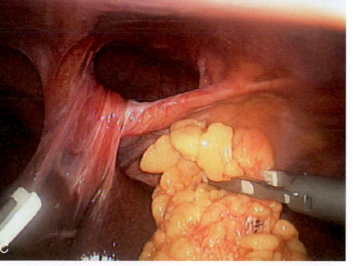

FIGURE 30-4 A to C, Sequential images showing a reduction of the hernia contents in a Morgagni hernia.

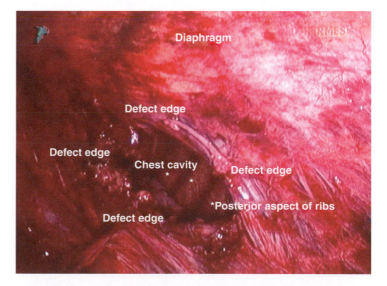

FIGURE 30-5 Defect of a diaphragmatic hernia after reduction of the hernia contents. The chest cavity with the ribs is visible through the defect.

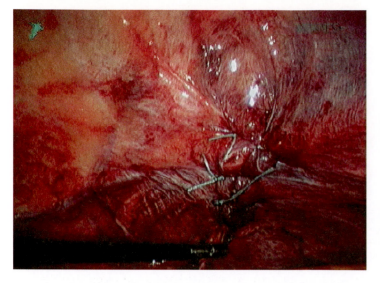

FIGURE 30-6 Suture repair of a diaphragmatic defect. This repair was under tension, so a mesh onlay was applied to complete the repair.

Generally speaking, the diaphragm is under constant physical stress, such as from respiratory and cardiac motion. In addition, coughing, sneezing, straining, and exercising also will stress the repair. Therefore, repair of diaphragmatic hernia with mesh makes sense considering these constant stressors.

Mesh Repair

Various types of mesh can be utilized for a diaphragmatic hernia repair. Polytetrafluoroethylene (PTFE) mesh is our choice for the repair of a diaphragmatic hernia in a noncontaminated field. Although polypropylene mesh has been suggested for these repairs, the risk for adhesion formation and erosion into the gastrointestinal tract outweighs the benefit of extensive tissue ingrowth. PTFE causes fewer adhesions and has been shown to follow the normal diaphragmatic motion under fluoroscopy. The major disadvantage of PTFE is poor resistance to infection; polypropylene is considered to be more resilient to infection than PTFE. In addition to single-component mesh products, there are mesh composites that utilize one side of polypropylene and a barrier on the other side to decrease the amount of adhesion formation. Furthermore, there are "biologic" mesh products, such as those employing cadaveric human skin or small intestine submucosa. These biologic meshes may be employed if a defect is present in a contaminated field.

Similar to minimally invasive ventral hernia repair, the mesh should overlap the defect on all sides with a minimum of 3 to 4 cm (see Chapter 29, on ventral hernia repair). Placement of the mesh typically involves at least two anchoring sutures at either end to facilitate orientation and manipulation of the mesh. The mesh then can be sutured, stapled, or tacked to the diaphragm. Tack fixation of the mesh near the tendinous portion of the diaphragm, which tends to be much thinner than the rest of the diaphragm, can be dangerous secondary to the risk of cardiac injury. Suturing of the mesh also can be done, but often the angles are quite awkward. Thus, the authors recommend the use of the laparoscopic hernia stapler. The stapler can be slowly activated which exposes the staple legs in a staged fashion. One leg then can grab the mesh (like a hook), while the other leg can bite into the diaphragm (see Fig. 29-5, which shows this technique). When utilizing the stapler in this manner, the surgeon is not required to use heavy pressure on the diaphragm in order to anchor the mesh; this should reduce the risk of cardiac injury. Staples are

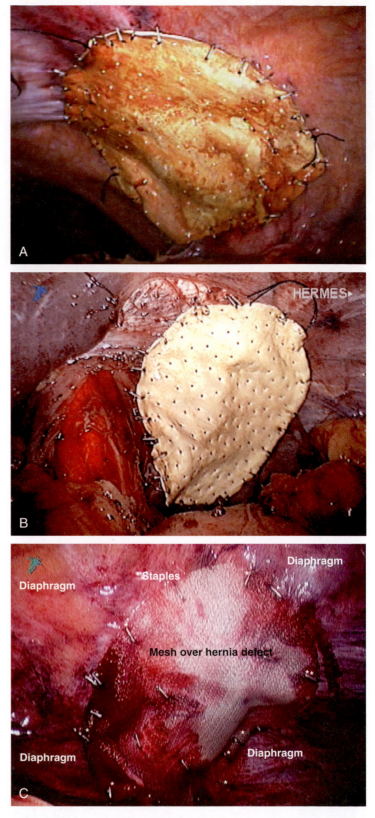

FIGURE 30-7 Completed diaphragmatic hernia repairs with PTFE mesh (A and B) or with polypropylene mesh (C). All three repairs underwent fixation with a stapler.

placed at 1-cm intervals around the mesh periphery. Completed diaphragmatic hernia repairs are shown in Figure 30-7.

POSTOPERATIVE CARE

The patient usually may be extubated on the operating room table. In the recovery room, an upright chest x-ray should be obtained; a small residual pneumothorax is not uncommon, and treatment is not necessary unless the patient is symptomatic. A baseline chest x-ray also is useful in case the patient later develops some respiratory symptoms. Aggressive respiratory toilet is indicated whether or not the patient has any symptoms. Most patients can be started on clear liquids and mobilized by the first evening. An elevated white blood cell count, fever, tachycardia, or severe abdominal pain in the postoperative period should raise the suspicion of a missed gastrointestinal injury. If the patient's pain is under control and there is no concern of missed injury, then the patient may be discharged the first postoperative day. For more difficult cases, discharge is usually delayed for several days.

PROCEDURE-SPECIFIC COMPLICATIONS

Intraoperative pneumothorax during laparoscopic diaphragmatic hernia repair can produce tachycardia, desaturation, and intra-abdominal protrusion of the hemidiaphragm. If the patient is hemodynamically stable, then the laparoscopic procedure can be continued following reduction of the intra-abdominal pressure to 10 mm Hg. The anesthesiologist can increase the respiratory frequency and closely monitor the patient. It usually is not necessary to introduce a chest tube, and the procedure can be finished without conversion. Prior to removal of the trocars, the pneumoperitoneum should be completely evacuated in order to minimize a residual pneumothorax. The anesthesiologist can perform a Valsalva maneuver with 40 cm water pressure while the trocar valves are open. If the patient develops hemodynamic instability secondary to the pneumothorax, then the pneumoperitoneum should be evacuated. If the patient does not dramatically improve after the evacuation of the pneumoperitoneum, then a thoracostomy tube or decompression needle should be utilized. Again, constant communication with the anesthesiologist is required throughout the whole case. Hypercarbia also may occur and may be aggravated by the decrease in the tidal volume after a pneumothorax. Hypercarbia can be compensated by increasing the respiratory rate (see Chapter 32).

Inadvertent visceral injury can occur during this procedure, and the best treatment is prevention. Gentle traction, use of atraumatic graspers, and possibly incising the rim of the defect may help prevent visceral injury. Any organ that was incarcerated should be carefully inspected. Any injury should be repaired or resected. If the gastrointestinal tract is entered, then PTFE mesh probably should not be utilized. Injury to the pericardium or the heart can result in hemopericardium with tamponade that may require emergent thoracotomy. Deep bites of sutures and excessive pressure while using the hernia stapler should be avoided during the repair.

RESULTS AND OUTCOME

Minimally invasive repair of diaphragmatic hernia not involving the esophageal hiatus is not a common procedure, and most centers do not have a large operative experience with this condition. The short-term results for this repair typically are quite good, though; most patients are able to leave the hospital within 1 to 2 days. No long-term recurrence data are available, but there is no evidence of a recurrence issue in the available literature. More important, the need for a laparotomy or thoracotomy is avoided with the laparoscopic repair.

Suggested Reading

Frantzides CT, Carlson MA: Laparoscopic repair of a penetrating injury to the diaphragm: A case report. J Laparoendosc Surg 1994;4(2):153–156.

Frantzides CT, Carlson MA, Pappas C, Gatsoulis N: Laparoscopic repair of a congenital diaphragmatic hernia in an adult. J Laparoendosc Adv Surg Tech A 2000;10(5):287–290.

Frantzides CT, Madan AK, O'Leary PJ, Losurdo J: Laparoscopic repair of a recurrent chronic traumatic diaphragmatic hernia. Am Surg 2003;69(2):160–162.

Frantzides CT, Madan AK, Zografakis JG: Laparoscopic repair of incarcerated diaphragmatic hernia. J Laparoendosc Adv Surg Techs 2007;17:39–42.

Huttl TP, Lang R, Meyer G: Long-term results after laparoscopic repair of traumatic diaphragmatic hernias. J Trauma 2002;52(3):562–566.

Matthews BD, Bui H, Harold KL, et al: Laparoscopic repair of traumatic diaphragmatic injuries. Surg Endosc 2003;17(2):254–258.

Yavuz N, Yibitbasi R, Sunamak O, et al: Laparoscopic repair of Morgagni hernia. Surg Laparosc Endosc Percutan Tech 2006;16(3):173–176.

SECTION

General Topics

IX

CHARLES E. EDMISTON, JR.

Antimicrobial Prophylaxis in the Era of Laparoscopic Surgery

31

Postoperative surgical site infections (SSIs) are associated with significant morbidity and mortality, especially in high-risk patient populations.[1-3] The probability of a patient developing a postoperative SSI is influenced by selected intrinsic and extrinsic risk factors present at the time of surgery.[1,4-7] It is estimated that 750,000 SSIs occur in the United States each year, resulting in increased patient morbidity and mortality rates and 3.7 million extra hospital days and costing over $1.6 billion in excess hospital charges each year.[6] Patients who develop an SSI have a greater likelihood of admission to the intensive care unit (60%), are more likely to be readmitted to the hospital (fivefold), and experience a higher mortality rate (twofold) than noninfected patients.[8] The fundamental cornerstones for reducing the risk of surgical site infection have included the following:

Exquisite surgical technique

Effective and persistent skin antisepsis

Timely and appropriate antimicrobial prophylaxis

Strategies for preventing postoperative surgical site infections require attention to infection control practices and appropriate patient care management. Three factors have been identified as influencing the development of a postoperative surgical site infection: (1) the patient's intrinsic risk factor, (2) extrinsic factors associated with the operation itself, and finally (3) virulence of selected microbial populations. The following discussion will focus upon these factors and the principles of antimicrobial surgical prophylaxis as emphasized by the current national initiatives, including the Surgical Care Improvement Project (SCIP) and its application to laparoscopic surgery.

MICROBIAL POPULATIONS ASSOCIATED WITH SURGICAL SITE INFECTIONS

Surgical site infections may be caused by endogenous or exogenous microbial contamination. Table 31-1 demonstrates the distribution of pathogens associated with surgical site infections in the United States. These data from the National Nosocomial Infection Surveillance (NNIS) program encompass two study intervals, 1986 to 1989 and 1990 to 1996.

Staphylococcus aureus is the most common surgical site pathogen at 20%, followed by *Staphylococcus epidermidis* (14%) and *Enterococcus* species at 12%. Overall, gram-positive pathogens are responsible for 53% of surgical site infections. *S. aureus* has been recognized to be a significant surgical pathogen since the late 19th century. Although *S. aureus* is recognized as the most virulent member of this genus, *S. epidermidis* is presently the most common pathogen recovered from biomedical device–related infections.[9] A recent study conducted in our laboratory has suggested that gram-positive microbial contamination of the surgical wound bed in vascular patients is likely a common occurrence and is more problematic during insertion of a biomedical device.[10] Presently, 73% of the *S. epidermidis* strains at our institution express resistance to the first-generation cephalosporins. This has potentially significant implications for the selection of a surgical prophylactic agent for patients undergoing clean (class I) surgical procedures and in some cases has prompted the substitution of a second-generation agent for selected surgical (cardiothoracic) procedures. According to data derived from the NNIS program, the incidence of methicillin-resistant *S. aureus* (MRSA) has increased from less than 2.5% in the mid-1970s to greater than 50% in 2005.[3,11] Furthermore, a recent study conducted by the Centers of Disease Control and Prevention (CDC) reported that the rate of hospitalization due to MRSA in the United States was highly variable, with the rate for MRSA hospitalization in patients under the age of 14 to be 13.1 per 1000 patient discharges, and the rate for patients older than 65 years of age was found to be 63.6 per 1000 patient discharges.[11] In addition, the emergence of community-acquired MRSA as colonizing flora in patients undergoing elective surgical procedures further threatens the potential efficacy of our current surgical prophylaxis regimens for clean/clean-contaminated procedures.[12]

The enterococci have been traditionally viewed as a second-class pathogen in surgery, often found as a component of normal flora and recovered in mixed infections. However, many enterococci express multidrug resistance, and drug susceptibility is highly variable, dependent upon the microbial species. In most institutions, *Enterococcus faecalis* is still highly sensitive to ampicillin (>90%), but greater than 80% of *Enterococcus faecium* strains will express resistance to ampicillin. Prior to 1994, the vast majority of hospital microbiology laboratories in the United States did not speciate the enterococci, but rather reported their results to genus level. It is obvious that with the emergence of these multiresistant strains greater efforts are needed to document the epidemiology of these organisms within the hospital environment. Susceptibility to other beta-lactam agents may also

Table 31-1 Predominant Microbial Pathogens Associated with Surgical Site Infections*

	Percentage of Isolates	
Organism	1986–1989	1990–1996
Staphylococcus aureus	17	20
Coagulase-negative staphylococci	12	14
Enterococcus species	13	12
Escherichia coli	10	8
Pseudomonas aeruginosa	8	8
Enterobacter species	8	7
Proteus mirabilis	4	3
Klebsiella pneumoniae	3	3
Streptococcus species	3	3
Candida albicans	2	3
Miscellaneous gram-positive organisms	—	4
Bacteroides fragilis	—	2

*National Nosocomial Infections Surveillance System, 1986–1996.
From Mangram AJ, Horan TC, Pearson ML, et al: The Hospital Infection Control Practice Advisory Committee: Guidelines for the prevention of surgical site infections. Am J Infect Control 1999;27:97–134.

demonstrate significant variation. While in some surveys sensitivities to piperacillin may exceed 90%, high rates or resistance (>95%) are demonstrated against many of the third-generation cephalsporins.[13]

Data from the NNIS hospitals suggest that gram-negative microorganisms continue to be a significant cause of illness and even death for surgical patients. *Pseudomonas aeruginosa* is currently responsible for approximately 9% of surgical site infections, while *Enterobacter, Escherichia coli* and *Klebsiella pneumoniae* occur as nosocomial SSI pathogens approximately 8.8%, 7.1%, and 3.5% of the time, respectively. Anaerobic bacteria, on the other hand, such as the gram-negative *Bacteroides fragilis*, occur as surgical site pathogens less than 3% of the time.[1]

ENDOGENOUS VERSUS EXOGENOUS SOURCES OF INTRAOPERATIVE CONTAMINATION

Historically, most SSIs have been viewed as derived from the patient's own endogenous flora, whether from the skin or the pharyngeal or gastrointestinal tract. For instance, vascular, orthopedic, or plastic surgical procedures often involve the skin or skin structures and therefore tend to involve a gram-positive flora if infection occurs; general surgical procedures involving the gastrointestinal tract have a more gram-negative focus. Alternatively, exogenous contamination may occur within the intraoperative environment as a result of contaminated instruments, breaks in aseptic technique, or from members of the surgical team. Studies conducted in our institution have shown that potential surgical pathogens, both gram-positive and gram-negative, are present in the air of the operating room environment.[10,14] As a result of these findings, a special effort needs to be undertaken to ensure that biomedical devices (orthopaedic implants, abdominal mesh, etc.) have limited exposure to operating room air during insertion.

The infecting dose required to produce a postoperative SSI in a clean surgical wound has been determined to be in the order of magnitude of 5 $\log_{10}$ colony-forming units or greater per gram of tissue.[15] This value was from studies conducted in experimental

animal models of infection. The inoculum size, however, required to produce an infection is diminished when an inert foreign body is present in the wound. It has been suggested that 100 microorganisms or less per gram of tissue may be sufficient to produce a biomedical-associated infection.[16] Unfortunately, patients presenting for surgery in 2008 are often high-risk, exhibiting multiorgan disease states and demonstrating varying levels of anergy. Therefore, it is likely that patients with diminished phagocytic cell function and poor wound healing characteristics, such as in the diabetic patient, are at higher risk for infection and that the microbial threshold dose for producing a postoperative infection is less well defined in this patient population.

PROBLEMATIC RISK FACTORS ASSOCIATED WITH SURGICAL SITE INFECTIONS

Univariate and multivariate analysis has been used to analyze the association of known risk factors to the subsequent development of surgical site infection. Table 31-2 identifies several factors that may influence the risk of developing a surgical site infection. Previous scientific studies have demonstrated that diminished leukocytic cell function and poor wound healing occurs in patients with hyperglycemia.[17–19] Recent studies have documented the relationship of hyperglycemia to infection in the critically ill patient population.[20–22] Advanced age has historically been viewed as a suggestive risk factor for infection following surgery; however, pragmatically it is difficult to separate the aging process from the various comorbid conditions that frequently occur in the elderly patient, predisposing one to infection.[23] The risk factors associated with surgical site infection can be categorized as either patient- or treatment-related.[24,25] Two recent publications have documented that obesity (body mass index > 30) is an important risk factor associated with occurrence of SSI.[26,27] The possible explanation for this increased risk likely resides with patient comorbidity (diabetes mellitus), physiologic factors such as hypoperfusion resulting in reduced blood flow, reduced oxygen tension in adipose tissues, and the large volume of distribution which may limit the distribution of perioperative antimicrobial prophylaxis.[28] Current efforts to reduce the risk of surgical site infections under the collaborative auspices

Table 31-2 Patient-Related (Intrinsic) and Treatment-Related (Extrinsic) Risk Factors for Surgical Site Infection

Patient-Related Factors	Treatment-Related Factors
Patient gender	Surgical wound environment
Patient age	Surgical scrub
Nutritional status	Surgical skin preparation
Diabetes/hypergylcemia	Hair removal
Smoking	Duration of surgery
Severity of disease—ASA score	Perioperative prophylaxis
Immunocompetence	Operating room ventilation
Weight	Drains and packs
Presence of other infections	Surgical attire and drapes
Perioperative hypothermia	Poor hemostasis
Malignancy	Dead space
Microbial host colonization	Tissue trauma

From Mangram AJ, Horan TC, Pearson ML, et al: The Hospital Infection Control Practice Advisory Committee: Guidelines for the prevention of surgical site infections. Am J Infect Control 1999;27:97–134.

of SCIP have focused on selective patient- and treatment-related risk factors such as glycemic control, proper hair removal, and appropriate antimicrobial prophylaxis.

Another area of continued controversy is the role that *S. aureus* nares colonization plays in the development of a postoperative surgical site infection. Mupirocin, a topical antibiotic, has been shown to be effective for eliminating *S. aureus* from the anterior nares of both patients and health care professionals. Recently, this agent has been used in selective surgical services in combination with active surveillance cultures to identify potential patients colonized with MRSA prior to elective surgical procedures.[29,30] The response to this phenomenon has been the implementation of decolonization protocol for selected patients. A study utilizing cardiothoracic patients has suggested that mupirocin when applied preoperatively to the nares resulted in reduced risk of SSIs.[31] However, a recent report from a Veterans Administration Hospital quite clearly demonstrated that the use of mupirocin to control endemic MRSA resulted in the recovery of MRSA *S. aureus* isolates exhibiting high-level resistance to mupirocin.[32] The precise role for this compound in the surgical patient population is yet to be determined. Clearly, *S. aureus* carriage appears to be a significant independent risk factor for surgical site infection following selected surgical procedures; however, further studies are needed to assess the most effective and judicious use of this agent in the surgical patient population.

Several treatment-related factors have also been suggested as contributing to the risk of surgical site infections. The environment within the surgical wound is an obvious factor; procedures involving the gastrointestinal tract will expose the wound to potential contamination involving a myriad of microbial population, yet a breast biopsy will have a much lower risk for contamination. An effective antimicrobial tissue (wound) concentration during the intraoperative period plays an obvious role in resolving potential wound contamination and is the current subject of a focused national initiative (SCIP).

LAPAROSCOPIC SURGERY VERSUS OPEN SURGICAL PROCEDURES: IS THE RISK OF INFECTION THE SAME?

For over 30 years, the NNIS system (now known as the National Healthcare Safety Network [NHSN]) has been an ongoing collaborative sponsored by the CDC to obtain national data on nosocomial infections.[33] The data are reported voluntarily by participating hospitals to estimate the magnitude of the nosocomial risk in the United States and to monitor trends in infections and risk factors. The data derived from this program are used to establish thresholds for selected hospital-associated infections, including SSIs. Detailed information including demographic characteristics, infections and related risk factors, pathogens and their antimicrobial susceptibilities, and outcome is collected on each infected patient. The goal of the NHSN is to use surveillance data to develop and evaluate strategies to prevent and control nosocomial infections. The data collected with the use of the surveillance components permit the calculation of risk-specific infection rates, which can be used by individual hospitals as well as national health care planners to set priorities for their infection control programs and to evaluate the effectiveness of their efforts. The risk index comprises three variables: operative time, American Society of Anesthesiologists (ASA) score, and wound class. For example, a patient who undergoes a surgical procedure that falls outside of the 75th percentile for operative time is deemed at risk for

wound infection and assigned a risk of 1. This same patient who at the time of surgery is assessed an ASA score of 3 or higher would receive another 1 risk point. Finally, if this patient is undergoing a surgical procedure that involves a potential contaminate or dirty wound he or she would be assigned an additional 1 risk point. In theory, therefore, our patient might have a risk index score ranging from 0 (no risk factors) to 3 (highest risk).[2] The higher the risk index, the greater potential for development of a surgical site infection.

The use of a laparoscope has been incorporated into the NNIS SSI risk index. It has been generally recognized that when other risk factors are controlled, selected laparoscopic cholecystectomy, appendectomy, and gastric procedures have a lower SSI rate compared to open procedures, especially at the low end of the risk index. The NNIS data in Table 31-3 illustrate this point, demonstrating that at the lowest risk strata (0) the mean threshold infection rate for a laparoscopically performed appendectomy, cholecystectomy, and gastric procedure is lower than the expected rate for a similar open surgical procedure. As the risk category increases, however, the open and laparoscopic threshold rates for these surgical procedures converge and are essentially the same. An exception, however, is noted for laparoscopically performed appendectomy, where the laparoscopic threshold rate is lower (3.3) with patients in risk category 2 compared to open cases (4.6) with the same risk index. Unfortunately, at present the laparoscopic NNIS data pool is limited to four operative procedure categories, but the future growth of hospital-based laparoscopic programs will likely increase this data set significantly.

Two publications in the early laparoscopic era suggested that one of the benefits associated with minimally invasive surgery was a reduction in the postoperative infection rate.[34,35] Several randomized clinical trials have documented reduced patient adverse events (morbidity) following laparoscopic cholecystectomy, colorectal resection, appendectomy, gastric resection and laparoscopic splenectomy.[36-38] Although minimally invasive surgery led to a revolutionary change in the way in which surgical patients are managed, infectious complications are still noted and when they occur are often problematic. A group in Buenos Aires reporting on 1577 laparoscopic cholecystectomies, documented 294 cases

Table 31-3 Surgical Site Infection (SSI) Rates and Risk Index Categories for Selected General Open and Laparoscopic Surgical Procedures

Procedure	Open Procedures		Laparoscopic Procedures	
	Risk Index	Mean SSI Rate (Pooled)	Risk Index	SSI Rate
Appendectomy	0	1.3	0	0.7
Appendectomy	2 or 3	4.6	2	3.3
Cholecystectomy	0	0.7	0	0.7
Cholecystectomy	2	3.3	2	3.3
Small bowel	1	7.1	—	—
Small bowel	2	8.6	—	—
Colon	1	5.7	1	5.6
Colon	3	11.3	3	11.2
Gastric	0	2.6	0	0.7
Gastric	2 or 3	8.3	2 or 3	8.3
Herniorrhaphy	0	0.8	—	—
Herniorrhaphy	2 or 3	4.5	—	—

From National Nosocomial Infections Surveillance (NNIS) System Report: Data summary from January 1992 through June 2004, issued October 2004. Am J Infect Control 2004;32:470–485.

(18.6%) of intraperitoneal bile spillage, which resulted in 15 (5.1%) umbilical surgical site infections. The infection rate in the cases without gallbladder effraction was 1.3% (17 cases). Wound healing in the group without gallbladder injury was uneventful, whereas 3 of the 15 cases involving bile leakage were associated with persistent infection of 2 to 8 months, requiring secondary operation to remove stones from the retroperitoneum or subcutaneous tissues.[39] An interesting paper recently published by investigators at the CDC looked at the impact of laparoscopic cholecystectomy on postoperative surgical site infections. An epidemiologic analysis was performed on data collected over a 7-year period by participating NNIS hospitals. Demographic data from 54,504 inpatient cholecystectomies were collected; there were 18,079 open and 36,425 laparoscopic procedures. The number of laparoscopic cholecystectomies performed at NNIS hospitals increased from 59% in 1992 to 79% in 1999. Overall there were 554 (1%) SSIs reported during the 7-year study period. The most common site for infection in both groups was superficial incisional; however, the number of organ-site infections was higher in the laparoscopic than in the open group (48% vs. 36%, $p < 0.006$). Overall, the site-specific infection rate was substantially lower in the laparoscopic group (0.15 per 100 operations) compared to the open (0.87 per 100 operations) group ($p < 0.001$). In both groups the major microbial pathogens were gram-positive. Most of the SSIs in the open groups were detected during hospitalization, but the majority of SSIs in the laparoscopic group were detected during postdischarge follow-up or readmission. Although overall risk of SSI was deemed low in the laparoscopic group, several risk factors were identified as independent predictors of postlaparoscopic surgical site infection: operation duration, age above 60, contaminated or dirty wound, ASA score 3 or more, and multiple procedures performed through the same incision ($p < 0.001$).[40] The results from this study have several implications for risk reduction in patients undergoing a laparoscopic procedure, not the least of which is the role of antimicrobial prophylaxis.

A French group conducted a meta-analysis to analyze the influence of open versus laparoscopic appendectomy on development of postoperative wound infections. In their analysis the incidence of wound infection ranged from 0% to 10% in the laparoscopic group as opposed to 2% to 14.3% in the open group. Overall, the incidence of infection was threefold lower in the laparoscopic group than in open appendectomy.[41] The incidence of biomedical device implantation has increased dramatically over the past 15 years on all surgical services and many of these devices are now placed endoscopically. The incidence of mesh infection during open hernia repair is highly variable and dependent on site and patient risk factors. The incidence of mesh infection during open hernia repair has been reported to range from 0.8% to 3% in some series. A group of surgical investigators from New York City reported an inguinal mesh infection rate of 0.17% following laparoscopic surgery. This group has suggested two possible reasons for this low rate. First, the device is introduced aseptically through a trocar, avoiding contact with the incision. Second, the mesh is implanted some distance from the incisional wound, which may also avoid incisional contamination.[42] These are interesting suppositions, which may bear merit. Studies conducted in our laboratory suggest that wound and device contamination may occur following microbial shedding (venting) from the traditional surgical mask.[10] Therefore, a theoretical benefit of laparoscopic device placement may be limited access through the wound incision and protection (sequestering) of the device from environment (OR) contamination at the time of implantation.

While the role of laparoscopic surgery for colorectal cancer has been viewed with some controversy, a recent meta-analysis of 2071 patients undergoing laparoscopic or open rectal surgery suggests selected benefits are associated with the laparoscopic technique. In addition to a better postoperative recovery as measured by return to normal bowel function and shorter hospital stay, there was a significant difference in the wound infection rate between laparoscopic (0%) and open abdominoperineal resections (13.9%).[43] Other miscellaneous applications from our own institutional experience would suggest that laparoscopic Roux-en-Y for morbid obesity, kidney harvesting, and splenectomy is clearly superior to standard laparotomy in terms of postoperative complication, such as urinary tract infection, surgical site infections, and respiratory complications. Although the vast majority of laparoscopic abdominal surgeons would subscribe to the argument that laparoscopic surgery is associated with a lowered infection rate, the data are less clear for other endoscopic practitioners. Data from the Cleveland Clinic (1996–1998) would suggest that there was no difference in the overall or deep incision infection rate in patients undergoing minimally invasive cardiac procedures (1.9 per 100 cases, $N = 1400$) compared to traditional open-heart surgery (1.7 per 100 cases, $N = 9633$).[44]

FUNDAMENTALS OF ANTIMICROBIAL PROPHYLAXIS: CONSIDERATION FOR LAPAROSCOPIC SURGERY

In 2002 the Centers for Medicare and Medicaid Services (CMS) with the cooperation of the CDC initiated the Surgical Infection Prevention (SIP) project in an effort to decrease nationally the morbidity and mortality associated with surgical site infections. Subsequently, this initiative has stimulated the development of a broad-based collaboration involving the participation of federal, scientific, and professional societies, the Surgical Care Improvement Project (SCIP), which has a focused objective of reducing surgical morbidity and mortality rates by 25% by the year 2010. A major objective of this initiative has been to foster improvement in surgical antimicrobial prophylaxis, and three performance measures have been developed for national surveillance and quality improvement:

1. The proportion of patients who receive antimicrobial prophylaxis 1 hour prior to surgical incision
2. The proportion of patients who receive antimicrobial prophylaxis consistent with current published guidelines
3. The proportion of patients in which antimicrobial prophylaxis is discontinued within 24 hours

It is important to note that in 2004 the Joint Commission for Accreditation of Healthcare Organization (JCAHO) accepted these three performance standards, and hospitals will be expected to demonstrate compliance. Individual hospital compliance (and comparison to other hospitals) to these and other quality initiatives can be viewed on the CMS Web site (www.hospitalcompare.hhs.gov). These three measures were developed for selected surgical procedures such as coronary artery bypass, vascular surgery, colorectal procedures, total joint arthroplasty, and abdominal/vaginal hysterectomy, but the performance measures have been embraced by other surgical services and are appropriate for procedures involving both laparoscopic and tradition (open) surgical procedures. It is important to note that for the future, failure to report adherence to these performance measures will result in a 2% withholding (penalty) in Medicare reimbursement.

The scientific merit for appropriate antimicrobial prophylaxis has been known for over 40 years.[45,46] The early effort of these investigators clearly documented what has become the "bottom line" for appropriate surgical antimicrobial prophylaxis: an effective concentration of the antibiotic must be present in the wound prior to incisional contamination. The classic clinical study conducted by Classen and colleagues in the early 1990s validated the impact of earlier studies by demonstrating how failure to deliver the prophylactic agent in a timely fashion resulted in an increased surgical site infection rate.[47] Appropriate antimicrobial prophylaxis requires that three separate but linked events must occur or else the tangible benefit of perioperative antibiotic administration is diminished. First, the antibiotic must be given within 1 hour of surgical incision or the maximal benefit is lost.[47] This component of timing is dependent upon the pharmacokinetics of the drug, and for agents like cefazolin, the 1-hour timeline is optimal.[48]

Second, the patient must be dosed based upon weight. The clinical data in this area are scant and few patients are dosed prophylactically based on their body weight (mg/kg). As a general rule, surgical patients in our institution who are less than 70 kg receive a 1-g prophylactic dose, whereas patients over 70 kg are given a 2-g dose perioperatively. This dosing strategy, however, may not be adequate for some patients, especially those patients whose body mass indexes (BMIs) are in excess of 40. A study conducted in our institution in patients undergoing laparoscopic and open Roux-en-Y for morbid obesity (BMIs ranging from 40 to 92) revealed decreasing serum and tissue concentrations of cefazolin following a 2-g dose delivered within the 1-hour window prior to wound incision. Even in those patients that required a second intraoperative dose, the intraoperative tissue and serum concentrations at wound closure were subtherapeutic for the majority of bariatric patients.[28] In general, there is a paucity of data on antimicrobial dosing in the obese patient population. It is apparent that the empiric dosing recommendations that most surgical practitioners have been using for the past 30 years (especially for bariatric patients) are likely inadequate for our higher BMI patient populatons.[49,50] It is possible that in selective patients (BMI > 50) a higher perioperative prophylactic dose (3 g) is required to provide adequate intraoperative serum and tissue levels.

A final consideration involves the duration of postoperative antibiotic administration. Are there any exceptions to the rule? Data from studies conducted in cardiothoracic, orthopaedic, peripheral vascular, and colorectal surgery demonstrate no benefit for continuing antibiotic prophylaxis beyond the intraoperative interval.[51–56] It would appear that even in the presence of insertion of a biomedical device such as a vascular graft, orthopaedic implant, or abdominal mesh there is no systematic benefit for continuing prophylaxis beyond the operating room. The third CMS performance measure (the proportion of patients in which antimicrobial prophylaxis is discontinued within 24 hours) represents a liberal extension of the antibiotic duration principle.[57] From a purely fiscal perspective, single-dose antimicrobial prophylaxis would also appear in most circumstances to result in a significant cost saving to the hospital formulary.[58]

When the National Surgical Infection Prevention Project performed a retrospective analysis of 34,133 Medicare surgical patients in 2960 acute care hospitals the finding suggested that substantial opportunities existed for improving the use of antimicrobial prophylaxis in surgical patients. The study determined that although guideline-based prophylactic agents were used in 92.6% of surgical patients, the prophylactic dose was administered within 1 hour of the incision in 55.7% of surgical patients, and only 40.7% of patients

had their prophylactic antibiotic discontinued within 24 hours of surgery.[59] Under these circumstances it would appear that the vast majority of U.S. acute care hospitals are failing to comply with the CMS performance measures.

Is antimicrobial prophylaxis a required component of all laparoscopic surgical procedures? This answer is highly dependent on several factors, some of which were discussed in a previous section. The decision whether to use antimicrobial prophylaxis during laparoscopic surgery should be determined by intrinsic patient risk factors, potential for wound contamination, patient comorbidity, and clinical experience. What of procedures that already have a relatively low infection rate, such as laparoscopic cholecystectomy? Several papers have explored the role of antimicrobial prophylaxis for laparoscopic cholecystectomy. In a well-controlled, prospective study by Higgins and associates, the findings suggested that the use of prophylactic antibiotic in patients undergoing laparoscopic cholecystectomy is not justified; administration of a single prophylactic dose of cefazolin or cefotetan did not lower an already low infection rate.[59] The majority of patients in this study fell within risk class 0 or 1. Three recent studies (two prospective, one retrospective) involving a total of 2063 patients have drawn a similar conclusion, suggesting that routine antimicrobial prophylaxis is unwarranted in most laparoscopic cholecystectomies.[60–62] However, the authors indicated that selected patient risk factors may necessitate the need for single-dose antimicrobial prophylaxis, such as in patients presenting with colic within 30 days of surgery, the diabetic patient, or other high-risk scenarios. Dellinger has defined the high-risk laparoscopic patient as an individual over age 60 years, presenting with common bile duct stones, bile duct obstruction, recent acute cholecystitis, or previous biliary tract surgery.[63]

A similar rationale would apply as to whether or not prophylactic antimicrobial prophylaxis is used during laparoscopic hernia repair. Again, patient risk factors should always influence the decision whether or not to use antimicrobial prophylaxis. As discussed in a previous section, obesity should always be viewed as a potential risk factor for infection, because it is often difficult to achieve thorough skin antisepsis in the obese patient. In the absence of obesity, diabetes or hyperglycemia would be another cause for considering a single dose of antimicrobial prophylaxis, because granulocytic cell function is diminished in the hyperglycemic state, altering the phagocytic properties of these cells with the wound bed. Finally, antimicrobial prophylaxis should always be considered during any laparoscopic surgery in which the potential exists for wound contamination, especially involving proximal or distal gastrointestinal procedures.

The antimicrobial drug selected for surgical prophylaxis should mirror those agents which are currently used for open surgical procedures with one important caveat. Selection of a prophylactic agent for traditional or laparoscopic surgery will in the future be influenced by CMS (JCAHO) performance measures. Table 31-4 lists the current agents and dosing schedule for antibiotics approved for open and laparoscopic surgical procedures. These agents are effectively the only agents which have been deemed appropriate for antimicrobial prophylaxis by both CMS and JCAHO and are based upon published (evidenced-based) guidelines.[64] In the past, the second-generation cephalosporins cefotetan and cefoxitin were used for clean/contaminated procedures because of their broad-spectrum activity. Unfortunately, limited supplies of these two agents have been noted in several regions of the country. Recently there has been some interest in using ertapenem as an alternative prophylactic agent as replacement for cefotetan. Ertapenem is a once-daily parenteral agent with broad-spectrum activity for both gram-positive and gram-negative, aerobic and anaerobic bacteria. A recent randomized, double-blind clinical trial conducted in 1002 patients undergoing elective colorectal surgery, comparing the safety and efficacy of ertapenem to cefotetan, demonstrated that ertapenem was a superior prophylactic agent compared to cefotetan.[65] In many ways ertapenem is an ideal prophylactic agent for colorectal, contaminated, or dirty surgical procedures. Its long half-life, which allows for 24-hour therapeutic coverage, fits within the CMS-JCAHO mandated performance measures. In 2007, ertapenem was recognized by CMS as an appropriate agent for antimicrobial prophylaxis in clean-contaminated, contaminated, and dirty surgical procedures. It is obvious that the results of this recently published clinical trial has stimulated broad support for including ertapenem as one of the logical choices for antimicrobial prophylaxis in abdominal or colorectal surgery.

The current national initiative to improve the delivery (timing, choice, and duration) of antimicrobial prophylaxis has broad support from public, professional, and governmental organizations. In the past, institutional (health care) compliance to the overwhelming body of evidence supporting the cardinal principles of appropriate antimicrobial prophylaxis have been given minimal attention. In part, the difficulty of implementing an effective program has resided within the question of ownership. Who will ensure that the patient receives the right antibiotic, at the right time, for the right duration? The problem can best be summed up as follows, the current delivery systems ensuring that patients receive appropriate antimicrobial prophylaxis are woefully inadequate and changing the process requires the willingness of hospitals to redesign the system such that antimicrobial prophylaxis becomes an institutional priority. This will require the broad collegiality of surgeons, nurses, pharmacists, and the hospital administrators.[66] The laparoscopic revolution has had a significant impact on the delivery of quality surgical care. Adverse outcomes, however, can rapidly negate the beneficial impact of innovative technology. Therefore, appropriate antimicrobial prophylaxis remains an important adjunctive strategy for reducing the risk of surgical site infection, even in the era of laparoscopic surgery.

Table 31-4 Antimicrobial Agents Appropriate for Laparoscopic Surgical Procedures*

Surgical Procedure	Preferred Antibiotic (IV once)	Alternative Antibiotic for Life-Threatening Penicillin Allergy (IV once)

Cardiothoracic
  Coronary artery bypass
  Valve replacement/repair
	Cefuroxime 1.5 mg	Clindamycin 900 mg
		or
		Vancomycin 15 mg/kg × ___kg = _____mg
		  (round to nearest 250 mg)

General
  Appendectomy
	Cefotetan 1 g (<70 kg)
	Cefotetan 2 g (≥70 kg)
		Metronidazole 500 mg + gentamicin 2.5 mg/kg ×
		  ____kg = ____mg (round to nearest 10 mg) (gram-negative coverage)

General
  Clean procedures
    Esophageal
    Gastroduodenal/stomach
    Small bowel
  Clean-contaminated/contaminated
  procedures
    Colorectal
	Cefazolin 1 g (<70 kg)
	Cefazolin 2 g (≥70 kg)
	
	Cefotetan 1 g (<70 kg)
	Cefotetan 2 g (≥70 kg)
	or
	Ertapenem 1 g
		Clindamycin 900 mg
		
		Metronidazole 500 mg + gentamicin 2.5 mg/kg ×
		_____ kg = ___ mg (round to nearest 900 mg)

General
  Pancreas/whipple
  Liver/biliary
	Ciprofloxacin 400 mg	Ciprofloxacin 400 mg

Ear, nose, and throat Clean procedure	Penicillin G 2 million units (<70 kg) Penicillin G 4 million units (≥70 kg)	Clindamycin 900 mg

Ear, nose, and throat
  Laryngectomy, other head and neck
  cancer
	Ampicillin/sulbactam 3 g
	or
	Cefotetan 1 g (<70 kg)
	Cefotetan 2 g (≥70 kg)
		Clindamycin 900 mg

Gynecology/obstetrics
  C-section
    Abdominal/vaginal
	Cefazolin or cefotetan 1 g (<70 kg)
	Cefazolin or cefotetan 2 g (≥70 kg)
	Cefazolin 2 g (≥70 kg)
		Clindamycin 900 mg

Neurosurgery
  Craniotomy/shunt
  Spinal surgery
	Cefazolin 1 g (<70 kg)
	Cefazolin 2 g (≥70 kg)
		Clindamycin 900 mg
		or
		Vancomycin 15 mg/kg × ___kg = _____mg (round to
		nearest 250 mg)

Oral surgery Mandibular fractures	Penicillin G 2 million units (<70 kg) Penicillin G 4 million units (≥70 kg)	Clindamycin 900 mg

Table 31-4 Antimicrobial Agents Appropriate for Laparoscopic Surgical Procedures—cont'd*

Surgical Procedure	Preferred Antibiotic (IV once)	Alternative Antibiotic for Life-Threatening Penicillin Allergy (IV once)
Orthopedics Spinal surgery Total hip/knee	Cefazolin 1 g (<70 kg) Cefazolin 2 g (≥70 kg)	Clindamycin 900 mg or Vancomycin 15 mg/kg × ____ kg = ____ mg (round to nearest 250 mg)
Orthopedics/trauma Fracture repair Open fracture	Cefazolin 1 g (<70 kg) Cefazfolin 2 g (≥70 kg) + gentamicin 2.5 mg/kg × ____ kg = ____ mg (round to nearest 10 mg) (gram-negative coverage)	Clindamycin 900 mg + gentamicin 2.5mg/kg × ____ kg = ____ mg (round to nearest 10 mg) (gram-negative coverage)
Plastics	Cefazolin 1 g (<70 kg) Cefazolin 2 g (≥70 kg)	Clindamycin 900 mg or Vancomycin 15 mg/kg × ____ kg = ____ mg (round to nearest 250 mg)
Thoracic Lobectomy, tracheostomy	Cefuroxime 1.5 g	Clindamycin 900 mg
Trauma—penetrating abdominal	Ampicillin/sulbactam 3 g or Ertapenem 1 g	Clindamycin 900 mg + gentamicin 2.5 mg/kg × ____ kg = ____ mg (nearest 10mg) (gram-negative coverage)
Transplant—kidney	Cefazolin 1 g (<70 kg) Cefazolin 2 g (≥70 kg)	Clindamycin 900 mg
Transplant—liver	Cefazolin 2 g or Ertapenem 1 g	Ciprofloxacin 400 mg
Transplant—kidney/pancreas	Imipenem/cilastatin 500 mg + vancomycin 18 mg/kg × ____ kg = ____ mg (round to nearest 250 mg) + fluconazole 400 mg PO (on the floor)	Ciprofloxacin 400 mg + vancomycin 18 mg/kg × ____ kg = ____ mg (round to nearest 250 mg) + fluconazole 400 mg PO (on the floor)
Transplant—heart/lung	Cefuroxime 1.5 g	Vancomycin 18 mg/kg × ____ kg = ____ mg (round to nearest 250 mg)
Urology—prostatectomy	Cefazolin 1 g (<70 kg) Cefazolin 2 g (≥70 kg) or Ciprofloxacin 400 mg	Ciprofloxacin 400 mg
Urology—stents/sphincters	Cefazolin 1 g (<70 kg) Cefazolin 2 g (≥70 kg)	Clindamycin 900 mg
Vascular/endovascular	Cefazolin 1 g (<70 kg) Cefazolin 2 g (≥70 kg) or Cefuroxime 1.5 g or Vancomycin 15 mg/kg × ____ kg = ____ mg (round to nearest 250 mg)	Clindamycin 900 mg IV once or Vancomycin 15 mg/kg × ____ kg = ____ mg (round to the nearest 250 mg)

*Antimicrobial selection based on Center for Medicare and Medicaid Services (CMS) and Joint Commission for Accreditation of Healthcare Organizations (JCAHO) approved agents used at Froedtert Hospital, Milwaukee, WI, 2008.
Selections, in part, based on Fry D: The surgical infection prevention project: Processes, outcomes and future impact. Surg Infect 2006;7:517; Bratzler DW, Houck PM: Antimicrobial prophylaxis for surgery: An advisory statement from the National Surgical Prevention Project. Clin Infect Dis 2004;38:1706.

References

1. Mangram AJ, Horan TC, Pearson ML, et al, The Hospital Infection Control Practice Advisory Committee: Guidelines for the prevention of surgical site infections. Am J Infect Control 1999;27:97–134.
2. Engemann JJ, Carmeli Y, Cosgrove SE, et al: Adverse and economic outcomes attributable to methicillin-resistance among patients with Staphylococcus aureus surgical site infection. Clin Infect Dis 2003;36:592–598.
3. National Nosocomial Infections Surveillance (NNIS) System Report, data summary from January 1992 through June 2004, issued October 2004. Am J Infect Control 2004;32:470–485.
4. Edmiston CE: Surgical site infection control in the critical care environment. In Rello J, Vanes J, Kollef M (eds): Critical Care Infectious Disease. Boston, Kluwer Academic Press, 2001, pp 817–831.
5. Shoemaker CP: Changes in the general surgical workload, 1991–1999. Arch Surg 2003;138:417–426.
6. Zhan C, Miller MR: Excess length of stay, charges, and mortality attributable to medical injuries during hospitalization. JAMA 2003;290:1868–1874.
7. Seal LA, Paul-Cheadle D: A systems approach to preoperative surgical patient skin preparation. Am J Infect Control 2004;32:57–62.
8. Kirkland KB, Briggs JP, Trivette SL, et al: The impact of surgical site infections in the 1990s: Attributable mortality, excess length of hospitalization, and extra costs. Infect Control Hosp Epidemiol 1999;20:725–730.
9. Edmiston CE: Prosthetic device infections in surgery. In Nichols RL, Nyhus LM (eds): Update Surgical Sepsis. Philadelphia, Lippincott, 1993, pp 444–468.
10. Edmiston CE, Seabrook GR, Cambria RA, et al: Molecular epidemiology of microbial contamination in the operating room environment: Is there a risk for infection? Surgery 2005;138:572–588.

11. Kuehnert MJ, Hill HA, Kupronis BA, et al: Methicillin-resistant Staphylococcus aureus hospitalizations, United States. Emerg Infect Dis 2005;11:868–872.

12. Kourbatova EV, Halvosa JS, King MD, et al: Emergence of community-associated methicillin resistant Staphylococcus aureus USA 300 clone as a cause of healthcare-associated infections among patients with prosthetic joint infections. Am J Infect Control 2005;33:385–391.

13. Gaynes RP: Surveillance of nosocomial infections: A fundamental ingredient for quality. Infect Control Hosp Epidemiol 1997;18:475–478.

14. Edmiston CE, Sinski S, Seabrook G, et al: Airborne particulates in the OR environment. AORN J 1999;69:1169–1183.

15. Krizek TJ, Robson MC: Evolution of quantitative bacteriology in wound management. Am J Surg 1975;130:579–584.

16. James RC, MacLeod CJ: Induction of staphylococcal infections in mice with small inoculum introduced on sutures. Br J Exp Pathol 1961;42:266–277.

17. Lilienfeld DE, Vlahov D, Tenney JH, McLaughlin JS: Obesity and diabetes as risk factors for postoperative wound infections after cardiac surgery. Am J Infect Control 1988;16:3–6.

18. Terranova A: The effect of diabetes mellitus on wound healing. Plast Surg Nurs 1991;11:20–25.

19. Talbot TR: Diabetes mellitus and cardiothoracic surgical site infections. Am J Infect Control 2005;33:353–359.

20. Zerr KJ, Furnay AP, Grunkemeier GL, et al: Glucose control lowers the risk of wound infection in diabetics after open heart operations. Ann Thorac Surg 1997;63:356–361.

21. Krinsley JS: Effect of an intensive glucose management protocol on mortality of critically ill adult patients. Mayo Clin Proc 2004;79:992–1000.

22. Sung J, Bochicchio GV, Joshi M, et al: Admission hyperglycemia is predictive of outcome in critically ill trauma patients. J Trauma 2005;59:80–83.

23. Richardson JD, Cocanour CS, Kern JA, et al: Perioperative risk assessment in elderly and high-risk patients. J Am Coll Surg 2004;199:134–146.

24. Barie PS: Surgical site infections: Epidemiology and prevention. Surg Infect 2002;3:9S–21S.

25. Cheadle WG: Risk factors for surgical site infection. Surg Infect 2006;7:S7–S11.

26. de Oliveira AC, Ciosak SI, Ferraz EM, Grinbaum RS: Surgical site infection in patients submitted to digestive surgery: Risk prediction and the NNIS risk index. Am J Infect Control 2006;34:201–207.

27. Anaya DA, Dellinger EP: The obese surgical patient: A susceptible host for infection. Surg Infect 2006;7:473–480.

28. Edmiston CE, Krepel C, Kelly H, et al: Perioperative antimicrobial prophylaxis in the gastric bypass patient: Do we achieve therapeutic levels? Surgery 2004;136:738–747.

29. Mori N, Hitomi S, Nakajima J, et al: Unselective use of intranasal mupirocin ointment for controlling propagation of methicillin-resistant Staphylococcus aureus in a thoracic surgery ward. J Infect Chemother 2005;11:231–233.

30. Fawley WN, Parnel P, Hall J, et al: Surveillance for mupirocin resistance following introduction of routine perioperative prophylaxis with nasal mupirocin. J Hosp Infect 2006;62:327–332.

31. Kluytmans JA, Mouton JW, Vandebergh MF, et al: Reduction of surgical site infections in cardiothoracic surgery by elimination of nasal carriage of Staphylococcus aureus. Infect Control Hosp Epidemiol 1996;17:780–785.

32. Vasquez JE, Walker ES, Franzus BW, et al: The epidemiology of mupirocin resistance among methicillin-resistant Staphylococcus aureus at a Veterans Affairs Hospital. Infect Control Hosp Epidemiol 2000;21:459–464.

33. Richards C, Emori TG, Edwards J, et al: Characteristics of hospitals and infection control professionals participating in the National Nosocomial Infection Surveillance System 1999. Am J Infect Control 2001;29:400–403.

34. Dubois F, Icard P, Berthelot G, et al: Coelioscopic cholecystectomy: Preliminary report of 36 cases. Ann Surg 1990;212:649–650.

35. NIH Consensus Conference: Gallstones and laparoscopic cholecystectomy. JAMA 1993;269:1018–1024.

36. Boni L, Benevento A, Rovera F, et al: Infective complications in laparoscpic surgery. Surg Infect 2006;7:S109–S111.

37. Steiner CA, Bass EB, Talamini MA, et al: Surgical rates and operative mortality for open and laparoscopic cholestectomy in Maryland. N Engl J Med 1994;330:403–408.

38. The Southern Surgeons Club: A prospective analysis of 1518 laparoscopic cholecystectomies. N Engl J Med 1991;324:1073–1078.

39. Diez J, Arozamena CJ, Ferraina P, et al: Relation between postoperative infection and gallbladder bile leakage during laparoscopic cholecystectomies. Surg Endosc 1996;10:529–532.

40. Richards C, Edwards J, Culver D, et al: Does using a laparoscopic approach to cholecystectomy decrease the risk of surgical site infection? Ann Surg 2003;237:358–362.

41. Meynaud-Kraemer L, Colin C, Vergnon P, Barth X: Wound infection in open versus laparoscopic appendectomy. Int J Technol Assess Healthcare 1999;15:380–391.

42. Moon V, Chaudry GA, Choy C, Ferzli GS: Mesh infection in the era of laparoscopy. J Laparoendoscopic Adv Surg Tech 2004;14:349–352.

43. Aziz O, Constantinides V, Tekkis PP, et al: Laparoscopic versus open surgery for rectal cancer: A meta-analysis. Ann Surg Oncol 2006;13:413–424.

44. Gordon SM: New surgical techniques and surgical site infections. Emerg Infect Dis 2001;7:217–219.

45. Miles AA, Miles EM, Burke JF: The value and duration of defense reactions of the skin to primary lodgement of bacteria. Br J Exp Pathol 1957;38:79–96.

46. Burke JF: Effective period of preventive antibiotic action in experimental incisions and dermal lesions. Surgery 1961;60:161–168.

47. Classen DC, Evan RS, Pestotnik SL, et al: The timing of prophylactic administration of antibiotics and the risk of infection. N Engl J Med 1992;326:281–286.

48. DiPiro JT, Vallner JJ, Bowden TA, et al: Intraoperative serum and tissue activity of cefazolin and cefoxitin. Arch Surg 1985;120:829–832.

49. Pories WJ, van Riji AM, Burlingham BT, et al: Prophylactic cefazolin in gastric bypass surgery. Surgery 1981;90:426–431.

50. Forse RA, Karam B, MacLean LD, Christou NV: Antibiotic prophylaxis for surgery in morbidly obese patients. Surgery 1989;106:750–757.

51. Galbraith U, Schilling J, von Segesser LK, et al: Antibiotic prophylaxis in cardiovascular surgery: A prospective, randomized comparative trial of one day cefazolin versus single dose cefuroxime. Drug Exp Clin Res 1993;19:229–234.

52. Kriaras I, Michalopoulos A, Michalis A, et al: Antibiotic prophylaxis in cardiac surgery. J Cardiovasc Surg 1997;38:605–610.

53. Mauerhan DR, Nelson CL, Smith DL, et al: Prophylaxis against infection in total joint arthroplasty: One day of cefuroxime compared with three days of cefazolin. J Bone Joint Surg 1994;76:39–45.

54. Hasslegren PO, Ivarsson L, Risberg B, Seeman T: Effects of prophylactic antibiotics in vascular surgery: A prospective, randomized, double-blind study. Ann Surg 1984;200:86–92.

55. Hall JC, Watts JM, Press L, et al: Single-dose antibiotic prophylaxis in contaminated surgery. Arch Surg 1989;124:244–247.

56. Scher KS: Studies on the duration of antibiotic administration for surgical prophylaxis. Am Surg 1997;63:59–62.

57. Fry D: The surgical infection prevention project: Processes, outcomes, and future impact. Surg Infect 2006;7:S17–S26.

58. Fonseca SNS, Kunzle SRM, Junqueira MJ, et al: Implementing 1-dose antibiotic prophylaxis for prevention of surgical site infection. Arch Surg 2006;141:1109–1113.

59. Higgins A, London J, Charland S, et al: Prophylactic antibiotics for elective laparoscopic cholecystectomy. Arch Surg 1999;134:611–614.

60. McGuckin M, Shea JA, Schwartz JS: Infection and antimicrobial use in laparoscopic cholecystectomy. Infect Control Hosp Epidemiol 1999;20:624–626.

61. Tocchi A, Leper L, Costa G, et al: The need for antibiotic prophylaxis in elective laparoscopic cholecystectomy: A prospective, randomized study. Arch Surg 2000;135:67–70.

62. Chang WT, Lee KT, Chuang SC, et al: The impact of prophylactic antibiotics on postoperative infection complication in elective laparoscopic cholecystecomy: A prospective, randomized study. Am J Surg 2006;191:721–725.

63. Dellinger EP, Gross PA, Barrett TL, et al: Quality standard for antimicrobial prophylaxis in surgical procedures. Infect Control Hosp Epidemiol 1994;15:182–188.

64. Bratzler DW, Houck PM: Antimicrobial prophylaxis for surgery: An advisory statement from the National Surgical Prevention Project. Clin Infect Dis 2004;38:1706–1715.

65. Itani KMF, Wilson SE, Awad SS, et al: Ertapenem versus cefotetan prophylaxis in elective colorectal surgery. N Engl J Med 2006;355:2640–2651.

66. Dellinger EP, Hausmann SM, Bratzler DW, et al: Hospitals collaborate to decrease surgical site infections. Am J Surg 2004;190:9–15.

JOSEPH W. SZOKOL AND
MARTIN NITSUN

Anesthetic Implications for Laparoscopic Surgery

32

The use of laparoscopy as an alternative to conventional open surgery began in the 1950s. Gynecologists were the first to use this method to aid in the diagnosis of pelvic pain. General surgeons began to employ this technique and soon came to realize that patients undergoing laparoscopic procedures had better cosmetic results, reduced hospital stays, less intraoperative bleeding, fewer postoperative wound infections, and better postoperative respiratory function.

Over the years the volume and breadth of laparoscopic procedures have exploded. Advanced technology and increased operator skill have allowed more complex procedures to be performed on increasingly older and sicker surgical populations. However, despite the distinct surgical advantages of laparoscopy over open surgery, there are significant anesthesia-related challenges that are pertinent to this burgeoning field.

PREOPERATIVE EVALUATION

The American Society of Anesthesiologists classification score provides a reasonable preoperative evaluation tool to assess for potential perioperative morbidity and mortality (Table 32-1). The patient's medical disease along with limitations in normal daily activity need to be identified preoperatively. In general, laparoscopy with pneumoperitoneum is contraindicated in patients with shock, increased intracranial pressure, ventriculoperitoneal shunt, peritoneojugular shunt, hypovolemia, severe myopia or retinal detachment, or congestive heart failure and in facilities with inadequate equipment and monitors.

PREOPERATIVE FASTING AND THE USE OF PHARMACOLOGIC AGENTS TO REDUCE THE RISK OF PULMONARY ASPIRATION

The American Society of Anesthesiologists has published a practice guideline to aid the clinician in deciding the appropriate period for individuals to fast before surgery. These practice guidelines are not standards. They may be adopted, modified, or rejected based on the clinician's judgment. Also, the practice guideline regarding perioperative fasting applies only to healthy patients undergoing elective surgical procedures. The guideline does not address patients who may have coexisting disease or other states that may affect gastric volume and emptying, such as pregnancy, obesity, diabetes mellitus, gastroesophageal reflux disease (GERD), hiatal hernia, bowel obstruction, or enteric feeding. Also, in the patient who may have a difficult airway the guidelines do not apply and do not recommend a specific airway technique.

The guidelines do recommend a pertinent history and physical examination to rule out GERD, dysphagia, or other issues related to gastrointestinal motility. The guidelines recommend that individuals have a minimum of 2 hours fast from clear liquids. Clear liquids are defined as water, fruit juices without pulp, carbonated beverages, clear tea, and coffee. The guidelines state that the "volume of liquid ingested is less important that the type of liquid ingested." The guidelines recommend that patients abstain from a light meal for a minimum of 6 hours before surgery, and longer for a meal that includes fried or fatty foods that may slow gastric emptying (Table 32-2).

The issue of routine use of gastric stimulants and pharmacologic agents such as histamine-2 receptor blockade and proton pump inhibitors is addressed in the guidelines. The recommendation is that neither the preoperative use of medications that block acid secretion nor the use of gastric motility—enhancing agents is recommended in the healthy patient undergoing elective surgery.

PNEUMOPERITONEUM

The physical characteristics of carbon dioxide gas approach the ideal properties for insufflation. These qualities include inability to support combustion and rapid excretion of absorbed gas. However, significant absorption across the peritoneum does occur, leading to the potential for hypercapnia with resultant acid-base disturbance, activation of the sympathetic nervous system, and potential cardiovascular instability. Additionally, pneumoperitoneum (PP)-induced increases in intra-abdominal pressure (IAP) may have significant cardiovascular, respiratory, and neurologic effects. Knowledge of the physiology of carbon dioxide PP is essential to providing safe anesthetic care to patients undergoing laparoscopic procedure.

CARBON DIOXIDE INSUFFLATION

Carbon dioxide is rapidly absorbed through the peritoneum resulting in hypercapnia and respiratory acidosis. End-tidal

Table 32-1 American Society of Anesthesiologists (ASA) Classification of Physical Status

ASA Rating	Description of Patient
Class I	A normal healthy individual
Class II	A patient with mild systemic disease
Class III	A patient with severe systemic disease that is not incapacitating
Class IV	A patient with incapacitating systemic disease that is a constant threat to life
Class V	A moribund patient who is not suspected to survive 24 hours with or without an operation
Class VI	A declared brain-dead patient whose organs are being removed for donor purposes
Class E	Added as a suffix for emergency operation

Table 32-2 Eating and Drinking Guidelines

Ingested Material	Minimum Fasting Time (in Hours)
Clear liquids	2
Breast milk	4
Infant formula	6
Nonhuman milk	6
Light meal	6

Summary of the American Society of Anesthesiologists Fasting Recommendations: The recommendations apply only to healthy patients presenting for elective surgery. The recommendations do not apply to the pregnant patients, morbidly obese patients, and patients with delay in gastric emptying or other conditions that might predispose to aspiration of gastric contents. Clear liquids include water, fruit juices *without* pulp, carbonated beverages, tea, and black coffee. A light meal is one that does not contain fried or fatty foods, which may prolong gastric emptying.

carbon dioxide increases with time if ventilation is kept constant. The absorption of carbon dioxide is especially enhanced by increased IAP. Hypercapnia can result in various cardiac perturbations, including cardiac arrhythmias, vasoconstriction of the pulmonary vasculature, and a mixed response in cardiac function. Hypercapnia may lead to increased sympathetic nervous system activation with resultant tachycardia and increased myocardial contractility. Acidosis may lead to depression of myocardial function. Avoidance of the deleterious effects of absorbed carbon dioxide is dependent on appropriate adjustments in ventilation to ensure elimination.

CARDIOVASCULAR EFFECTS

Major hemodynamic shifts may occur during laparoscopic procedures. These changes are the result of the confluence of multiple factors. These include the magnitude of increased IAP, the degree of hypercapnia, the ventilatory technique, the patient's intravascular volume, surgical conditions, patient positioning, and anesthetic agents.

At IAP below 15 mm Hg, cardiac output is increased as a result of increased venous return from the splanchnic bed. Additionally, hypercapnia-induced sympathetic stimulation and peripheral vasoconstriction can augment cardiac output. Further increases in IAP result in compression of the vena cava with resultant decreased venous return and decreased cardiac output. Significant bradyarrythmias due to vagal stimulation have been reported during insufflation and include bradycardia,

atrioventricular dissociation, and asystole. Vagal stimulation may be triggered by insertion of an insufflating needle or trocar by peritoneal stretch or by carbon dioxide embolization. Removing the inducing stimulus typically results in resolution of the problem. Tachyarrhythmias and hypertension may occur as a result of increased levels of carbon dioxide and catecholamines. Preoperative volume loading may prevent the decreased cardiac output associated with high IAP and extreme reverse Trendelenburg positioning. Slow carbon dioxide insufflation may decrease the likelihood of significant carbon dioxide embolism and may prevent significant vagal stimulation. The lowest IAP possible should be used to avoid many of the hemodynamic consequences of carbon dioxide pneumoperitoneum.

Carbon dioxide embolism is a rare and potentially devastating complication of laparoscopic procedures. Carbon dioxide embolism is usually caused by inadvertent placement of the insufflating needle into the vasculature or intra-abdominal organ. Clinically significant gas embolism may present as cardiovascular collapse with hypotension, cyanosis, arrhythmia, and asystole. Treatment is supportive and includes deflation of pneumoperitoneum, institution of 100% oxygen therapy, increasing minute ventilation, aspiration of air via a central line, placement of the patient in left lateral head-down position to prevent gas from entering the pulmonary artery, and cardiopulmonary resuscitation if necessary.

Pneumothorax can occur from gas entering the thoracic cavity via a tear in the visceral peritoneum or breach of the parietal pleura. Pneumothorax can be asymptomatic or life threatening. Treatment is based upon severity and may involve only observation or may necessitate emergent chest tube insertion and cardiopulmonary resuscitation.

Typically, healthy patients with normal cardiovascular function tolerate laparoscopic procedures without incident. Those with an altered volume status or underlying cardiovascular disease and those subjected to extreme positioning require meticulous vigilance in their management.

PATIENT POSITIONING

Extreme patient positioning during laparoscopic procedures may result in altered cardiorespiratory function and potentially may result in nerve damage. Reverse Trendelenburg or head-up positioning results in decreased venous return with resultant decreased cardiac output, decreased mean arterial pressure, and increased peripheral and pulmonary vascular resistance. Trendelenburg or head-down position has the opposite effects, resulting in increased venous return and normalization of blood pressure. Respiratory mechanics are affected by pneumoperitoneum and patient positioning.

ANESTHESIA AND LAPAROSCOPIC BARIATRIC SURGERY

Bariatric surgery was developed in the late 1960s; however, it was not until the late 1990s that there was a significant growth in these types of procedures in the United States. This rise in popularity was due in part to the advancement in laparoscopic techniques. According to the 1999–2000 National Health and Nutrition Examination Survey, 4.7% of U.S. adults are morbidly obese. Studies have demonstrated that laparoscopic gastric bypass (GBP) offers advantages over open GBP, including less blood loss, shorter hospital stay, faster convalescence, and equal weight loss at 1 year with better quality of life. Despite advances in technique and technology, by virtue of their habitus, morbidly obese patients are predisposed to a variety of systemic disease processes that impact the safe delivery of anesthesia care and ultimately their health and survival.

Preoperative Evaluation and the Morbidly Obese

Data indicate that there is a direct correlation between extent of obesity (body mass index [BMI]) and the likelihood of perioperative morbidity and fatality. Obesity predisposes patients to a variety of significant pathologic conditions including hypertension, coronary artery disease, diabetes, obstructive sleep apnea, and hypercoagulability. Preoperative evaluation should include a thorough review of the patient's medical chart, a detailed history and physical examination, and a discussion with the patient's primary care provider and surgeon to ensure that all preexisting conditions are optimized.

Sleep Apnea and the Morbidly Obese

It is estimated that 4% of men and 2% of women in the United States have clinically significant obstructive sleep apnea (OSA). Between 60% and 90% of patients with OSA are obese, and 70% to 80% of patients with OSA are undiagnosed. Preoperative identification of these patients is essential because difficulty in securing the airway and postoperative airway obstruction and respiratory depression can result in significant perioperative morbidity and even death. Additionally OSA is associated with multiple systemic disease processes including hypertension, coronary artery disease, stroke, arrhythmia, pulmonary hypertension, and metabolic syndrome. The standard diagnostic test for OSA is polysomnography. Apnea is defined as cessation of airflow for more than 10 seconds, and hypopnea is defined as diminished airflow by 50% for more than 10 seconds. The apnea-hypopnea index (AHI), the sum total of apneas and hypopneas per hour, is a method of quantitating the severity of OSA. An AHI of 6 to 20 indicates mild OSA, an AHI of 21 to 40 indicates moderate OSA, and an AHI of greater than 40 indicates severe OSA. In the absence of a formal polysomnogram, clinical criteria may be used to judge the presence and severity of OSA (Table 32-3).

OSA is characterized by repetitive episodes of airway obstruction during sleep. During deep non-REM sleep and REM sleep a loss of airway muscle tone occurs, resulting in airway obstruction. These episodes are characterized by hypoxemia and hypercarbia resulting in arousal from sleep and return of airway musculature tone. Multiple episodes of apnea and arousal result in poor quality sleep with daytime hypersomnolence. Activation of the sympathetic nervous system and an inflammatory response to these episodes may contribute to the cardiovascular consequences associated with OSA.

Most anesthetic agents may exacerbate symptoms of OSA by affecting the airway musculature. These drugs include all sedative-hypnotics, narcotics, muscle relaxants, and inhalation agents. Narcotics may also decrease the ventilatory response to hypoxemia and hypercarbia, thus further exacerbating apneic episodes.

Preoperatively, elective surgery for patients with suspected but undiagnosed OSA should be postponed pending polysomnography. Alternatively these patients can be treated presumptively as if they had OSA. Postoperative follow-up with a sleep specialist is advisable in this subgroup of patients. Because of numerous reported benefits, continuous positive airway pressure (CPAP) and other airway stenting devices should be considered preoperatively in patients with moderate to severe OSA. Intraoperatively, it is postulated that there is a correlation with severity of OSA and a higher incidence of difficult mask ventilation and tracheal intubation. However, there does not seem to be a correlation with BMI and difficult intubation.

Airway Management in the Bariatric Patient

The obese patient may be more difficult to mask after induction of anesthesia, and the laryngoscopic view may be less than the ideal found in normal size patients. The difficult airway is one in which a trained anesthesiologist experiences problems with either mask ventilation or tracheal intubation. Difficult intubation is encountered when the view of the glottic opening is inadequate. More than one factor needs to be assessed preoperatively to determine if intubation may be difficult and other methods of intubation might be considered (e.g., awake fiberoptic intubation). Factors that may predict a difficult intubation include a short sterno- or thyromental distance, large neck circumference, limited neck extension, small mouth opening, receding mandible, and prominent upper incisors. The Mallampati Score as modified by Samsoon and Young is also used during the evaluation of the airway. The score was designed as a predictor of ease of laryngoscopic view (Fig. 32-1). However, the Mallampati score has a low sensitivity and specificity and must be utilized with other parameters of the airway examination. Neck circumference may be one of the best indicators of a potential difficult intubation. Increasing neck circumference has been associated with increasing odds of a patient having OSA. Studies have demonstrated that patients with OSA have a higher likelihood of difficult intubation. The incidence of difficult intubation in these patients may be as high as 17%, whereas it is only 3.3% in patients without OSA.

In morbidly obese patients presenting for surgery proper, patient positioning may lead to a higher likelihood of ease of intubation. It is important that these patients have their head, upper body, and shoulders placed above their chest. Simply placing the chin higher than the chest is not adequate. Alterations in pulmonary physiology in morbidly obese patients in general and those with OSA specifically lend to rapid decompensation when rendered apneic even for short periods of time.

Oxygenation

The obese patient has a reduction in expiratory reserve volume and functional residual capacity. The decreases are 60% and 80%, respectively. If the expiratory reserve volume decreases below closing capacity, dependent alveoli may be underventilated or

---

Table 32-3 Clinical Signs and Symptoms Suggesting Possibility of Obstructive Sleep Apnea

Predisposing physical characteristics
  Body mass index $\geq$ 35 kg/m^2
  Neck circumference greater than 17 inches (men), 16 inches (women)
  Craniofacial abnormalities affecting the airway
  Anatomic nasal obstruction
  Tonsils nearly touching or touching midline
History of apparent airway obstruction during sleep
  Snoring (loud enough to be heard through a closed door)
  Frequent snoring
  Observed pauses in breathing during sleep
  Awakens from sleep with choking sensation
  Frequent arousals from sleep
Somnolence
  Frequent somnolence or fatigue despite adequate "sleep"
  Falls asleep easily in a nonstimulating environment

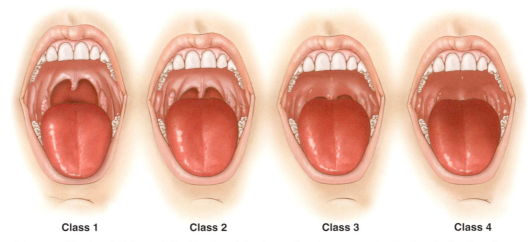

| **Class 1** | **Class 2** | **Class 3** | **Class 4** |

FIGURE 32-1 Samsoon and Young modification of Mallampati Classification of the airway. Class 1 represents visualization of soft palate, fauces, uvula, and pillars. Class 2 represents the soft palate, fauces, and uvula. Class 3 shows the soft palate and base of uvula. Class 4 depicts only the hard palate.

nonventilated, leading to hypoxemia. Placing the obese patient in the supine position may further decrease lung volume. The expiratory reserve volume is the main source of oxygen during periods of apnea. Therefore, preoxygenation of the obese patient is more difficult to accomplish and the time to desaturation is shorter. If it becomes difficult to mask ventilate the patient or intubate the patient, a hypoxemic disaster may ensue.

Hypoxemia has many causes, including a low inspired oxygen concentration, elevated arterial carbon dioxide, ventilation-perfusion mismatch, right-to-left shunt, and diffusion nonequilibrium. Main stem intubation may occur when the patient is placed in the Trendelenburg position and cephalad shift of the carina and mediastinum occur.

It is important to preoxygenate patients before induction of anesthesia. Preoxygenation can be accomplished by applying a tight-fitting face mask for 5 minutes with 100% oxygen. Alternatively, having the patient take four vital capacity breaths, though not as efficacious as the aforementioned technique, can also delay the time to desaturation in the event of an inability to ventilate/oxygenate the patient. In the nonobese patient without significant cardiac or respiratory disease, the time to desaturation (oxygen saturation less than 90%) may be up to 10 minutes.

Intrapulmonary shunt leads to lower arterial oxygen content. The main cause of intrapulmonary shunt is atelectasis. Atelectasis occurs within minutes in almost all patients under general anesthesia. The amount of atelectasis is higher in the obese patient, compared to the nonobese patient. Therefore, the obese patient will desaturate faster than a nonobese patient. One strategy that may help to limit atelectasis after induction of anesthesia is the application of CPAP at 10 cm H_2O for 5 minutes followed by ventilating the patient for another 5 minutes with the application of 10 cm H_2O of positive end-expiratory pressure (PEEP). The one caution is that morbidly obese patients have a larger residual gastric volume and the risk of aspiration under such conditions may be higher.

Atelectasis is the most common cause of postoperative hypoxemia. Arterial oxygenation is decreased during anesthesia more in obese than lean patients, and the decrements in oxygenation are directly proportional to the patient's BMI. A 50% reduction in functional residual capacity occurs in obese patients after induction of general anesthesia as compared to a 20% fall in lean patients. The intrapulmonary shunt is also increased in obese patients as compared to normal weight patients. The shunt may

be as high as 25% in obese patients versus 5% in lean patients. The reduced oxygen reserve combined with a higher metabolic rate in obese patients may result in rapid oxygen desaturation. Strategies to reduce postoperative hypoxemia may include the use of a vital capacity maneuver (manual lung inflation to 40 cm H_2O for 15 seconds in the patient without hemodynamic compromise), followed by 40% oxygen, with 100% oxygen immediately before extubation. If a patient is ventilated with 100% oxygen, atelectasis formation after a vital capacity maneuver can recur within 5 minutes. Decreasing the inspired oxygen concentration to 40% or adding PEEP may limit the amount of atelectasis encountered and increase the postoperative arterial oxygen content. The use of larger tidal volumes (15–20 mL/kg) has been recommended as one method to improve functional residual capacity and therefore arterial oxygenation but in and of itself does not improve oxygenation to any significant extent. Larger tidal volumes may also lead to hypocapnia or increased inspiratory pressures, and the excessive lung expansion potentially may create volutrauma (though this may not be clinically significant). Moderate tidal volumes (10–12 mL/kg) and the application of PEEP may be the best strategy to preserve oxygenation during laparoscopy.

The use of reverse Trendelenburg position may improve gas exchange and respiratory mechanics. After induction of anesthesia the alveolar-arterial oxygen difference increases. It increases more in the obese than the lean patient. Placing a patient in a 30-degree reverse Trendelenburg position may improve the alveolar-arterial difference. The reverse Trendelenburg position increases lung compliance and may lead to a recruitment of alveoli and thus functional residual capacity. It must be kept in mind that the reverse Trendelenburg position may lead to decrease venous return and decreased cardiac output. However, in patients with normal cardiac reserve this should not be clinically relevant.

Neutrophils are an important mechanism to avoid postoperative wound infections. Neutrophils work by oxidative killing and the infection risk is increased in areas of low tissue oxygen concentration. In awake obese and nonobese volunteers the subcutaneous wound tissue oxygenation ($Psco_2$) is around 60 mm Hg. In the obese surgical patient the $Psco_2$ slightly increases during surgery with an 80% inspired oxygen concentration, whereas in the lean patient the $Psco_2$ nearly doubles. Part of the reason is that the arterial oxygen content is reduced in the obese compared to the nonobese patient. Mild hypercapnia (an arterial Pco_2 of around 58 mm Hg) leads to an increase in tissue oxygenation from approximately 56 mm Hg to 78 mm Hg. A $Psco_2$ near 80 mm Hg greatly reduces the risk of wound infection.

Pneumoperitoneum causes changes in pulmonary function during laparoscopy. These effects are a decrease in lung volumes, increase in peak airway pressures, and decrease in pulmonary compliance due to increased intra-abdominal pressure. The increase in intra-abdominal pressure leads to a reduction in diaphragmatic movement and also shifts the diaphragm headward, which results in earlier closure of small airways, resulting in atelectasis and lower arterial oxygenation. These changes can be exacerbated if the patient is placed in the Trendelenburg position. In rare cases, the higher intra-abdominal pressure can cause pneumothorax or pneumomediastinum due to increased alveolar pressures. If peak intraoperative airway pressures are encountered or hypoxemia from increased pulmonary shunting, the insufflation pressure may need to be reduced or ceased to see if the adverse effects are attenuated.

Because obese patients and those with OSA are prone to airway obstruction after tracheal extubation and because of the dangers inherent in their compromised respiratory physiology, tracheal extubation should be performed only when the patient is wide awake and following purposeful commands, the muscle relaxant has been fully reversed, and the patient has demonstrated adequate strength. Extubation should be performed in the nonsupine position. OSA coupled with the respiratory effects of narcotics and sedatives place these patients at increased risk of airway obstruction postoperatively. The severity of OSA coupled with the patient's comorbid conditions and need for postoperative narcotics should dictate whether the patient requires closer postoperative monitoring in an intensive care or "step-down" unit.

URINE OUTPUT DURING LAPAROSCOPY

A reduction in urine output has been well demonstrated in laparoscopic surgery. An increase in antidiuretic hormone, aldosterone, and plasma rennin activity is evident during laparoscopy. Intra-abdominal blood flow during laparoscopic surgical procedures is affected by three factors: intra-abdominal carbon dioxide insufflation pressure, intra-abdominal pressure, and patient position. Laparoscopic manipulation may also cause renal artery vasospasm, which may lead to a decrease in urine blood flow. Renal cortical perfusion pressure can decrease as much as 60% with a peritoneal insufflation pressure of 15 mm Hg. This perfusion abnormality abates when the insufflation is stopped. Increased intra-abdominal pressure has a direct compressive effect on the kidney parenchyma and renal blood vessels. Increasing the intra-abdominal pressure from 0 to 20 mm Hg can usually decrease renal blood flow and glomerular filtration by 23% and increase renal vascular resistance sixfold. Hypercapnia during insufflation causes systemic effects that may impact significantly on hemodynamics and intra-abdominal organ blood flow. One may encounter reduced venous return, which leads to renal vascular insufficiency. Urine output falls dramatically during the first hour of laparoscopic insufflation and remains lower during the rest of the insufflation period. Once insufflation pressure is released, the urine output returns to baseline in patients with normal renal function. Patients who have undergone laparoscopic cholecystectomy have an increase in urinary excretion of N-acetyl-β-D-glucosaminidase, a subtle indicator of renal function. However, this perturbation in renal function is unimportant clinically.

Intravascular volume expansion may prevent some of the decrease seen in urine output during carbon dioxide insufflation. However, renal creatinine clearance is still diminished with volume expansion. Creatinine clearance is improved once the pneumoperitoneum is released. The one caveat with volume expansion is that this technique may be hazardous in patients with limited cardiac reserve and may lead to congestive changes and ischemia.

Intra-abdominal pressure greater than 15 mm Hg may lead to oliguria, and pressures greater than 30 mm Hg may lead to a state of anuria. Special attention may need to be given to patients with a poor baseline renal function. The precise creatinine or creatinine clearance at which one should consider not subjecting the patient with limited renal reserve to laparoscopic insufflation has not yet been defined in the literature.

Plasma arginine vasopressin (AVP) is elevated during laparoscopic surgical procedures. AVP causes an antidiuretic effect by activating renal vasopressin receptors, which promote the reabsorption of water in the distal tubules and collecting ducts. This in turn leads to more concentrated urine. Vasopressin receptor antagonists work by blocking the ability of vasopressin to reabsorb water in the distal tubule and collecting duct and antagonize the antidiuretic effect of AVP. However, carbon dioxide insufflation leads to a reduction in glomerular filtration rate, which diminishes the creation of free water in the ascending limbs. This causes increased water permeability in the collecting ducts and therefore augments water reabsorption, which can occur even in the absence of AVP.

NEUROMUSCULAR BLOCKING AGENTS

The use of neuromuscular blocking agents (NMBAs) is necessary to prevent high intrathoracic and intra-abdominal pressures during laparoscopic procedures. The use of NMBAs may also lead to improved surgical conditions. NMBAs may be even more essential in the patient undergoing a laparoscopic procedure than in the patient undergoing an open surgical procedure in that high intra-abdominal pressure may make laparoscopic surgery difficult, if not impossible. The adequacy of pneumoperitoneum for trocar placement may be improved in the paralyzed and ventilated patient, and the intra-abdominal pressure may be higher in general anesthesia patients who do not have adequate neuromuscular blockade. However, it is important not to overuse NMBAs. Residual neuromuscular blockade is a common event in the postanesthesia recovery room. Residual neuromuscular blockade can lead to impaired airway protective reflexes, upper airway obstruction, decreased hypoxic ventilatory response, and postoperative hypoxemia. This may be even more hazardous in the obese patient who is still partially paralyzed in conjunction with lower arterial oxygen content due to increased atelectasis. The duration of NMBAs is prolonged when given based on real body weight versus ideal body weight.

HYPOTHERMIA

Mild hypothermia has been described as a core temperature between 34°C and 36°C. Hypothermia has significant perioperative adverse effects. Postoperative shivering may increase oxygen consumption up to 400%, but rarely exceeds 200% in healthy volunteers. Elderly patients, who may be most at risk, do not shiver as much as younger patients, and the increased oxygen consumption imposed by shivering may not play a significant role in perioperative ischemia. However, patients at high risk have been found to have a threefold risk of adverse myocardial outcomes with as little as 1.3°C core hypothermia. The mechanism may be related to a significant increase in plasma norepinephrine levels, which may in turn augment cardiac irritability and lead to perioperative arrhythmias.

Mild hypothermia also leads to increased blood loss. Platelet function, clotting factor function, and fibrinolytic activity are all adversely affected by hypothermia. A small decrease in core body temperature has been found to lead to a 30% increase in blood loss in patients undergoing total hip arthroplasty. Hypothermia may also predispose the patient to decrease wound healing and a greater risk of infection. Hypothermia triggers compensatory vasoconstriction that decreases subcutaneous tissue oxygen tension. Also, hypothermia adversely impacts immune function, in particular T-cell-mediated antibody production, and neutrophil function. Hypothermia also interferes with metabolism of drugs. In particular, neuromuscular blocking agents may have their duration as much as doubled by a 2°C drop in body temperature. This may lead to the inadequate reversal of these drugs in the recovery room and may lead to pharyngeal incoordination, which might predispose the patient to aspiration and need for reintubation. The hypothermic patient may awaken slower due to increased tissue solubility of anesthetic agents.

Hypothermia results initially from the distribution of relatively warmer blood from the core to the periphery, which is cooler. This gradient is dependent on peripheral temperature, which in turn is established by the patient's vasomotor status and thermal environment (Fig. 32-2). Anesthetic agents decrease thermoregulatory control by 2°C to 4°C. Patients become relatively poikilothermic, similar to cold-blooded animals that have their body temperature regulated by the environment.

Ninety percent of metabolic heat is lost through the skin. The most effective way to prevent heat loss is to have a warm environment (i.e., operating room) for anesthetized patients, administer warm intravenous fluids (a liter of normal saline at room temperature decreases body temperature by 0.25°C), and use active cutaneous warming. Cutaneous warming is most effectively and safely accomplished by utilization of forced air through a warming blanket. The use of a warming blanket can increase core body temperature by 1°C per hour.

High-flow insufflators may lead to intraoperative hypothermia. Many reports exist that describe intraoperative hypothermia secondary to carbon dioxide pneumoperitoneum. Some authors have found that unheated insufflated gas as opposed to heated insufflated gas lead to a greater loss in body temperature, while others have demonstrated no difference between the two techniques. The most important consideration is that the patient should have intravenous fluids warmed, and forced air warming methods should be employed. These techniques can help ensure that patients do not suffer the adverse consequences of hypothermia.

SUMMARY

Laparoscopy has revolutionized the care of the surgical patient. It has also created new challenges for the anesthesiologist. These challenges can be met if the cardiovascular and respiratory alterations of pneumoperitoneum and extremes of positioning are understood and appreciated.

Suggested Reading

American Society of Anesthesiologists (ASA) Task Force on Preoperative Fasting: Practice guidelines for preoperative fasting and the use of pharmacologic agents to reduce the risk of pulmonary aspiration: Application to healthy patients undergoing elective procedures. Anesthesiology 1999;90:896–905.

American Society of Anesthesiologists: Practice guidelines for patients with OSA. Anesthesiology 2006;104:1081–1093.

Benoit Z, Wicky S, Fischer J, et al: The effect of increased FIO$_2$ before tracheal extubation on postoperative atelectasis. Anesth Analg 2002;95:1777–1781.

Berber E, String A, Garland A, et al: Intraoperative thermal regulation in patients undergoing laparoscopic vs. open surgical procedures. Surg Endsoc 2001;15:281–285.

Brodsky JB, Lemmens HJ, Brock-Utne JG, et al: Morbid obesity and tracheal intubation. Anesth Analg 2002;94:732–736.

Coussa M, Proietti S, Schnyder P, et al: Prevention of atelectasis formation during the induction of general anesthesia in morbidly obese patients. Anesth Analg 2004;98:1491–1495.

Flegal KM, Carroll MD, Ogden CL, Johnson CL: Prevalence and trends in obesity among US adults, 1999–2000. JAMA 2002;228:1723–1727.

Gerges FJ, Kanazi GE, Jabbour-Khoury SI: Anesthesia for laparoscopy: A review. J Clin Anesth 2006;18:67–78.

Hager H, Reddy D, Mandadi G, et al: Hypercapnia improves tissue oxygenation in morbidly obese surgical patients. Anesth Analg 2006;103:677–681.

Henny CP, Hofland J: Laparoscopic surgery, pitfalls due to anesthesia, positioning and pneumoperitoneum. Surg Endosc 2005;19:1163–1171.

Kim JA, Lee JJ: Preoperative predictors of difficult intubation in patients with obstructive sleep apnea syndrome. Can J Anesth 2006;53:393–397.

London ET, Ho HS, Neuhaus A, et al: Effect of intravascular volume expansion on renal function during prolonged CO$_2$ pneumoperitoneum. Ann Surg 2000;231:195–201.

Nguyen NT, Perez RV, Fleming N, et al: Effect of prolonged pneumoperitoneum on intraoperative urine output during laparoscopic gastric bypass. J Am Coll Surg 2002;195:476–483.

Schäfer M, Krähenbühl L: Effect of laparoscopy on intra-abdominal blood flow. Surgery 2001;129:385–389.

Sessler DI: Complications and treatment of mild hypothermia. Anesthesiology 2001;95:531–543.

Williams MT, Rice I, Ewen SP, Elliott SM: A comparison of the effect of two anaesthetic techniques on surgical conditions during gynaecological laparoscopy. Anaesthesia 2003;58:574–578.

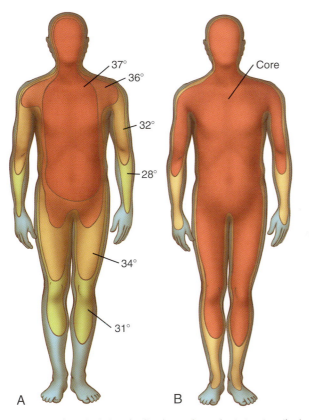

FIGURE 32-2 Hypothermia during the first hour of anesthesia is primarily due to core-peripheral redistribution of blood. **A,** A patient with a significant gradient between core and peripheral temperatures (in Celsius). **B,** After induction of anesthesia, vasodilatation occurs and core blood mixes with cooler peripheral blood, which produces a drop in core body temperature.

TALLAL M. ZENI, CONSTANTINE T. FRANTZIDES, AND
RONALD E. MOORE, JR.

Instrumentation in Laparoscopic Surgery

33

VIDEO MONITOR SYSTEM AND CAMERA

In 1985 the charge-coupled device (CCD) three-chip camera was developed such that visualization on a video monitor allowed freedom of the surgeon's hands to perform therapeutic surgery. Furthermore, it allowed the assistance of other members of the surgical team. Certainly, performance of advanced laparoscopic procedures, in which at least four or more trocar sites are used at any particular instant, would not have been achievable without this major advancement.

Continued advancements in imaging have now progressed to include high-definition signal boxes and monitors. Fundamentally, the system has five main components: the laparoscope, the fiber-optic light cable and light source, the camera head and video signal box, the insufflator, and the monitor. Thorough familiarity on the part of the surgeon and operating room staff can minimize poor and inadequate imaging.

The laparoscopes now in use vary from the typical 10-mm size to 5-mm scopes and the smaller micro 2-mm scopes. Newer 5-mm scopes provide images that are full screen and comparable to 10-mm laparoscopes. Although the imaging provided by a 2-mm scope is limited, it can be used in some instances such as the placement of a peritoneal dialysis catheter. Varying degrees of angled laparoscopes are also available including 0, 30, and 45 degrees. Most advanced laparoscopic cases are performed primarily using a 30-degree angled scope. Extraperitoneal surgery such as inguinal hernia repair is facilitated by use of the 45-degree scope to compensate for the limited space. The dual-channel laparoscopes used by the Da Vinci robotic system provide a three-dimensional (3D) view.

The light sources typically now utilize a xenon bulb but previously halogen bulb or metal halide bulbs were used. The fiberoptic cable transmits the light from the light source to the laparoscope and can become degraded over time. Replacement is incumbent in those cases to preserve picture quality.

Camera systems utilize the three-chip devices. A prism in the camera head splits the laparoscopic image into its three primary colors—red, blue, and green—and each color falls onto its own CCD chip. This provides the most accurate color reproduction available. Current high-definition systems are capable of producing more than 1080 lines of resolution provided that a high-definition monitor is connected. Currently, cables have become long enough to conduct the high-definition signal. Flat panel monitors are ideal for endosuite room construction.

Endosuites, through the presence of fixed equipment placement upon booms that do not require significant manipulation, ultimately preserve the equipment in the long term and ensure an efficient operating room environment (Fig. 33-1). Monitors can then be manipulated to a position at the eye level of each individual surgeon. This can avoid neck strain and cervical disk injury.

In addition, current systems (Stryker, San Jose, CA) may capture infrared emissions (for example, a bougie used for Nissen fundoplication or ureteral stents used for sigmoid colectomies). Also important, and particularly well illustrated in this book, is the capability to record surgical procedures. Multiple methods of final storage exist whether it be onto a DVD, CD (older versions), or USB flash drives.

The pneumoperitoneum provided by insufflators can be provided via high-flow tubing allowing for 40 L/minute, which is ultimately limited by the caliber of the connection to the trocar. The air can also be heated and humidified, although most studies do not show significant benefit. It should be noted that vigilance to ensure adequate patient paralysis by anesthesia and patient positioning to facilitate visceral retraction by gravity also assist significantly in visualization and performance of the intended procedure. Liver retraction can be done via many devices (Fig. 33-2) including the Soft-Wand balloon retractor (Gyrus-ACMI, Southborough, MA) or Nathanson retractor (Cook, Bloomington, IN) among others. This is frequently critical particularly in gastric bypass and other procedures performed at the hiatus. The balloon retractor can also be used to retract the mesocolon (in identifying the ligament of Treitz) or other structures atraumatically.

TROCARS AND ABDOMINAL ACCESS

Although Jonas Veress described his blunt spring-loaded needle in 1938, it was not until the 1980s that the Veress needle became routinely employed to achieve access into the abdominal cavity. After the needle enters the peritoneal cavity, the resistance to entry of the Veress needle subsides, resulting in protrusion of the blunt obdurator shielding the sharp outer sleeve. Most often it is placed in the infraumbilical position, but it can be placed in the left or right upper quadrants immediately below the costal margin, making it especially useful in patients who have undergone prior surgeries. Although theoretically this will prevent injury to intra-abdominal viscera, in fact there still exists a low but significant risk. It is important to lift away the abdominal wall

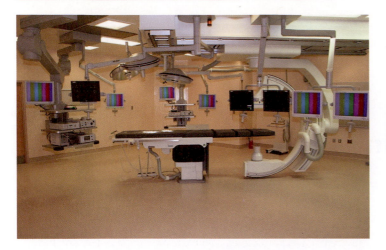

Figure 33-1 Endosuite configuration.

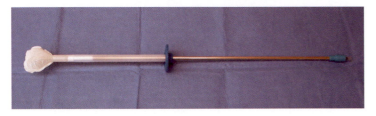

Figure 33-2 Balloon retractor (Gyrus-ACMI, Southborough, MA).

during placement to attempt to create a space between the peritoneum and intra-abdominal viscera. A negative aspiration after placement and low intra-abdominal pressures obtained after insufflation may signify atraumatic placement. However, verification of the absence of bile, blood, succus, or mesenteric emphysema is required upon visualization.

Hasson described his open technique for entry into the abdominal cavity in 1970. A vertical incision through the umbilicus or more commonly an infraumbilical curvilinear incision is made. The umbilical raphe is incised after being elevated followed by incision of the linea alba. Preperitoneal fat is usually thin or absent in this location and the peritoneum is usually adherent to the linea alba. Stay sutures are usually placed to secure the cannula and ease closure of the fascia at the conclusion of the procedure. The Hasson blunt trocar is then inserted under direct visualization. The Hasson technique can be difficult in obese patients, and if a large fascial incision is made, subsequent leakage of carbon dioxide may result in difficulty maintaining the pneumoperitoneum and thus exposure.

Optical access trocars involve placement of a 5- or 10-mm, 0-degree laparoscope through a transparent blunt tipped trocar (Fig. 33-3). This allows visualization of trocar placement as the trocar traverses the layers of the abdominal wall by a rotational twisting movement into the peritoneal cavity. Experience is required to discern the various layers of the abdominal wall and avoid visceral injury. In most cases the safest location for initial placement is the left upper quadrant below the subcostal margin. Other locations may include the right upper quadrant followed by the lateral abdomen in some instances. Staying away from the midline, especially in cases of prior surgeries, reduces the incidence of iatrogenic injury. Avoidance of umbilical insertion should be emphasized so as to avoid major vessel injury. Although umbilical blind insertion has been described in the gynecologic literature, we feel that this is not the safest option.

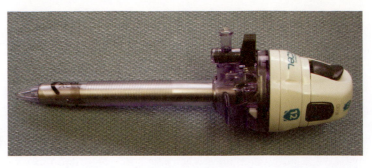

Figure 33-3 Optical bladeless trocar (Ethicon Endo-Surgery, Cincinnati, OH).

Particular care should be exercised, regardless of the location of entry, in thin patients. We also anecdotally feel that use of 5-mm Optiview may result in a higher incidence of iatrogenic visceral injuries and should thus be avoided. It is the opinion of the authors that the new Excel bladeless optical trocar (Ethicon Endo-Surgery, Cincinnati, OH) is not as well designed as their previous version. It appears that there is a 3- to 4-mm disparity in the relationship between the obturator and the sheath of the new Excel trocar compared to the previous version; thus, introduction of the sheath into the abdominal cavity requires deeper protrusion of the sharp edge (obturator). This may increase the likelihood of intra-abdominal organ injury.

After placement of the initial trocar, the surgeon may choose among many varieties of trocars. The selection of the trocar is based on many factors that are beyond the scope of this chapter. Reusable trocars are available and usually have a sharp conical tip or have a shielded blade. Disposable trocars may be bladed or bladeless. The bladeless type has been reported to be associated with a much lower rate of incisional hernias even without closure compared to closure after bladed trocar insertion. Radial expansion after insertion of a modified Veress needle is a variant of the bladeless trocar insertion technique that may also reduce abdominal wall bleeding. Bladeless trocar insertion often requires more force, and therefore, care must be taken to avoid uncontrolled rapid entry into the abdominal cavity. A two-handed technique is therefore recommended. Threaded cannulas reduce the likelihood of uncontrolled forceful entry into the abdominal cavity and also reduce outward slippage of the cannula during the surgery.

Cannula sizes that are typically used range from 5 to 15 mm. Miniature ports 2 to 3 mm in size may be used to improve even further the cosmetic results and lessen postoperative pain. Minilaparoscopic instrument failures are not uncommon and studies are mixed on reduction of postoperative pain; however, minilaparoscopic techniques may be beneficial in those individuals in whom cosmesis is particularly important.

The Endo GIA (U.S. Surgical, Norwalk, CT) staplers require at least 12-mm cannulas (Fig. 33-4) for introduction into the

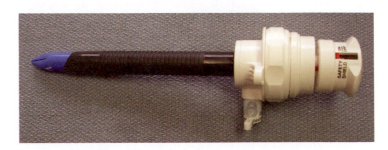

Figure 33-4 Bladed 12-mm trocar (U.S. Surgical, Norwalk, CT).

abdomen. The 4.8-mm Endo GIA stapler requires a 15-mm cannula. Larger cannulas (18 to 33 mm) can be used for end-to-end anastomotic (EEA) stapler placement or placing large pieces of mesh. The Endo Stitch (U.S. Surgical) device requires a 10-mm trocar. Often it is a variety of cannula sizes in specific locations as dictated by the particular procedure that is used to complete the surgery.

Extraperitoneal approaches for performance of inguinal hernia repair, nephrectomy, and spinal fusion, among other procedures, typically require creation of a working space by balloon dissectors. Progressive balloon dissection under direct laparoscopic visualization separates the tissue planes which then allows for pneumopreperitoneum and establishment of the working space.

Hand-assisted laparoscopy may be done using hand-assisted devices such as the Gelport (Applied Medical, Rancho Santa Margarita, CA) (Fig. 33-5) or LapDisc (Ethicon Endo-Surgery). Benefits often include a faster learning curve in performing advanced laparoscopic cases, reduced operative time in lengthy or complex procedures (such as a total colectomy), removal of an intact specimen (such as in nephrectomy), provision of a wound barrier in cases of malignant specimen removal, an alternative to open conversion when the totally laparoscopic technique is inadequate, and rapid digital control of hemorrhage. Detractions may include increased incision size (usually 7–8 cm), increased postoperative pain, hand fatigue, and interference with visualization depending on the location of hand port placement, particularly if triangulation is not utilized. The hand port incision should also be made in such a way that if the need arises to convert to open procedure, it can be extended appropriately. Typically the nondominant hand is used through the hand port.

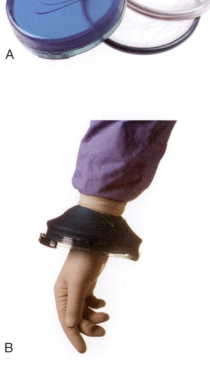

A

B

FIGURE **33-5** **A** and **B**, Gelport assembly for hand-assisted surgery.

ELECTROSURGERY

Monopolar cautery utilizes electrosurgery via an alternating current with a high frequency of 500,000 to 2 million Hz to heat tissues. Depending on the resistance of the tissue and the setting of coagulation/cutting, then heat is subsequently produced. Because excellent hemostasis is critical to maintaining good picture quality in laparoscopic surgery, the importance of hemostasis cannot be underestimated. The cutting current provides relatively poor hemostasis and thus should be avoided except in avascular tissue. The blend current is an intermediate current between the cutting and fulguration currents and represents the most commonly used setting. Breaks in insulation along the length of the instrument can result in injury to adjacent tissues that may be outside the view while performing laparoscopic surgery. The smaller the break in insulation and the smaller the area of contact, the higher the current density resulting in a more severe injury to the adjacent viscera. The cannula also may be a source of capacitive coupling. Visceral injuries may result from improper use of electrosurgery. Electrosurgery should be avoided to control bleeding at staple lines so as to avoid necrosis which may result in subsequent leak. Typically bowel thermal injuries become clinically apparent 3 to 7 days postoperatively. Instead of electrocautery, hemostasis at the staple line should be controlled using sutures, clips, or topical agents such as thrombin/Gelfoam. Arching may also occur with monopolar cautery but is usually limited to less than 3 mm. Unprepped bowel may also contain methane or hydrogen that may result in a potentially explosive mixture of gases in the presence of monopolar cautery. Use of ultrasonic devices to create enterotomies, for instance, in Roux limb creation, is thus a safer option.

Bipolar cautery can avoid some of the inadvertent injuries that may be associated with monopolar cautery. The current flow is limited to the two electrodes that are about 3 mm apart, thus reducing significantly the depth of penetration. In addition, less energy is needed in bipolar cautery, thus also reducing the likelihood of significant injury to adjacent viscera. Bipolar devices, such as the LigaSure (Valleylab, Boulder, CO), can control vessels up to 7 mm and are particularly useful in transecting the mesocolon or short gastric vessels, for instance.

ULTRASONIC ENERGY

Ultrasonic waves represent a newer method of maintaining hemostasis without the use of electrosurgery, clips, or staplers. The harmonic scalpel (Ethicon Endo-Surgery) (Fig. 33-6) and Autosonix (U.S. Surgical) both operate at a frequency of 55.5 kHz. A piezoelectric crystal is used to convert electrical energy to mechanical energy that denatures protein and produces heat from internal tissue friction. Because the heat production is lower than in electrosurgery, there is less tissue charring and less

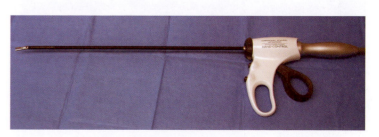

FIGURE **33-6** Harmonic hand-activated ultrasonic shears.

depth penetration, making it safer unless activated for more than 10 seconds. Typically, blood vessels up to 5 mm can be controlled with the harmonic scalpel. In contrast to electrosurgery, the harmonic scalpel will fail if it is placed in contact with metal (which prohibits blade vibration) or if there is too much exerted pressure. Care must be taken to allow appropriate time for the harmonic scalpel to complete hemostasis and cutting. A slight progression away from the closed vibrating blade results in quicker and more efficient dissection.

Ultrasonography has been used in many facets in the setting of laparoscopic surgery. The laparoscopic transducer transmits ultrasound waves and then measures the time it takes for those waves that are reflected back to travel. The amplitude of the reflected waves is depicted as a gray-scale two-dimensional image (B-mode). Color Doppler capabilities can also be added with the use of a second transducer.

Laparoscopic ultrasound probes are available operating between 5 to 10 MHz. This usually provides excellent resolution with an adequate penetration depth. Typical uses include detection and treatment of liver masses using radiofrequency ablation, for instance, detection of choledocholithiasis, staging and diagnosis of pancreatic and other aggressive tumors, and in adrenal surgery.

STAPLING TECHNOLOGY

The introduction of staplers in the late 1960s has facilitated the performance of general surgery in an efficient manner. Clearly, without the availability of staplers in laparoscopic surgery many advanced procedures, such as Roux-en-Y gastric bypass, could not be performed in an expeditious fashion. Therefore, detailed knowledge of staplers and their uses is essential to the advanced laparoscopic surgeon.

Staplers are mainly manufactured by two companies: U.S. Surgical Company produces the Endo GIA (Fig. 33-7) and Ethicon produces the EndoPath ETS. The Endo GIA staplers uniformly lay down three rows of staggered B-shaped staples on each side of the transected tissue. The width of these staples is variable. The smallest width of 0.75 mm corresponds to a gray load of staple length 2.0 mm. This gray load is typically used for transection of the mesentery or of blood vessels such as the renal or splenic vein and artery.

A white load lays down a 1.0-mm wide formed staple that corresponds to 2.5-mm staple length. Often this size is used for transection of vasculature and for transection of the bowel and appendix. Other uses include liver and pancreatic resection. It routinely allows for a more hemostatic bowel anastomosis without creating undue ischemia.

The blue load 1.5-mm width corresponds to a 3.5-mm staple length. It is often used for proximal gastric resection, colon resection, and bowel resection if felt to be thicker than normal. In cases of dis-

tal gastric resection (antrum) or rectal resection the green load of 4.8 mm, laying down a 2.0-mm staple width, is necessary. In even some cases of antral resection the green load can be inadequate. Again, one should always check staple lines for intactness. If inadequate, then suturing will be necessary to close the defect (see later discussion). The capability to suture laparoscopically is a necessary adjunct for those performing advanced laparoscopic surgeries and often prevents unnecessary conversion to open surgery.

Circular staplers are also frequently used, particularly in gastric bypass and low anterior resections (Fig. 33-8A). Two staggered rows of staples are fired to create the anastomosis. The anastomotic diameter varies according to the size of the circular stapler and manufacturer. For instance, a U.S. Surgical 21-mm EEA stapler results in an 11-mm anastomosis, and a 25-mm EEA stapler leads to a 15.4-mm anastomosis. A 21- or 25-mm EEA stapler is typically used in Roux-en-Y gastric bypass. Placement of the anvil can be done either transabdominally or transorally (Fig. 33-8B).

Typically, colorectal surgery requires a 25-mm EEA stapler for an ileorectostomy and a 29-mm stapler for a colorectal anastomosis. Staple width is only 2.0 mm with the previous generation of U.S. Surgical EEA staplers but newer DST series circular staplers have varying staple widths similar to linear staplers (see Fig. 33-8A).

Linear staple line closures can be reinforced using Seamgard (WL Gore & Associates, Flagstaff, AZ) or Peri-Strips Dry (Synovis, St. Paul, MN). This reinforcement can also be used with circular stapler loads. In some cases staple line reinforcement is needed by use of suturing. This can be due to shearing of a staple line or inadequate closure for whatever reason. In these cases the ability to suture in an intracorporeal fashion is necessary to avoid conversion to open. For those who are novices, practicing in a laparoscopic

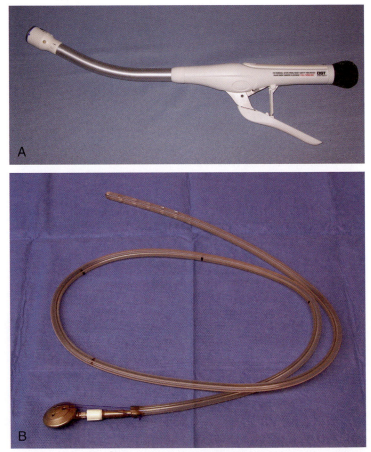

FIGURE 33-8 A, EEA DST series (U.S. Surgical, Norwalk, CT) 25-mm circular stapler. B, Anvil for transoral placement.

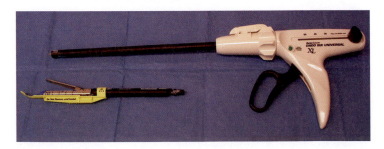

FIGURE 33-7 Linear Endo GIA (U.S. Surgical, Norwalk, CT) with 3.5-mm staple load.

trainer box is invaluable. Hours spent fine-tuning one's technique should not be underestimated. Triangulation of port placement allows for ergonomic and reproducible placement of sutures. A curved needle holder allows easier placement of sutures in a perpendicular fashion to the line of closure. The principles of open surgery should be similarly applied. Placement of sutures should be perpendicular to the tissue and should achieve approximation without undue tension to avoid ischemia. Typically, a 4- to 5-inch length of suture allows for efficient knot tying.

When one is comfortable with intracorporeal sutures, then mechanical devices can be used such as the Endo Stitch device. In some cases, the use of the Endo Stitch is more reasonable such as in hiatal hernia closure and Nissen fundoplication where the angles necessary for intracorporeal suturing can be difficult. Extra- or intracorporeal tying may be used with the Endo Stitch device.

Many fascial closure devices exist including the Carter-Thomason fascial closure device (Inlet Medical, Trumbull, CT), which is quick and efficient. It utilizes a cone to allow for a guided tract through which the needle is introduced, resulting in an adequate fascial closure. Longer cones are available for morbidly obese patients.

GRASPERS

Gentle dissection is critical and necessary in any surgery. In open surgery the hands are atraumatic and tension can be gauged easily to avoid excessive pulling or tearing. In laparoscopic surgery, on the other hand, this may be more difficult. Therefore, atraumatic instrumentation is even more necessary. Atraumatic grasping instruments are clearly the most essential. The Atraugrip (Specialty Surgical Instrumentation, Nashville, TN; Fig. 33-9) 10-mm grasper is useful to avoid serosal or deeper injury to tissues while handling them. It is available in a 45 cm length.

Bowel graspers also are useful in that they are relatively atraumatic. On the other hand, wavy or Babcock graspers can be fairly traumatic to tissues and should preferentially be limited to those applications in which resection of the particular organ will occur (for instance, in sleeve gastrectomy) or where more aggressive grasping/retraction is necessary. Dissection also may be accomplished by the use of some graspers such as a Maryland grasper or right-angle dissector. Another instrument that we find useful in dissecting around large vessels or difficult structures is the gastric banding retractor (Karl Storz, Germany).

MESH PROSTHESIS

An extensive discussion regarding mesh selection is beyond the scope of this chapter. Meshes may be simply stratified according to whether they are absorbable or not, synthetic or biologic,

and whether they incite adhesion formation. Clearly, when choosing mesh for intra-abdominal procedures, one should utilize mesh that minimizes adhesion formation. Commonly used intra-abdominal meshes include polytetrafluoroethylene (PTFE) mesh, and more recently introduced is Parietex (U.S. Surgical). Although studies are limited, some biologic meshes, although absorbable, may form a platform for collagen deposition. These may suffice for long-term repair of a hernia, whether ventral or hiatal. One advantage may be placement in a contaminated field, although infection of the mesh may still occur even in these cases. Examples include porcine small intestinal submucosa-derived mesh (Cook) and Alloderm (Lifecell, Branchburg, NJ). Extraperitoneal use may utilize Prolene and similar meshes. One should be cautious though to avoid tears in the peritoneum that may allow bowel-mesh adhesions. Parietex may be an alternative to account for this possibility, although studies are limited.

ROBOTICS

Robotic systems have been developed that allow for more efficient conduct of laparoscopic surgery in many cases. AESOP preceded other therapeutic robotic devices as it allowed for camera manipulation. Initially hand/foot activated, it subsequently became voice activated. It is most used in the context of laparoscopic Nissen fundoplication but can be applied in many other laparoscopic surgeries.

The ZEUS robotic system, initially approved in 2001 by the Food and Drug Administration has been replaced by the Da Vinci (Intuitive Surgical, Sunnyvale, CA) system, which allows for two robotic arms. These arms are controlled by a separate console. Manipulation of the instruments mimics wrist movement in that one has a similar 7 degrees of freedom. Room setup is initially time consuming but becomes progressively more efficient. The Da Vinci robotic system has been applied in many advanced laparoscopic surgeries such as gastric bypass, low anterior and abdominoperineal resections, and Heller myotomies. Its most consistent and widespread use has been in the performance of radical prostatectomies. Although initially developed for performance of minimally invasive cardiac surgery, acceptance has been slow. It may also have a role in hysterectomy among the gynecologic surgeons. The advantages of Da Vinci assisted laparoscopic surgeries over other laparoscopic procedures are difficult to assert at the present time. Only time will show whether the Da Vinci or any other robotic system will be a flash in the pan or will find its niche in general surgery.

NATURAL ORIFICE TRANSLUMINAL ENDOSCOPIC SURGERY

The progression from open to advanced minimally invasive surgery may continue even further. Although still in the research stage, natural orifice transluminal endoscopic surgery (NOTES) is a potentially exciting field that may revolutionize surgery once again. Access into the peritoneal cavity may be obtained via the stomach or less likely via the colon or vagina. Dual-channel endoscopes allow for therapeutic interventions. Appendectomies and some other limited procedures have been performed successfully. Quite clearly, closure of the gastrotomy, for instance, must be secure once the procedure is completed. Further developments may allow this to occur in a reliable and reproducible fashion. Again, NOTES is still in its infancy and its future is uncertain at this stage.

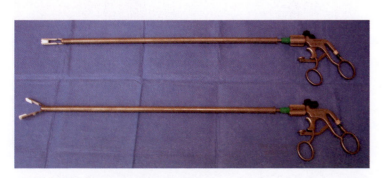

FIGURE 33-9 Atraugrip grasper (Specialty Surgical Instrumentation, Nashville, TN).

Index

Note: Page numbers followed by f indicate figures and those followed by t indicate tables.

DISCOVERY LIBRARY
LEVEL 5 SWCC
DERRIFORD HOSPITAL
DERRIFORD ROAD
PLYMOUTH
PL6 8DH